SMALL BITES

SMALL BITES

BIOCULTURAL DIMENSIONS OF CHILDREN'S FOOD AND NUTRITION

Tina Moffat

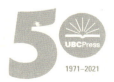

© UBC Press 2022

All rights reserved. No part of this publication may be reproduced, stored in a retrieval system, or transmitted, in any form or by any means, without prior written permission of the publisher, or, in Canada, in the case of photocopying or other reprographic copying, a licence from Access Copyright, www.accesscopyright.ca.

31 30 29 28 27 26 25 24 23 22   5 4 3 2 1

Printed in Canada on FSC-certified ancient-forest-free paper (100% post-consumer recycled) that is processed chlorine- and acid-free.

Library and Archives Canada Cataloguing in Publication

Title: Small bites : biocultural dimensions of children's food and nutrition / Tina Moffat.
Names: Moffat, Tina, 1967– author.
Description: Includes bibliographical references and index.
Identifiers: Canadiana (print) 20210388935 | Canadiana (ebook) 20210389370 |
    ISBN 9780774866880 (hardcover) | ISBN 9780774866903 (PDF) |
    ISBN 9780774866910 (EPUB)
Subjects: LCSH: Children—Nutrition. | LCSH: Children—Nutrition—Social aspects. |
    LCSH: Nutrition—Social aspects. | LCSH: Nutritional anthropology. |
    LCSH: Food security—Social aspects. | LCSH: Food habits—Social aspects.
Classification: LCC GN407 .M64 2022 | DDC 613.2083—dc23

Canada

UBC Press gratefully acknowledges the financial support for our publishing program of the Government of Canada (through the Canada Book Fund), the Canada Council for the Arts, and the British Columbia Arts Council.

This book has been published with the help of a grant from the Canadian Federation for the Humanities and Social Sciences, through the Awards to Scholarly Publications Program, using funds provided by the Social Sciences and Humanities Research Council of Canada.

Printed and bound in Canada by Friesens
Set in Segoe and Warnock by Apex CoVantage, LLC
Copy editor: Joanne Richardson
Proofreader: Sarah Wight
Indexer: Noeline Bridge
Cover designer: Michel Vrana

UBC Press
The University of British Columbia
2029 West Mall
Vancouver, BC V6T 1Z2
www.ubcpress.ca

To Tom, Tara, and Lucas

Contents

List of Figures and Tables / viii

Acknowledgments / ix

Introduction / 3

1 Baby Steps: Prenatal, Infant, and Young Child Feeding / 17

2 Biocultural Variation in Child Feeding and Eating / 44

3 Children's Food in the Age of the Industrial Diet / 64

4 It Takes a Village: School Feeding Programs / 95

5 Global Malnutrition and Children's Food (In)security / 116

6 Childhood Obesity: A Twenty-First-Century Nutritional Dilemma / 137

7 New Directions in Children's Food and Nutrition / 163

Notes / 182

References / 184

Index / 224

Figures and Tables

Figures

I.1   Food systems map depicting the modern agri-food system / 10
1.1   Earthenware spouted jar (infant feeding cup), c. 1750–1550 BC, excavated at Dakhleh Oasis, Egypt / 26
5.1   Linear growth rate of Nepali children from birth to five years compared to the WHO 50th and WHO 5th growth references / 121
5.2   The food security continuum / 136
7.1   The *Canada Food Guide* / 175
7.2   USDA's *Choose My Plate* / 176

Tables

3.1   Recommended dietary allowances (RDAs) for calcium / 67
3.2   Inventory of snack foods specifically marketed to children found in one Canadian supermarket / 79

Acknowledgments

This book is the product of a journey that began over twenty years ago when I started doing anthropological research in child food and nutrition. I have many people to thank for supporting me along the way. I begin by thanking my Nepali friends Rhade Shyam Duwadi, his wife Nanu, and their family, who supported me graciously with their Nepali language instruction, research assistance, and delicious food and hospitality. As well, my research assistants (Maya Sherpa, Tsering Sherpa, Ang Tsering Sherpa, and Lakhpa Lama), the medical personnel at the Ramhiti and Dakshin Dohka clinics, and the research participants working in the carpet-making industry who generously shared with me their time and their stories.

In Hamilton, I am indebted to the many organizations that have assisted me in my research, in particular the Hamilton Wentworth District School Board, Hamilton Public Health Services, and the Hamilton Community Food Centre and Neighbour to Neighbour, with special thanks to Claire Wagner and Krista D'Aoust.

In Paris, I want to thank Eloise Gaillard for assisting me in my school meal research as well as the administrators, educators, and dietitians I interviewed. Michel Le Guernic was particularly generous with his time and expertise.

I am grateful to my long-standing and dear friends and colleagues at McMaster University and the Canadian Association for Biological Anthropology. A special thank you to Ann Herring and Patangi Rangachari (Chari) for their generous intellectual mentorship and friendship over the years. And to the graduate and undergraduate students I have had the privilege to advise and who have assisted me in my research – I'm quite sure they have taught me as much as I have them.

James MacNevin, acquisitions editor, and Meagan Dyer, production editor, both at UBC Press, skillfully guided me through the publishing process. Thanks to the two anonymous reviewers, who critiqued previous drafts with excellent insight and advice, and enabled me to create a much stronger manuscript.

Finally, I reserve my deepest gratitude for my parents, my sister, and my husband and children, who have taught me many life lessons about kids and food and who have nourished both my body and soul.

SMALL BITES

Introduction

Feeding children is seemingly one of the most natural things we do as humans. Yet a perusal of media accounts indicates a crisis in children's nutrition, either real or perceived depending on your viewpoint. Since the 1980s, child obesity rates have risen steadily around the globe (Lobstein and Jackson-Leach 2016). Headlines abound about child obesity, and it has been predicted by some researchers that, due to increases in diet-related diseases, children will not live as long as the previous generation (Olshansky et al. 2005). Parents, caregivers, educators, and concerned citizens worry about what food children should be eating, and public health dietitians respond by stating that children are being fed too much sugar and fat and that they're not eating enough fruit and vegetables.

Despite an abundance of concern among health professionals, there is at the same time widespread apathy among many policy-makers and the general public. Canadians and Americans feed children food full of refined grains, fat, sugar, salt, and chemical additives. They eat a steady stream of fast-food burgers and fries, sugary breakfast cereals, cheese sticks, soda pop, highly sugared fruit drinks, chicken nuggets and fingers, and instant macaroni and cheese in a box, just to name a few of the ultra-processed, commercial food products that are marketed to children. Many children grow up believing that this is tasty food, never having eaten fresh fruit or vegetables and home-cooked meals. This is a product of socioeconomic inequalities and a food system that produces processed food more cheaply than fresh food. It is, as well, a story of constructing North American children as fussy eaters, who require different foods from adults, so-called "children's foods." So too, children, through the machinations of food industrialists and marketers, exert agency within their families so that they can consume these foods.

At the same time child obesity is on the rise, there are children going hungry. These disparities in access to food are seen most drastically in low-income countries – where there are still many children who experience malnourishment and hunger as a daily reality. But these food access inequities exist in high-income countries too; there is an unconscionably large proportion of children in Canada and the United States who live in food-insecure households.

How did we get to this state? How can an understanding of human evolution inform paediatric nutrition? How do we parse the need for special nutrition for young children from the manufacture of children's food by the industrial food system? How are children paradoxically fed so well and so poorly nourished at the same time? How do we protect children from the food industry while at the same time navigate the reality of a commodity-driven system in which food is part of a billion-dollar industry? Is it only parents' responsibility to feed children or should we collectively share the duty to make sure it's done well? How do our values about children and feeding them become embodied in our children through our sociocultural approaches to childhood and their food? How do we make sure there is equitable access to food and nourishment for all children?

Throughout this book I attempt to answer these questions to forge a path towards improving children's nutritional well-being. I do this using an anthropological approach that looks back to our evolutionary heritage and continues historically through time and space to the twenty-first century. I focus on the evolutionary underpinnings of infant and young child feeding, parsing biological from sociocultural factors, which require equal attention and ultimately cannot be disentangled. I examine the rise of the industrial food system that began in North America and spread worldwide through the increasing globalization of multinational food corporations and food commodities. I then take a cross-cultural approach by examining children's food in several particular and contrasting settings around the world – Nepal, France, Japan, Canada, and the United States – exploring how we feed our children as a reflection of our cultural approaches to childhood and food in these societies. While the scope of the book is international, there is a strong Canadian lens through which I compare and contrast child food and

Introduction   5

nutrition in Canada to other countries. Finally, I address current social and paediatric nutrition dilemmas – namely, undernutrition and obesity.

This book is based on my scholarly and community-based research over the past twenty-five years. As an anthropologist, I have worked in various settings, including in the nations of Nepal, Canada, and France. In Nepal, my focus was on child growth and the health of the children of carpet-making workers living just outside of Kathmandu. I researched rural-to-urban migrants who had moved to the city to do wage labour. These families raised their children in this impoverished, urban environment, and I examined the effects of this environment on children's nutritional health. On the upside they had wage earnings to enable them to access some health care and to buy food, but, on the downside, they lived without clean water and sanitation, and relied on market food instead of freshly grown village foods. In Canada I studied elementary school children's diets and school environments in relation to child overweight and obesity. Though a very different setting from Nepal, there were similar themes of disadvantage affecting the nutritional health of children living in food-insecure households, resulting in malnutrition, sometimes in the form of overweight and obesity. Finally, I conducted research in France, in collaboration with a co-investigator working in Japan, to consider the place of school meal programs in addressing child nutrition and obesity prevention. Through this work I also explored the place of school meal programs in France and Japan as a site of social and cultural reproduction through culinary nationalism, a phenomenon I call "gastro-citizenship."

~

The other hat I wear, in addition to being an anthropologist, is that of a white, middle-class parent who has raised two children in an urban setting from the beginning of the twenty-first century and who has found feeding children to be as fraught these days as any other aspect of raising a child. With all the parenting manuals and media advice from pregnancy right through to negotiating daycare and school food, parents are constantly being supplied and admonished with conflicting advice. I have personally endured this and thus can relate to the wider experiences of other caregivers who also face these challenges. My experiences also connect with those of educators and health care and food/nutrition providers, who are concerned about the nutritional health and well-being of children and future generations. I realize, however, that my personal experiences of feeding my children are filtered through a privileged lens, which I try to point out throughout the book, but ultimately this lens biases the perspectives I present.

I present these personal and research experiences using a variety of theoretical approaches that are academic but that I believe are relevant to how we frame the problems and the solutions we propose.

Theoretical Approaches

In this book I employ multiple theoretical approaches from anthropology and other social sciences that complement and at the same time intersect with one another. I begin with a foundational evolutionary approach, in particular life history theory, which hypothesizes the evolution of species-specific key life history phases and traits related to reproduction, growth and development, mortality, and ecology that has also been applied to *Homo sapiens* (Chisholm 1993; Hill and Kaplan 1999). For example, unlike other mammals, and even other primates, human children mature slowly and depend on adults for most of their childhood, with adolescence as a transitional stage that is unique in delayed maturation (Reiches 2019). *Homo sapiens* engage in a long period of learning and apprenticeship; thus, we have always had the profound privilege and responsibility to nurture our children. For much of our evolutionary history this nurturing rested not only on parents but also on grandparents, older siblings, and various extended relatives (Blaffer Hrdy 2009).

Today that responsibility extends to some institutions such as daycares and schools. Feeding children is one of the most vital aspects of this care and yet perhaps one of the most challenging. In the past the simple act of having enough food to feed children posed a major difficulty for many people. That is still the case for many in the contemporary world but now with added complications for those with abundance in determining what and how to feed children. There are no simple answers to current dilemmas in child nutrition. I believe, however, that the holistic perspective of anthropology allows us to step back from the hype described above to critically consider where our species came from, where we are situated in this current capitalist and global food system, and how we want to shape our future societal approaches to feeding children.

My hope is that by understanding the bigger picture we can get away from making children little nutrition projects, as we are apt to do in this era of "nutritionism" (Scrinis 2012), where we count nutrients in every mouthful. To counter nutritionism in this book, I consciously make a distinction between children's food/child feeding and children's nutrition, as inspired by the understanding of the distinction between foods and nutrients eloquently outlined by Rozin and Vollmecke (1986, 434, emphasis mine).

> *People eat food, not nutrients.* Although foods stimulate the chemosensory, visual, thermal and tactile senses, it is the mental representation invoked by this stimulation that is critical to humans' response: we respond to the mental representation of foods in order to identify particular items as either edible or not. The food itself is at once a source of nutrition, a source of harmful microorganisms or toxins, a great source of pleasure and satisfaction, and a vehicle for the expression of social relations and values.

In keeping with this understanding that the practice and thought humans put into food/eating and human nutrition at the biological level are both separate and yet intertwined, I employ a biocultural approach.

Biocultural Framework

The biocultural framework, more commonly referred to as "biosocial" in Europe and the UK,[1] is at its most basic level the recognition that human biology, health, and nutrition are fundamentally shaped by the biophysical, social, cultural, political, and economic environments in which we live. As humans we are extremely adaptable to different environments, and that is reflected in the wide variety of diets we have consumed as a species from the Arctic to the extreme southern latitudes (Leonard 2002). Human biology – particularly our genetic inheritance, our microbiota, our requirements for certain nourishment – may also shape our social and cultural worlds, so the relationship among these factors is interactive and dialectical. In anthropology the biocultural approach has been most explicitly formulated among American biological, medical, and nutritional anthropologists. A review of biocultural approaches used by anthropologists in scholarly research demonstrates, however, that the approach is often defined very loosely or not at all (Wiley and Cullin 2016). I suggest this looseness is convenient as it enables researchers to use it flexibly in their studies.

Biocultural approaches began in the 1970s in biological anthropology with a focus on population adaptations to environmental stressors such as high altitude, malnutrition, and disease risk. They were also taken up by bioarchaeologists studying past populations (Zuckerman and Martin 2016), and, more recently, anthropologists have conceptualized resource insecurities such as food and water as environmental stressors (Brewis, Piperata, and Thompson 2020). Writing from the perspective of nutritional anthropology, Pelto, Dufour, and Goodman (2013, 2) describe ecological studies of food and nutrition as paying holistic attention to "biological and social forces in shaping human food use and the nutritional status of individuals and population," but they go on to say that "the hallmark of a biocultural approach is the examination of interactions among them." Since the 1990s, some scholars have been actively developing the biocultural approach in more explicit ways. Andrea Wiley (1992) emphasizes the importance of considering evolutionary context and the concept of adaptation to changing environments as a fundamental aspect of the biocultural approach. In *Medical Anthropology: A Biocultural Approach*, Wiley and Allen define the biocultural perspective as a consideration of "the social, ecological, and biological aspects of health issues, and how these interact within and across populations," while still maintaining that "the body has also been shaped by a history – an evolutionary history – during which it has been molded by changing environmental conditions" (Wiley and Allen 2013, 8). Hicks and Leonard (2014) extend this definition by arguing that, though our biology constrains specific patterns of growth and development that have been inherited through our human evolution, as a species we experience developmental plasticity that is linked to and shaped by our political economy and culture. Goodman and Leatherman (1998) imprint the biocultural approach with a critical and Marxist analysis, arguing that human health and biology are fundamentally shaped by access to material resources; their description of the approach, while not fundamentally different from those described above, pays close attention to the social processes of power and structural constraints at both local and global levels on individuals and populations. This focus on political economy has led to labelling these approaches as "critical biocultural" because they elucidate how local and global political economic processes are literally embodied as they "get under the skin" (Goodman and Leatherman 1998; Hertzman and Boyce 2010; Leatherman and Goodman 2019).

Some key features of the biocultural approach include the focus on "local or situated biologies," as opposed to the standardized or universal body, which recognizes the entanglement of sociocultural and biological processes through embodiment (Brewis, Piperata, and Thompson 2020; Krieger 2005; Lock 2017). Critical biocultural studies of embodiment include investigating health disparities due to social and cultural inequalities linked to race, gender, indigeneity, colonialism, and poverty (Gravlee 2009; Krieger 2016; Kuzawa and Sweet 2009; Leatherman, Hoke, and Goodman 2016;

Introduction

Schell 2020). Related to the concept of embodiment, and relevant to a focus on children's food and nutrition, is consideration of the lifecourse or early origins, which is fundamental to understanding the developmental origins of health and disease. This approach focuses on stressors in the maternal environment (nutrition, stress, toxins) that affect the unborn baby and its health throughout the lifecourse and even beyond to the next generation (Ellison 2005; Kuzawa and Quinn 2009). As Nicholas Nisbett (2019, 10) states: "In sharing socio-structural determinants as well as being inherited from maternal nutrition, malnutrition can therefore be considered as an intergenerational form of embodied poverty: a key way of transmitting the conditions of poverty through the generations." This critical approach to nutrition within the biocultural framework aligns with those in critical food studies described next.

Critical Food Studies

Scholars of critical food studies apply interdisciplinary approaches – including social, nutritional, and environmental sciences – to understand how food systems work and to imagine alternative futures for those systems (Koç, Sumner, and Winson 2012). In this book I reference "the food system" and "food systems" repeatedly. The "food system," as described by Sobal, Khan, and Bisogni (1998), is often metaphorically described as "from field to table," which is a quick way of characterizing a conceptually complex system that involves multiple intersecting sectors of food production, consumption, maintenance of human nutritional health, and social relationships involving food. Within the food system there are smaller complex systems, including agriculture, industry and trade, economics, health, politics, and sociocultural practices and values. While there have been multiple food systems through time and space, based on a variety of food production methods (including gathering and hunting/ fishing) as well as distribution systems (subsistence and communal food sharing), the modern food system, which now feeds most of the 9 billion people on the planet and is highly integrated, is based on industrial agriculture and distribution through a capitalist economic system. This is depicted in Figure I.1.

As with the critical biocultural approach, scholars of critical food studies aim to reveal structural forces and barriers to nutritional health and well-being by taking a systems approach with a focus on political economy. This approach is nicely illustrated by Kate Cairns and Josée Johnston in their

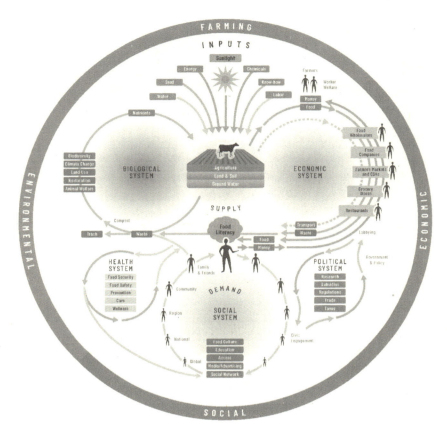

FIGURE I.1 Food systems map depicting the modern agri-food system. | Courtesy WorldLink, www.nourishlife.org.

discussion of how the state applies hegemonic strategies to disinvest itself from taking responsibility for nutritional health and well-being:

> Food is commonly framed through the lens of individual choice: you can *choose* to eat healthily; a mother *chooses* to make dinner each evening because cooking is an activity she enjoys. This individualized framing appeals to a popular desire to experience agency, but draws attention away from the structural obstacles that shape and stratify individual food choices – especially in a neoliberal context where the state has transferred responsibility for food onto individual consumers (e.g. the expectation that mothers seeking to protect their children from pesticides and chemicals must purchase expensive organic produce). (Cairns and Johnston 2015, 13)

Similarly, Raj Patel (2012), in his book *Stuffed and Starved*, investigates the neoliberal and capitalist basis of the global food system to understand current nutritional problems and dilemmas through a critical food studies lens. Patel argues that the global food system, with its main goal as profit, has shaped and constrained our access and appetites for certain types of food that are in overabundance for some and not available for others. In considering food systems we must remember that food and nutrition systems are connected to and affected by many other complex and adaptive systems, including environmental, governmental, transportation, health care, and political-economic systems, and within all of these systems we must be attuned to social inequities that become embodied in individuals and communities (Nisbett 2019). Scholars working within the critical food studies framework are not only focused on understanding how food systems and biological and nutritional outcomes have come to be but also on how they can take an activist stance to improve systems going forward. This is relevant to children's food and nutrition since children's ability to gain access to nutritious foods necessary for their growth and development depends on adults' willingness to fight for their right to food and to protect them from ultra-processed food items that are driven by food industry profits.

Researchers using a critical food studies lens also examine widely used concepts such as "healthy food/eating." Though national food/dietary guides are perceived to be authoritative guides to healthy food/eating, they are also influenced by the food industry and food politics. The US Food Pyramid, for example, was heavily shaped by lobbying by the meat and dairy industries (Nestle 2002). As well, lay definitions of "healthy food" vary by individual sociodemographic backgrounds. In a qualitative study of 105 Canadians from various ethnic and socioeconomic backgrounds, Ristovski-Slijepcevic, Chapman, and Beagan (2008) found three predominant though overlapping discourses in discussions of "healthy eating": cultural/traditional, mainstream, and complementary/ethical. The cultural/traditional discourse is held by those who identify with a specific ethnicity and who hold that food from their ethnic traditions or what they ate in their home/countries is healthiest; similarly, those who think about food in ethical terms (e.g., local/ environmental and/or vegetarian/vegan) have very different conceptualizations of healthy food from what is found in mainstream discourses. In North America, gender, age, ethnicity, and socioeconomic status all factor into peoples' values and cognition attached to "healthy eating/food" that revolve around multiple concepts such as "low fat," natural versus unprocessed foods, balance, disease prevention or managing an existing disease, and controlling weight (Winter Falk et al. 2001).

Throughout *Small Bites*, I am mindful that what constitutes healthy food/eating will depend on the reader's perspective, which may vary considerably from mine. Nevertheless, as there is a need to make some differentiation between "healthy" and "unhealthy" food/eating when discussing children's food and nutrition, for the purposes of this book I define "healthy food/eating" as an approximation of the most recent *Canada Food Guide* (Government of Canada 2019a), which emphasizes high consumption of fresh plant foods and a variety of other foods that are minimally processed. Whether everyone can or wants to eat this kind of diet is another issue that I address throughout the book.

Social Studies of Children and Childhood

While not as relevant to studies of food and nutrition as the other theoretical approaches explained above, perspectives from social studies of children and childhood are fundamental to the study of children's food and nutrition. Though my conception of infancy and childhood is rooted in the physiological and developmental phenomena that are shaped by evolutionary forces (Bogin 2010) as a starting point, it is further enlightened by the understanding that childhood as an institution and our treatment of children is modified by social and cultural forces. This latter point is articulated in Allison James and Alan Prout's edited volume *Constructing and Reconstructing Childhood*. In this volume they call attention to children and childhood as subjects of serious scholarly recognition, and they set out "central tenets of the emergent paradigm" in childhood sociology, which begin with an understanding of the institution of childhood as a social and cultural construction that varies through time and across cultures (James and Prout 1997, 3).

Since that publication, there has been a re-emergence of anthropology in the study of children and childhood (Bluebond-Langner and Korbin 2007), with a number of volumes related to children and childhood in present and past societies (Beauchesne and Agarwal 2018; Lewis 2006; Panter-Brick and Smith 2000). Though anthropological ethnographies of contemporary societies have often considered children, most of them have considered children and childhood from afar, as opposed to gaining children's own perspectives as research participants. Anthropological research about children's food and consumption from this former perspective is exemplified by a

Introduction

collection of studies in *Feeding China's Little Emperors: Food, Children, and Social Change*, edited by Jun Jing (2000). There are, however, researchers who have worked with children as active participants. Janet Patico's (2020) ethnography of an Atlanta charter school community, *The Trouble with Snack Time*, for example, though mainly focused on parents' voices about children's snack food at school, does include some children's voices in the mix. No matter how the research is approached, however – whether children are active participants or whether they are understood through the eyes of adults – the concept that children and the institution of childhood are malleable to social and cultural forces is fundamental to considering how we feed our children and how children themselves may be agents in shaping the food they eat.

The Book's Menu

The structure and content of *Small Bites* is driven by the central argument that children's food and nutrition cannot be considered in isolation from larger understandings of food, environmental, social, cultural, political, and economic systems. Contemporary nutrition problems such as child obesity and undernutrition must be addressed as societal issues that are linked to current problems with the industrial food system as well as social inequities that are embedded in the global capitalist food system. Using an anthropological lens, I advocate for a wider perspective, moving from the usual focus on children and their families, mostly their mothers, to a concern for children's food and nutrition that extends beyond the individual and household unit to larger institutional organizations such as schools, community organizations, and governments. This includes the recognition that children grow up to become adults who reproduce the next generation, and so our view of children's nutrition and malnutrition must be dynamic and intergenerational. It also includes the recognition that what we feed children is literally an embodiment of social inequities and societal perspectives on children and childhood.

The first two chapters focus on prenatal nutrition, infant, and young children's feeding followed by attention to older children and adolescents. Chapter 1 is an overview of how we feed infants and young children in relation to human evolutionary history and more recent histories. Within this review I also explore how prenatal diet can affect a person's health through their lifecourse and how evolutionary understandings of infant and young child feeding is relevant to contemporary paediatric debates, such as breastfeeding versus bottle-feeding and complementary first foods and their potential impact on allergies and growth, as well as longer-term impacts on child/adult obesity and diet-related diseases. It becomes clear from this historical review of infant and young child feeding that a trait unique to our species is flexible feeding practices that are influenced by both the constraints on mothers as well as their agency; and, in turn, these are affected by the presence or absence of supports for infant and young child feeding in the wider society.

Chapter 2 explores biocultural variation in child feeding and eating within the context of life history parameters that include the long period of childhood unique to the human species. I present cross-cultural and ethnographic accounts of child feeding and eating among hunter-gatherer children as well as families living in postindustrial societies to explore the parent-child feeding relationship and self-feeding as part of the transitional phases of late childhood and adolescence. While human children display evolved traits such as neophobia (fear of new foods), I parse biologically based from culturally constructed understandings of the way children eat through a comparison of North American versus French approaches to child feeding and eating to interrogate well-known axioms such as "children are picky eaters."

The subsequent chapters of the book examine issues related to the way we feed children in societies through space and time. They take as a point of departure that childhood is an institution constrained by biological parameters of growth and development but that it is socially and culturally experienced in ways that vary through time and space; the way we feed children at the household, community, national, and international levels reflects sociocultural values that we attach to children's lives and their well-being. Chapter 3 begins with a review of the nutritional needs of children from a physiological perspective, taking into account children's growth and development with a reminder that, although children have special nutritional requirements, they do not require "special foods" per se. I then move to a historical and cross-cultural review of children's food that problematizes the creation of "special children's food," which, I argue, has been socially and materially constructed by the industrial food system. I describe in detail specific categories of processed foods – fast foods, breakfast cereals, and snack foods – that are not uniquely children's foods but have been heavily marketed to them. With an eye to an activist approach towards improving food systems and children's nutrition, I address the issue of marketing and advertising to children, the impact they have had on North American children's diets, and how we can begin to disrupt and fight back against these commercial forces.

Introduction   15

In Chapter 4, I focus on school food and feeding programs as a site of cooperative breeding and caregiving that goes beyond the focus on parents and the immediate family context. Schools are where most children in the world spend much of their lives each day, and they are important sites in the institutionalization of childhood and children's food. Understanding the sociocultural construction of school feeding programs that go back almost a century in some countries is central to considering current approaches to child feeding. Schools, moreover, are increasingly viewed as important sites of child nutrition interventions both for under- and overnutrition. I present two international case studies of children's school meal programs – in France and Japan – and then go on to address the unusual situation that holds in Canada, where there are to date no state-funded school meal programs in place.

The problem of children's food insecurity and malnutrition in both international and North American contexts is presented in Chapter 5. I argue that these problems are rooted in the current global food system, where social and economic inequalities unfairly burden children, the most vulnerable members of society. To that end, I review global statistics on child malnutrition in some of the most troublesome spots in the world: sub-Saharan Africa and South Asia. I then discuss child malnutrition as measured through growth and nutrition in Nepal, with reference to the improvement of these indicators over the past twenty years. While the situation is far from perfect in Nepal, improvements there – mainly a result of economic growth, national policy, and international aid – make that nation an exemplar of what can be done to reduce the harmful effects of social inequalities on children's nutritional health and well-being. The second half of the chapter returns to North America to investigate why, in two of the wealthiest nations in the world, Canada and the United States, children still experience food insecurity and malnutrition.

Chapter 6 examines the late twentieth- and twenty-first-century phenomenon of child overweight and obesity. I begin with a primer that reviews the medical categorization and measurement of child overweight and obesity and the underlying biological basis of adiposity. I then review the so-called childhood obesity epidemic, specifically addressing some of the current prevalence data but also reflecting on how we have come to view this issue through a lens of crisis and moral panic about children. I argue that the focus on child obesity as a problem of individuals and families is not helpful in ultimately moving us forward to address underlying determinants of child obesity. These underlying determinants include social inequities rooted in poverty, racism, and social as well as biophysical environmental deficits where children live, grow, and develop. As an alternate way of viewing the determinants of child obesity that helps us move away from framing it as an issue related to individual diet and physical activity behaviour, I review two scientific theories that link rising obesity to exposure to obesogenic toxins and antibiotics during prenatal and early childhood periods. As part of this paradigm shift in preventing child and adult obesity, I revisit lifecourse theory with a focus on the developmental origins of health and disease and the importance of pregnancy nutrition and infant feeding. Attention to the early origins of life (conception through the first few years) results in treating obesity and nutrition-related diseases as multigenerational problems, removing the blame from individuals and families and placing it on larger societal structures and systems managed by governments.

In conclusion, in Chapter 7 I review the book's main arguments and introduce concrete examples of new directions to address the problems and dilemmas of children's food and nutrition, with a focus on policy and community-level change. I also briefly consider some new challenges for children's food and nutrition (such as climate change) as well as new approaches to youth food activism (such as food justice movements).

1

Baby Steps

Prenatal, Infant, and Young Child Feeding

One of the central premises of this book is that, as human primates, we are biologically compelled to feed our children in certain ways – lactation, weaning, and child reliance on adult caregivers – and yet our biology is modulated by our culture, which varies and changes through space and time. This chapter is a biocultural overview of how we feed infants and young children. As part of this, I demonstrate how an evolutionary understanding of child feeding is relevant to contemporary paediatric issues such as breastfeeding versus bottle feeding, introduction of first foods, and their potential impact on allergies and on growth and development. I begin with the current understanding of the importance of the prenatal environment to children's nutritional status and then proceed to breastfeeding and alternatives. I then go on to discuss the weaning period, which includes the decrease in milk consumption and addition of complementary foods in the infant's first year of life. Here, I draw on evolutionary frameworks, such as life history theory, that highlight our species-specific and unique human phase of complementary feeding, as well as highlight the sociocultural variation in complementary feeding and weaning.

In the final consideration of the biocultural aspects of infant and young child feeding, I discuss politics and feminist theory. Since ancient times, women in many societies have been told (often by men) how they should feed their children. Women are often blamed for the nutritional outcomes of their children and bear the brunt of the responsibility for infant and child feeding. How do we get past this? I suggest that *both* evolutionary and feminist theory can guide us to more equitably distribute resources – income, knowledge, and support – to women and their families.

Prenatal Nutrition and the Lifecourse Approach

Let's start at the very beginning – and it turns out that the "beginning" may go back even before the conception of a baby. This is known as the lifecourse, or early origins, approach (Godfrey, Gluckman, and Hanson 2010). Within this framework there is a focus on the mother and what they are eating when the baby is in utero. One hypothesis, called the predictive adaptive response, argues that, through the placenta, the mother sends signals to the foetus to predict the type of environment (resource-rich or -poor) that the offspring may expect in its lifetime (Kuzawa and Quinn 2009). As Godfrey, Gluckman, and Hanson (2010) explain, however, there may be a mismatch in one individual's lifetime, such that the individual could be conceived and carried to term in a resource-poor environment but then grow up in a resource-rich environment, as has been the case for many people living in countries with rapidly developing economies. This exposure to more high-energy and high-fat foods results in a higher risk for noncommunicable diseases (NCDs) such as type 2 diabetes and heart disease later in life. An alternative hypothesis to the predictive adaptive response is the idea of "maternal capital," whereby the mother's nutritional status before and during pregnancy, among other factors, signals to the foetus the size of the offspring she is able to support (Wells 2012a).

The influence of the intrauterine environment on long-term health outcomes is now called the developmental origins of health and disease. This area of study was first developed by David Barker, an epidemiologist in the UK who used various databases of retrospective birthweight and mortality records to examine the onset of adult diseases, namely, cardiovascular disease and type 2 diabetes (Barker 1995; Barker et al. 2002 ; Barker and Osmond 1986; Hales and Barker 1992). One seminal study was based on birthweight and later medical records of the children of pregnant women living during the Dutch Winter Famine that occurred in the Netherlands at the end of the Second World War, from 1944 to 1945, when the Germans blockaded that nation's food supplies (Ravelli et al. 1998). An examination of a birth cohort from 1943 to 1947 with detailed prenatal and birth records served as a "natural" experiment to compare the adult glucose and insulin response, an indicator of type 2 diabetes, of those who were severely malnourished in utero to those who were not. Adult participants born to low birthweight babies with mothers of low body weight, those exposed to famine, had the highest glucose concentrations, suggesting insulin resistance, and thus were at higher risk of developing NCDs in their adult lives. While animal models have been the mainstay for testing the effects of maternal diet on the metabolic health of offspring – feeding rodents, sheep, or non-human primates high-fat or low-fat diets, for example, to study the offspring outcomes (Li, Sloboda, and Vickers 2011) – there are now a number of human cohort studies under way that will help us to further understand the implications of the in utero nutritional environment on children's health and nutrition (Huang et al. 2015). It is clear from these studies that both low and high birthweight, as proxies for under- and over-nutrition, can increase the risk for development of NCDs (Godfrey, Gluckman, and Hanson 2010).

In addition to a consideration of under- or over-nourishment in utero, there are some specific micronutrient deficiencies during pregnancy that can have very detrimental effects on the baby. A deficiency in folate, one of the B-complex vitamins (B9), has been well documented to substantially increase the risk of neural tube defects (NTDs) in the developing foetus (Pitkin 2007). NTDs occur when the neural tube does not close during embryonic development, causing damage to underlying tissues. The most deleterious NTD is anencephaly (absence of the brain) resulting in death; another NTD, spina bifida, causes physical impairments of the lower limbs, including paralysis and urinary and fecal incontinence (Crider, Bailey, and Berry 2011). Though in randomized control trials folic acid supplementation early in pregnancy (within the first twenty-eight days) was shown to be effective in reducing or eliminating the risk altogether, almost half or more of all pregnancies are unplanned and many women do not know they are pregnant until they have passed the first month of pregnancy. As a result, many countries, including Canada, the United States, South Africa, Costa Rica, Chile, Argentina, and Brazil, instituted mandatory folic acid (the synthetic and stable form of folate) fortification of commercially available wheat flours. Women are advised, if they are trying to get pregnant, to take folic acid supplements. This has been one of the most successful public health programs in the past century; since the initiation of mandatory fortification in 1998, NTDs have decreased in these countries by anywhere from 19 to 55 percent (Crider, Bailey, and Berry 2011).

If we subscribe to the developmental origin of health and disease perspective, are we forced into a reductionist position, where a person's nutritional lifecourse is set before birth? Does it mean that we might as well not worry about what we feed children after they are born because their nutritional pathway is set in stone? Absolutely not. The in utero environment and the nutrition they obtain from their mother sets children on a biological trajectory, but that trajectory can be modified throughout an individual's life depending on their postnatal environment. In fact, one of the very important feeding stages happens right after birth and through the first years of life with the first food – milk.

Milk Is Life: Breastfeeding

As mammals are altricial newborns (meaning that we are born relatively helpless compared to other animals), there is only one food that we can ingest and thrive on from birth, and that is milk. Not only is milk a complete food, from birth to approximately six months of age, but it is the only food that infants are equipped to consume, given their very undeveloped chewing muscles and lack of teeth, along with a gastrointestinal system that cannot really process any other foods. Mammary glands are one of the sine qua non features of the Mammalia class of animals, and, as part of that class, humans lactate just like other mammals. As members of the order *Primate*, we are a very social sort of animal, and many of our behaviours are learned, as opposed to driven by instinct, as is the case for the class *Aves* (birds). As such we must in part learn how to look after our children.

Sarah Blaffer Hrdy (2009) discusses the gusto with which many monkey females seek out other monkeys' infants – a behaviour called alloparenting – to develop and practise mothering skills that will enhance the survival of their own offspring. One of those learned mothering skills is lactation, which is a more difficult operation for humans, whose infants are even more physically and developmentally helpless at birth than are those of monkeys. The necessity to learn lactation skills through observation and modelling may explain why so many women complain about the difficulty of learning to breastfeed, especially with their first child. This becomes even more of a challenge in postindustrial contexts. The challenge of breastfeeding in these contexts became very apparent to me soon after embarking on my PhD fieldwork to study young infant and child feeding in Kathmandu, Nepal. In an excerpt from my field notes I comment: "Everyone seems so comfortable about breastfeeding here. Women feed their babies freely with children, youth, young men and women watching and interacting with the breastfeeding mother. No one seems embarrassed or looks away."

Baby Steps 21

I remarked on this fact because it was so different from my own experience growing up in Canada, where seeing a woman breastfeed was extremely rare – I personally can't remember ever seeing a woman breastfeed a baby until I was in my twenties at least – and even when I did see it, it was a strange and almost embarrassing sight. I felt I had to look away and not stare in case I might (gasp) see the woman's nipple. I don't mean to imply that no woman in Nepal has challenges with learning to breastfeed her infant. However, the act of learning to breastfeed – and it is a learned rather than an instinctual practice – is disrupted in postindustrial contexts by the inability of women to watch other women while they breastfeed, to learn through example and observation. Part of the reason for this is that in postindustrial, high-income nations, most families live in nuclear units, whereas in much of the rest of the world families continue to live in extended households where there are a variety of age cohorts of women living under one roof. This affords more opportunity for girls and women to observe their mother, aunt, sister-in-law, and so on feeding their infants.

As primates we learn by watching other individuals around us. Think of Jane Goodall's (1964) observations of chimpanzees fishing termites and ants using a twig – the juvenile by an adult chimp's side, mimicking the behaviour, maybe not successfully, but learning through experiential practice and observation. Think of the young child sitting in the kitchen, perhaps playing with a toy, but watching their parent cooking and understanding at a deep level how to prepare and cook a daily meal. So now think of the young woman who has a baby for the first time and is expected to perform a practice that is both mechanically complicated and at the same time emotional and deeply embodied. But she's never seen it done before because it's been cloaked in secrecy, something she's never seen practised in either real life or in the media. No wonder she can't perform this act, and often it goes awry.

A British woman described this experience in Williamson and colleagues' (2011, 439) study of new mothers' accounts of breastfeeding.

> Try and get him in the right position, try and get his arms out of the way ..., you're trying to hold and support his head which wobbles, and getting him to open his mouth wide, and it's just so much to do. I know it sounds pathetic, it must be, it should be the most natural thing in the world, but ... so difficult isn't it, baby boy? (Queenie, diary, day 1)

The authors of the study, using daily audio-diaries from first-time mothers during the early days after the birth of their children, found that women who struggled with breastfeeding were surprised at how difficult it was given the discourse that surrounds breastfeeding as "natural." In other words, because it is expected to be instinctual, when women are unable to perform it effortlessly, they are confused and frustrated.

So why is breastfeeding not instinctual, at least not for the mother, even though it's rooted in mammalian biology? Let's review the biology of lactation, the word used to denote the purely physiological aspects of producing milk in the mammary glands. Lactation is to some extent a mechanical process that is directed by various hormones within the mother's body. The two main hormones made in the pituitary gland that are involved in breastfeeding are prolactin and oxytocin. Prolactin is produced in response to stimulation of the nipple and promotes the production of milk. Oxytocin promotes the squeezing of the cell lining of the milk ducts, making milk flow along and fill the ducts, sometimes ejecting milk in fine streams. The oxytocin reflex is also known as the "letdown reflex." Oxytocin works when a mother has sensations, like the touch, feel, and smell of her baby; if she is in pain or emotionally upset, the reflex can be interrupted (WHO 2009).

The instinctual part of lactation and breastfeeding is the newborn's suckling and rooting reflexes that enable them when placed skin-to-skin on the mother to locate through smell and vision the mother's nipple, and to "crawl," albeit slowly, to the breast in the "awakening and active phases" shortly after birth (Widstrom et al. 2011). Widstrom and colleagues recommend that infants stay skin-to-skin with their mothers for the first hours after birth so that they can crawl to the mother and initiate their own latch with as little interference (e.g., weighing the baby) as possible and, preferably, with the umbilical cord attached.[1] What becomes the "learned" part of breastfeeding is the mother's practice, which, as those who subscribe to an evolutionary framework argue, can be messed up by "modern-day" medical interventions or even a regular medically assisted birth. Breastfeeding on some level must be an instinctual behaviour or our hominin ancestors and early humans would not have survived. Having said that, even our hominin ancestors, just like contemporary apes, would have had role models and support from other females.

What we know about breastfeeding patterns in non-agricultural and non-industrial societies is based on twentieth-century anthropological studies of hunter-gatherer foragers around the world. The groups that have been most researched in terms of infant and young child feeding include the !Kung San, living in the Kalahari desert in Botswana (Konner 2005), and the

Hadza in Tanzania (Marlowe 2010). A generalized overview of hunter-gatherer infancy and early childhood written by Melvin Konner (2005) describes a pattern of continual and frequent breastfeeding (through day and night) from birth to approximately the first year and then continued breastfeeding, though with less frequency, to the second to fourth year. Based on these models of breastfeeding, James McKenna and colleagues have hypothesized why human lactation in postindustrial settings some-times goes awry. Initially, McKenna focused on the prevention of sudden infant death syndrome through the practice of maternal-infant co-sleeping, demonstrating through careful monitoring of sleeping infant-mother dyads in a laboratory setting that the close contact with a mother's respiratory system actually regulates the baby's breathing and prevents sudden respira-tory failure (McKenna and McDade 2005; McKenna, Ball, and Gettler 2007). McKenna's co-sleeping research, however, also demonstrates why sleeping with an infant facilitates breastfeeding and why the separation of mother and infant can interrupt the initiation and continuation of breastfeeding (McKenna and Gettler 2016). Our human ancestors, of course, for sheer survival would have slept in very close proximity, both for warmth and for protection from predators. Historically and today in many low-income countries around the world, families sleep together out of necessity, due to close living quarters; if there is an extra room available, it's not going to the infant! But it turns out that having the option to give a new baby their own room, separate from mom, may not be the best choice after all. McKenna and Gettler (2016) have coined the term "breastsleeping" to underscore, in part, both the physiological and behavioural need for early and sustained maternal-infant contact throughout the day and night.

It is noteworthy that most of the biomedical research about breastfeeding has not been based on the types of anthropological studies described above but, rather, on WEIRD (Western, educated, industrialized, rich, and democratic) (Henrich, Heine, and Norenzayan 2010) study populations that do not repre-sent the behaviours or perspectives more common throughout much of the world. For example, biomedical caregivers from the early twentieth century advised breastfeeding mothers to schedule their feeds rather than to feed "on demand," though this is changing more recently with the move to baby-led breastfeeding (Fallon et al. 2016). And the practice of co-sleeping continues to be debated in the medical community with some medical doctors condemning it as a dangerous practice (Vennemann et al. 2012).

What of breast milk as a food, apart from the practice of breastfeeding? The first milk, much more diluted than mature breast milk and emitted from the mammary glands from days three to seven postpartum, is called colostrum. Apart from being a source of water, it has its most value in non-nutritive ways. Colostrum aids in clearing meconium (a green, dark tar-like substance) from the infant's gastrointestinal tract and is full of antimicrobial agents, such as immunoglobulins, that confer passive immunity to the infant's developing immune system. This immunity can be lifesaving for infants, especially those living in an environment with a heavy pathogen load (Andreas, Kampmann, and Mehring Le-Doare 2015). Even mature breast milk has many bioactive agents, in addition to microbial agents, some of which include hormones like ghrelin and leptin that are active in regulating hunger and appetite suppression, and may be implicated in preventing paediatric obesity, though this is still in early research development (Thompson 2012).

Of course, the main importance of breast milk is to nurture the growing child. Milk, coined by Andrea Wiley (2016) as the "special food," is constituted from macronutrients – fats, sugars, and proteins – as well as a range of micronutrients (vitamins and minerals). It is thus a complete food for infants, at least until about four to six months postpartum, at which point infants require more nutrients through complementary foods. Human milk is constitutionally unique to human nutritional requirements, as is every other mammalian milk, each with different proportions of macro- and micro-nutrients. Human milk, relative to, say, cow's milk, has less protein and fat and more sugar (lactose), specific to our life history as long-living, slow-growing, and relatively large mammals (Wiley 2016). It is important to note that the milk that is delivered to infants through lactation is dynamic in its makeup in that it differs not only between individuals but also within an individual, varying by feed throughout the day (peaking in mid-morning) and with the developmental trajectory of the child. Fat, for example, increases from the beginning (fore milk) to the end of the feed (hind milk), while the lactose content is inversely correlated with fat content, with further frequency and duration of feeds increasing through the day (Andreas, Kampmann, and Mehring Le-Doare 2015). There is evidence from research done in Kenya by Masako Fujita and colleagues (2012) that fat content may even differ depending on the sex (male or female) of the infant and the socioeconomic circumstances of the mother and child. Thus, human milk is specifically tailored to the needs of the individual baby, and the baby is to some extent agentic in terms of their control of suckling frequency and duration changing the quantity and quality of the milk (Pike and Milligan 2010).

Lactation is, simply put, a dance between maternal and infant feedback systems, supply and demand, as well as demand and supply, since both infant and mother mediate the activation of the milk production through suckling and access to the breast. There are, however, competition and trade-offs between infant demands and maternal ability to synthesize milk. Hinde and Milligan (2011, 20), in their review of primate lactation, note that there is always "a compromise between infant energy requirements for growth, development, and behavioral activity on the one hand, and maternal abilities to access and mobilize dietary energy and bodily reserves during lactation on the other." I argue later in this chapter that these "trade-offs" go beyond the biological aspects of lactation – or breastfeeding, a term that incorporates more fully the biocultural nature of human lactation – into the cultural realm, where reproducing women are constantly negotiating their environmental, cultural, and economic activities when it comes to nourishing their infants.

Breastfeeding and Beyond

The biocultural practice of infant feeding has mirrored the human evolution of food systems, from Paleolithic gathering and hunting right through to industrialized food systems. Alternatives to the mother-infant feeding dyad have always existed, for example in the form of "wet nursing," "milk sharing," or "cross-nursing" (i.e., breastfeeding another individual's baby). Early humans would no doubt have wet-nursed to take the place of another mother in the case of illness or death, or just for sheer convenience if the mother needed to be temporarily absent. The practice of wet-nursing has been documented in ancient civilizations with accounts among the elite classes of ancient Greeks and Romans, including textual evidence in the form of wet-nursing contracts and treatises by medical writers Galen and Soranus on the best types of wet nurse and their qualities (Fildes 1986). In early modern Europe, from 1500 to 1800, and especially in France and Central Europe, wet-nursing was de rigeur among the upper classes. Breastfeeding was frowned upon as disfiguring, leading to premature aging, and interfering with fashion, and many men were publicly against the practice for their wives.

With the development of agriculture in the Neolithic, the possibility of feeding a baby milk from domesticated animals – cows, goats, sheep, camels, pigs, or horses – arose (Stevens, Patrick, and Pickler 2009), and there are numerous accounts of infants feeding directly from animal teats in ancient Greek, Roman, and Arabic texts, as well as archaeological evidence from Neolithic Europe of ceramic drinking vessels with organic residue analyses

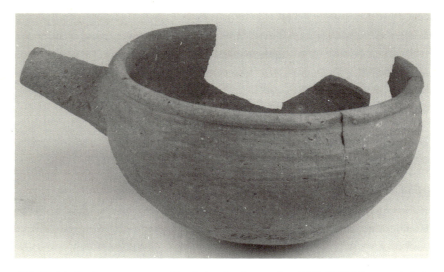

FIGURE 1.1 Earthenware spouted jar (infant feeding cup), c. 1750–1550 BC, excavated at Dakhleh Oasis, Egypt. | Courtesy Royal Ontario Museum.

indicating that they were used for feeding infants milk from domesticated ruminants – cows, sheep, and goats (Dunne et al. 2019). Figure 1.1 shows an example of an infant feeding cup excavated from the Dakhleh Oasis in Egypt, circa 1750–1550 BC. While breastfeeding was valued in many societies, as evidenced by medical texts from ancient Greece, Rome, and Islam, the mother's death or illness sometimes required that breast milk alternatives be used from birth. Alternatives included infant paps made from animal milk and grain flour, what Valerie Fildes (1986) calls "dry nursing." Dry nursing was common for those who could not afford to contract a wet nurse as well as for institutional foundling settings if wet nurses could not be found. Dry nursing became so common in preindustrial Europe that in many parts of central and northern Europe it became customary.

The ability to feed infants alternatives to breast milk accelerated in the first part of the industrialization of the food system – beginning around 1870 – when food products began to be patented and advertised (Winson 2013). The first baby bottles made of glass were developed in France in 1851 (Stevens, Patrick, and Pickler 2009) and were used for feeding babies cow's milk, which was becoming more commonly marketed in urban areas in North America and Europe (Wiley 2016). With the development of sterilizing food in sealed containers, products such as evaporated milk, patented in 1853 by William Newton, became available as an infant feeding alternative

(Stevens, Patrick, and Pickler 2009). The use of artificial feeding was not without a downside; many more infants died prematurely due to either malnutrition, infection from unsterilized feeding bottles, or a combination of the two. A historical demographic study done by John Knodel and Etienne van de Walle documents the deleterious effects of bottle feeding from 1870 to 1940 in the south of Germany (Bavaria), where bottle feeding was more commonly practised than in northern Germany. They found much higher rates of infant mortality in the south relative to the north, with a clear infant mortality gradient depending on the age in months at which the infant was weaned from the breast (Knodel and van de Walle 1967).

It wasn't until the mid-twentieth century that artificial feeding became safer for humans, with the understanding of the germ theory of disease ushering in the era of pasteurization of milk (from Louis Pasteur's discovery in 1862 that bacteria could be killed by heating liquids to high temperatures), sterilization of feeding bottles, and the development of infant formula. In the 1920s, formula was scientifically rendered to mimic as closely as possible human milk as it was understood at the time. Also developed were alternatives to cow's milk formula such as soy-based formula for infants with milk allergies. In 1929, the American Medical Association began to oversee the safety and efficacy of infant formula, and over the years there have been many improvements and enhancements on the original recipe in the form of fortification of micronutrients such as iron and vitamin D (Stevens, Patrick, and Pickler 2009). Indeed, by the time of the intensification of the industrial diet from 1945 to 1980 (Winson 2013), infant formula was considered, at least in North America, to be superior to breast milk, and many biomedical professionals recommended that mothers should not even initiate breastfeeding; infant formula was considered more scientific and modern, and was normalized as best for baby (Bentley 2014). This medical advice along with the increasing numbers of women entering the formal economic workforce led to a sharp decline in the initiation of breastfeeding for women in the US between 1955 and 1978 (Martinez and Nalezienski 1979).

The rise of bottle feeding had profoundly detrimental effects in low-income countries, where Nestlé and other companies were promoting their products aggressively, due to the large potential market. As had been the case historically in Europe and North America, bottle feeding in low-income countries was at best a recipe for malnutrition and at worst a death sentence for many infants. Lack of clean water to make infant formula and sterilize bottles precipitates a cycle of infant diarrhea, sometimes leading to mortality from dehydration. Infant formula, prohibitively expensive for many families in low-income countries, is in practice often incorrectly prepared or watered down to make it go further. Penny Van Esterik (1989), an anthropologist and advocate, outlines the "infant formula controversy" that took place in the 1970s and into the early 1980s. After the 1974 translation of a publication by a German non-governmental organization (NGO) titled "Nestlé Kills Babies," Nestlé filed a libel suit against the organization. Though the NGO was found guilty, the judge recognized the unethical aspects of Nestlé's conduct, and this galvanized the public and other NGOs to rally behind a boycott of all Nestlé's food products. This boycott lasted from 1977 to 1984 and was deemed the most successful consumer boycott to date, though rather than curbing its promotion of infant formula Nestlé spent most of its efforts on improving public relations by sponsoring paediatric research into infant feeding and conferences. In 1981, however, the boycott did precipitate the development of the World Health Organization's (WHO) code for the marketing of breast milk substitutes. The code included an end to mass marketing and free gifts to health care providers and retailers, as well as labelling to indicate the superiority of breast milk over infant formula (Van Esterik 1989, 11).

Back to Breast

As with other cultural influences on human food systems, infant feeding changed with the times: in the 1970s, with the growing awareness of environmentalism, the growth of the health-food industry, and back-to-the-land movements, the promotion of "breast is best" began. At this time, as well, biomedical researchers were "discovering" some of the benefits of breastfeeding, both for babies and for women, in terms of postpartum recovery and even lower rates of breast cancer (Labbok 2001). From this growing evidence base of the benefits of breastfeeding, the Baby-Friendly Hospital Initiative was launched by WHO and UNICEF in 1991, following the Innocenti Declaration of 1990 (WHO/UNICEF 2018). The Innocenti Declaration was signed in Florence, Italy, at a WHO/UNICEF policy-makers' meeting. The declaration includes statements about the benefits of exclusive breastfeeding during the first six months, and complementary breastfeeding continued beyond, as optimal for maternal and child health, as well as commitments to support women to enable them to breastfeed through nourishment and health care, and national policies to "protect, promote and support breastfeeding" in perinatal, nutrition, and family planning services. The declaration also includes the need to promote a "breastfeeding culture" that empowers women to have the confidence to breastfeed. Finally, the declaration states that all governments (by the year 1995) should have "enacted imaginative legislation protecting breastfeeding rights of working women and established means for its enforcement."

It was from this point on that the familiar mantra "breast is best" was heard in the public health domain. Feeding babies with infant formula had taken hold, however, in large part due to the multi million-dollar infant formula industry, with multinational formula companies, like Nestlé, investing huge amounts in the research, development, and advertising of these products. Many hospitals around the world were receiving funding to promote infant formula in paediatric wards, and thus hospitals had to divest themselves of that investment from infant formula companies to certify as baby-friendly hospitals. Hospitals certify by following the WHO International Code of Marketing of Breast Milk Substitutes as well as by following other practices, such as training staff about breastfeeding and helping mothers to initiate breastfeeding within a half-hour after birth through skin-to-skin contact (Breastfeeding Committee for Canada 2017). Canada now has a growing number of baby-friendly hospitals, but not all of them are certified (Yourex-West 2017).

Despite the promotion of breastfeeding by health care professionals, the WHO (in addition to many other government and non-governmental organizations) and many advocacy groups (like the La Leche League International), mothers have not stopped using infant formula. Infant formula promotion by multinational organizations like Nestlé is only part of the story of why women do not always breastfeed their infants. The other parts are diverse, but one important theme that resonates for all women around the globe is the complicated dance of reproduction and production that directly affects how women nurture their infants.

Women's Productive and Reproductive Work: An Uneasy Tension

Perhaps because we are so focused on how breastfeeding is circumscribed by women's productive labour or work (Leslie 1988; O'Gara 1989; Moffat 2002), we rarely consider, as Van Esterik (1995) points out, the impact of breastfeeding on productive work – that is, are women's work opportunities and productive lives limited by breastfeeding?[2] The view of breastfeeding as an impediment to work may also be a result of many researchers' postindustrial perspective, according to which the two forms of labour are viewed as incompatible.[3] Thus, we are either stuck in an old-fashioned view of women's work being primarily and most importantly reproductive in nature (Ball and Swedlund 1996), or we adopt an existentialist feminist perspective, originating in Simone de Beauvoir's writings, that posits that women must free themselves from reproduction to be truly liberated (Rosser 1997).

One way of attempting to break this dichotomy is to define breastfeeding as work in so far as women are expending energy for the growth and development of their offspring (Vitzthum 1994; McDade and Worthman 1998). All women work in that they "expend energy for a purpose" (Van Esterik and Greiner 1981, 185). Unless one sets out to study the relationship between women's work and breastfeeding, however, it is often forgotten that women are productive workers, even if they are not engaged in formal wage labour. Exceptions to this are the studies that examine breastfeeding in relation to women's subsistence agricultural work (Levine 1988; Panter-Brick 1992) as well as the focus on the informal wage sector in urban and peri-urban centres in low-income countries (Rogers and Youssef 1988; Joekes 1989; O'Gara 1989; Moffat 2002). The approach to breastfeeding and work is nicely captured by O'Gara, Canahuati, and Moore's (1994, S33) plea that we consider "every mother a working mother." Instead of asking if breastfeeding and work can be combined, we should ask: "What kind of work are mothers doing? In what settings are they working? Have there been changes in recent years that have made breastfeeding and working less compatible? What trade-offs do mothers make? How important is breastfeeding for working women? What support do they need? What full range of infant feeding options are a minimum for working mothers?" Van Esterik (1995) further interrogates this issue by asking if we can even really separate women's productive and reproductive work and whether breastfeeding is always work. Breastfeeding is not only work; there are enjoyable aspects to it, as in spending time with an infant. It may also be a respite from work for many women. This is an important point because, though it is useful from feminist and evolutionary perspectives to consider breastfeeding as work, it is also a rather limiting view of it.

My PhD dissertation focuses on young children's nutritional well-being, but it is also about the nature of women's reproductive and productive work (Moffat 1998). I did my fieldwork in 1995–96 just outside of the capital city of Nepal, Kathmandu, in an area where the Tibetan/Nepali carpet-making industry had taken hold and was booming. Migrants came from all regions of the country, moving from their natal villages to Kathmandu to pursue work in the carpet-making industry. The industry sprang up at the edge of the city, where land was cheapest and was available for establishing larger factories. After Nepal's democratic revolution in 1990, and with the hope of growing economic development, the carpet-making industry was born out of a small cottage industry that, with the help of mostly foreign partners and a large European market, became the second biggest industry in Nepal after tourism (O'Neill 1997). This offered an economic opportunity for women – who have traditionally been weavers – since they were valued as employees rather than just for their supposed docility and hard work. Unfortunately, due to unfair labour standards, they were paid at lower wages than their male counterparts, but they were still earning wages.

Many of these working women had young infants and children, and it was on these women and children that I focused my research. One of my research questions concerned how women in this context were able to combine their productive and reproductive work and what impact this had on the health of their children. During my fieldwork, I began to question some of my own assumptions and biases, such as that productive and reproductive work was a "natural" dichotomy. It was my fieldwork with carpet workers in Nepal that led me to understand the possibility of blurring these two spheres. In my study I set out to compare breastfeeding practices and the health of children whose mothers worked in the more formal, though flexible, setting of the carpet factory versus those who spun wool in their homes in an informal work setting. Initially believing that women in the factory setting would be *less* likely to breastfeed their infants, I hypothesized that home workers would be *more* likely to exclusively breastfeed their infants and for a longer duration. What I found, however, was that, due to lack of distinction between productive and reproductive work, there was no difference between women's breastfeeding practices in the factories and in the homes. Thus, women in both home and factory freely breastfed while working or when taking a break from spinning or weaving (Moffat 2002). Breastfeeding and productive work were blurred, and breastfeeding was also a pleasurable break from productive work. While this was not necessarily the ideal setting for young children – there were hazards in the factories, such as sharp metal implements and an abundance of airborne wool fibres – this was a flexible solution to the problematic dichotomy that we have created in industrial and postindustrial settings.

We need to approach these studies from the perspective that it is not necessarily "normal" to split productive and reproductive work, and we need to examine how, through gender discrimination, women's intentions and bids for equality are often thwarted by structural barriers within society. As Van Esterik (2002, 266) points out: "Breastfeeding and women's work cannot be examined independently of the economic and political context of maternity entitlements, health insurance, wages, and child-care arrangements." Medical professionals can preach about the benefits of breastfeeding and "educate" women about appropriate practices, but if the workplace environment or working hours are such that women are not flexibly able to maintain breast milk supply through regular feeding (and/or expressing), then breastfeeding will cease (Yimyam, Morrow, and Srisuphan 1999) and women will become frustrated and exhausted (Shao Mlay, Keddy, and Noerager Stern 2004). As Maher (1992, 173) points out, the inability for women to breastfeed in the postindustrial world of wage labour is not a problem of "work itself," or even of "work outside the home," but of capitalist industrial relations.

Here I am reminded of an amusing video by Naya Health called *If Men Breastfed* (If Men Breastfed – Bing video) that was brought to my attention by one of my students. The video is a delightful sendup of the male-dominated workplace with working men sitting in a beautiful breastfeeding lounge at the office equipped with state-of-the-art breast milk pumps. This parody effectively communicates the message that if women had more power and influence in the workplace, they could potentially combine more of their reproductive and productive work. In Canada there are fairly generous federally mandated parental leaves to extend shorter private-sector parental benefits for up to sixty-one weeks (roughly fifteen months) postpartum (Government of Canada 2019b). However, the Canadian government's parental leave payments are a fraction of a woman's full-time wages, and thus women must have savings or a partner with full employment to support parental leave from work. In the US, by contrast, there are no federally mandated parental leaves, and workplace leaves generally range from six weeks to three months. Contrast this with Denmark, where mothers get eighteen weeks of parental leave, all at full pay, after which parents can split an additional thirty-two weeks of leave however they choose (Weller 2016).

But if you look at responses to questions in the Canadian Community Health Survey regarding why women breastfeed for less than six months, in 2011–12 the top responses were: they have insufficient breast milk (44 percent) or had difficulty with breastfeeding technique, followed by "returned to school or work" (10 percent) (Gionet 2013). So there is more than the challenge of combining work and breastfeeding, though the answers shown above may not be mutually exclusive, since a mother, in anticipation of returning to work, may introduce the occasional bottle of formula to an infant, thereby setting up a cycle whereby the decrease in nipple suckling precipitates a reduction in breast milk volume. This can result in the mother feeling, and rightly so, that she does not have enough breast milk for her infant. This hypothesis is supported by understandings of autocrine control of breast milk production in addition to endocrine (hormonal) control from the pituitary gland. Autocrine control refers to local glandular control of lactation in the breast, where frequent and, perhaps as important, complete emptying of the breast is necessary to maintain an adequate breast milk supply. Breast milk that remains in the breast after a feed acts as a negative feedback signal, inhibiting further breast milk production (De Coopman 1993; Woolridge 1995). Regular emptying of the breast is usually experienced with on-demand breastfeeding as opposed to scheduled feeds (e.g., every four hours) that may not be frequent enough to keep up with infants' breast milk requirements (Woolridge 1995). Mothers' claims of insufficient breast milk are frequently labelled as "perceived insufficiency" (cf. McCann and Bender 2006), assuming that the mind is separate from the body's mechanical capacity to lactate. There is a clear mind-body interaction, however, where "letdown" and breast milk supply can be influenced by a myriad of emotions and states, including chronic illness, fatigue, depression, and anxiety.

Interestingly, during my research on breastfeeding in Nepal many women also cited "insufficient milk" as a problem. Without the means to bottle feed, however, because they were too poor to afford either formula or bottles, insufficient milk resulted in supplementing their infants early (before the recommended six months) with weaning foods like rice pabulum. But these Nepali women continued to breastfeed up to, on average, two and a half years, so claiming that they had insufficient breast milk certainly did not precipitate an end to breastfeeding. It is possible that insufficient breast milk, though expressed similarly by mothers in both high- and low-income countries, is a result of different processes. I conjecture that it is possible that insufficient breast milk among the Nepali mothers I interviewed, whether real or perceived, was a result of maternal malnutrition, perhaps in the form of iron deficiency, all too common among women in Nepal and South Asia generally, resulting in fatigue, weakness, and a decrease in the production of breast milk (Moffat 2002).

Young Child Feeding

Though the first six months of an infant's life is one of the most crucial periods for survival, growth, and development, there is more to infant feeding beyond breastfeeding. Kennedy (2005) and Sellen (2001, 2007) have both considered the evolutionary aspects of human lactation and weaning vis-à-vis non-human primates and argue, using a life history theory lens, that the pattern of early weaning for humans may be a strategy to support larger brain growth and higher fertility relative to other primates, particularly the great apes. Daniel Sellen (2007, 2010) goes on to further articulate complementary feeding as a uniquely human transitional feeding strategy that is not observed among any other mammals or even non-human primates. We humans are unique in our early and flexible weaning. As part of that early weaning, we have a special phase in our human lifecourse during which our parents feed us complementary foods while we are still altricial, meaning that we are incapable of procuring our own foods and that our dental formation is still too immature to handle chewing completely solid and adult forms of food. These are described by Sellen (2010, 67) as "special transitional foods." Though chimpanzee mothers have been documented as sharing food with their infants during the transitional period between exclusive suckling and independent foraging, only humans specifically prepare and provision complementary foods that are often cooked or processed in some way to make them healthful and digestible for infants.

The human weaning process has been documented through anthropological studies based in contemporary settings, mostly in predominantly agricultural, low-income countries, as well as historical studies based on bioarchaeological evidence (Van Esterik 2002). One can distill from these ethnographic studies a basic pattern for the weaning process, which includes a period of exclusive breastfeeding from birth to approximately four to six months of age, followed by the introduction of complementary foods accompanied by the continuation of breastfeeding. Most children are weaned (i.e., breastfeeding has stopped completely) by about three years of age, though some may continue into the fourth year. This pattern of complementary feeding while accompanied by breastfeeding for up to three years is quite different from infant feeding practices in industrialized countries, where breastfeeding is often replaced by complementary foods rather than accompanied by it.

Thus, there is no universal pattern of infant and young child feeding, and as humans we tend to complicate the way we eat and feed our young. Sellen's (2010) descriptor "flexible" is key here. Indeed, just as we have seen with early infancy and breastfeeding, there are permutations in the variety as well as in the timing of the introduction of complementary foods fed to infants during the weaning process. What complementary foods and when to introduce them are hotly debated topics, dating back at least to ancient Rome, when medical experts like Galen and Soranus wrote infant feeding guidelines. Galen suggested that the introduction of solid foods should occur around the time when the deciduous (baby) teeth start to emerge (around six months of age). Soranus suggested a period when the infant's body was "ready" to accept more solid food and criticized the common Roman practice of feeding infants cereal as early as forty days after birth (Prowse et al. 2008). Direct studies of infant feeding practices in the ancient Roman Empire indicate that, for the most part, Romans followed these medical guidelines (Moffat and Prowse 2018). Evidence from the analysis of stable isotopes of carbon and nitrogen found in infant skeletal material and teeth in a variety of locales across the Roman Empire indicates that the introduction of complementary foods started from about six months of age and that breastfeeding continued to approximately two to three years of age (Dupras, Schwarcz, and Fairgrieve 2001; Keenleyside et al. 2009; Prowse et al. 2008).

While guidelines and practice sometimes converge, this is not always the case, as is seen in many contemporary low-income countries. The WHO stipulates that infants should be breastfed exclusively (that means no water or non-breast milk food) until six months of age (WHO 2002). This is based on both the physiological understanding of when the infant's digestive system is mature enough to process non-milk food and the reality of many mothers and infants living in low-income countries, where sanitation systems and clean water are not available to most, and the risk of morbidity and mortality due to diarrheal diseases is high. Despite strong recommendations to practise exclusive breastfeeding till six months postpartum, I found in my surveys of mothers with infants and young children in Nepal that there is variation in the introduction of complementary foods. In my sample of mother-infant dyads, infants were first fed rice pabulum anywhere from three to eight months of age. As stated above, the most common reason for introducing non-breast-milk food to infants before six months was mothers' perceptions that their babies were not getting enough breast milk. It is hard to know without further investigation whether the perception of insufficient breast milk was "true" or not; mothers may have wanted to move the weaning process along faster, though, as I argue above, this was probably not the case since they continued to breastfeed their infants up to, on average, two and a half years. Alternatively, they were sensing a slow-down in their infants' growth, a well-known phenomenon of growth retardation, common in many low-income countries, that spurred them to supplement their infants' diets (Moffat 2001, 2002). An argument that breast milk alone may not completely meet the energy needs of infants up to six months of age has also been made by Reilly and Wells (2005). In my sample of infants from Kathmandu, there appeared to be no significant difference in the growth or the occurrence of morbidity in the form of diarrhea and/or respiratory infections for those fed non-breast-milk foods before six months versus those exclusively breastfed until six months or later (Moffat 2002). These findings have also been documented by other authors in different populations in low-income regions of the world, indicating that the six-month mark may not be as crucial a target for exclusive breastfeeding as is stipulated by the WHO. There may be room for more flexibility, perhaps as early as four months in some cases (Wilson et al. 2006; Qasem, Fenton, and Friel 2015). The consideration of local ecologies and biologies when stipulating universal guidelines is certainly warranted here.

The question of which foods are best to feed infants is, to a large degree, a matter of which available foods can be rendered soft for them. Prior to the advent of agriculture or in hunter-gatherer/fisher populations, infants would have been fed meat, cooked tubers, and mashed berries. Premastication (adult chewing of the food to soften it before feeding) was probably also commonly practised and still is in some hunter-gatherer and horticultural populations (Konner 2005; Pelto, Zhang, and Habicht 2010). With the development of agriculture, cereal grains became preferred weaning food. As documented by texts in ancient Rome, for example, complementary foods fed to Roman infants included animal milk (i.e., sheep, goat, or cow), eggs, bread mixed with milk, and soft cereals. In Europe between 1500 and 1800, medical writers weighed in on the best time to introduce complementary foods, basing it mostly on the age of the child and the eruption of the first incisors. Fildes's (1986) analysis of these texts shows changing recommendations: in the sixteenth century it was seven to nine months, whereas in the seventeenth and eighteenth centuries two to five months was favoured. First foods were usually pap – consisting of milk, cereal, and flavourings like spice or sugar and sometimes eggs – or panada (made from breadcrumbs and a liquid like broth).

Today, with postmodern diets that range from Paleodiets to veganism, standards for complementary feeding are diverse, though in most agricultural societies grain cereals are normatively the first foods fed to a baby. As an alternative to grains, Paleo Mom blogger Sarah Ballantyne (2012) recommends first foods such as mashed ripe avocado, banana, cooked sweet potato, squash, pureed liver (preferably pastured/grass-fed) and pastured egg yolk. For babies at least six months old: very well-pureed, well-cooked meats (pureed with broth or breast milk) and whole milk yogurt (especially from grass-fed cows). Yogurt is an incongruous dietary item for someone who subscribes to a Paleodiet since dairy food was not available before the advent of agriculture and is therefore not normally part of a Paleodiet. But according to PaleoPlan, some dairy, preferably goat milk, is safe for children under two or three years, assuming they have no allergies or sensitivities to it (McNew 2016).

There is merit to offering babies a range of vegetables, fruits, and high-protein, fat, and iron-rich foods. Though most commercially prepared infant pabulums are iron-fortified, one of the failings of many weaning foods, especially those prepared in low-income countries, is that they may be deficient in protein and iron; young children during this period can become iron-deficient and anemic (Pelto 1987). Iron is one of the essential micronutrients needed for healthy growth and development; deficiencies in it can result in severe cognitive impairments and a depressed immune system (Zimmermann and Hurrell 2007). This Paleo approach has become more mainstream recently and has spawned a trend in "baby-led weaning," whereby as soon as infants can sit up on their own with good head control, they are offered "solid" food (i.e., not pureed or pabulum), and they self-feed with their fingers, eating ground meat, a chicken leg, an avocado, a sweet potato, and so on (Gregory 2017).

I am not a fan of the Paleodiet, in part because of the anthropological and evolutionary inaccuracies on which most of it is based (see Marlene Zuk 2013 for an excellent critique of the Paleodiet), and because we can never go back to the Paleolithic in any form. The examples above, however, have illustrated, I believe, that there is some benefit to understanding human evolution and its relationship to modern paediatric nutrition. For example, recent recommendations for young child feeding related to allergy prevention have completely overturned previous ideas that infants and young children must be prevented from eating common allergen-inducing foods like peanuts and eggs. It is now recommended that earlier exposure, as early as four to six months, and even in utero through the pregnant mother, may prevent these food allergies from occurring later in life (DuToit et al. 2016; Abrams et al. 2019). This is certainly in keeping with "Paleobaby" feeding described above, where the baby is fed foods that the older members of the household are eating. As well, an understanding of how breastfeeding and weaning occur in other parts of the world may help us to get a clearer understanding of how patterns of infant feeding in postindustrial societies have been more aberrant than "normal" as many of us assume.

Infant and Young Child Feeding Politics

The topic of infant and young child feeding is like most food-related topics fraught with politics, as food and feeding are always political. The breastfeeding versus bottle feeding debate is sensitive, since some women do not wish to breastfeed for reasons related to career, body, or otherwise. In an article by Hanna Rosin (2009) in the *Atlantic Monthly*, this debate is clearly articulated from a mother's perspective. Rosin, herself a breastfeeding mother, questions the over rating of the health benefits of breastfeeding for children living in high-income countries with access to clean water and sanitation. In high-income countries the three big paediatric health issues linked to breastfeeding are atopy, diabetes, and obesity (Stevens, Patrick, and Pickler 2009). Atopy includes eczema, asthma, and allergies. The prevalence of these conditions has been increasing among children for the past ten to fifteen years. Atopy might be prevented through breastfeeding because breast milk contains factors that actively stimulate the infant's immune system, though more research is required to fully understand the relationship among breastfeeding, the infant immune system function, and atopy. A large meta-analysis study of breastfeeding and these conditions indicates that there is some low-grade quality evidence that longer duration of breastfeeding is associated with a reduced risk of asthma and the reduced risk of allergic rhinitis and eczema in children up to two years of age, but there is no association found between breastfeeding and either increased or decreased risk for food allergies (Lodge et al. 2015). There is some evidence for a lower risk of developing type 1 (formerly known as juvenile onset) diabetes among infants who are breastfed for twelve months or longer among genetically predisposed children (Lund-Blix et al. 2015). But unfortunately, breastfeeding is not a panacea for any of these conditions.

Rosin (2009) goes on to argue that there are valid reasons women may not want to breastfeed, including the desire to co-parent equally (with bottle feeding both parents can equally accept the responsibility for feeding right from birth). Rosin humorously and pointedly explains her position:

> In Betty Friedan's day, feminists felt shackled to domesticity by the unreasonably high bar for housework, the endless dusting and shopping and pushing the Hoover around – a vacuum cleaner being the obligatory prop for the "happy housewife heroine," as Friedan sardonically called her. When I looked at the picture on the cover of Sears's *Breastfeeding Book* – a lady lying down, gently smiling at her baby and *still in her robe*, although the

Baby Steps

sun is well up – the scales fell from my eyes: it was not the vacuum that was keeping me and my 21st-century sisters down, but another sucking sound.

And Rosin goes on to point out that breastfeeding, especially for the middle-class, educated woman, has become the sine qua non of respectable parenting. Rosin deviously tried out a line in her local playground, telling other mothers about how she had decided to stop breastfeeding her young infant. "The reaction was always the same: circles were redrawn such that I ended up in the class of mom who, in a pinch, might feed her baby mashed-up Chicken McNuggets."

I present these provocative passages from Rosin's (2009) article to drive home the complexity of breastfeeding politics. How do we ensure a woman's right to breastfeed – with full access to well-paid parental leave, the freedom to breastfeed in public places without being subjected to derision, recognition and accommodation among employers to breastfeed/breast pump in the workplace – and at the same time allow women the freedom to choose *not to* breastfeed without stigma? There are many structural barriers to breastfeeding, so at this moment in time whether a woman breastfeeds or not is not always a "choice." But sometimes it *is* a choice, and as long as the infant has adequate means to a safe breast milk alternative then this issue can be considered to be in the realm of reproductive rights, akin to the right to bear a child or not, the right to give birth at home under the care of a midwife or in a hospital, and so on.

To address this debate within the biocultural approach to infant feeding that I take in this book, I consider several theoretical paradigms. The first and foremost is feminism. Starting from the fundamental premise that feminism considers gender as a key variable of analysis, its theoretical palette is diverse, coming in a variety of shades from liberal feminism – the early first and second waves of feminism that sought to alleviate women's oppression and foster equality in the workforce – through to third wave postmodern feminism (see Rosser 1997 for a review). Feminism's multivocality is healthy as it allows for a certain freedom of perspectives, and thus I draw from several of its multiple strains. As a "white," highly educated woman living in a high-income country, in an attempt to avoid the universalizing tendencies of liberal feminism I for the most part employ an intersectional feminist framework that considers gender as only one form of oppression with multiple identities (Rosser 1997, 34; see also Mohanty 1991 for a critique of Western feminism's production of the "oppressed third world woman"). In conceiving of postmodern feminism, I refer to Moore's (2006, 23) point that "gender can no longer be analyzed as distinct from other forms of difference. The lived experience of gender is that it is already class, already race or any of the other differences through which people construct a sense of self and engage with the world."

We must then re-examine the public health goal to promote universal, exclusive breastfeeding. While I believe this goal is laudable and well-meaning, it falls prey to failings similar to those of liberal feminism (Rosser 1997; Mohanty 1991). It assumes that every woman is capable of breastfeeding, despite overwhelming structural and social barriers that are often overlooked or ignored. This is not to say that it is not desirable nor that every woman does not have a right to breastfeed her children, just as it is every woman's right to be treated equally with men. I believe we should hold to this as an ideal. However, in research we must foreground the multitude of class, ethnic, and globalizing factors that make it clear that there is no such thing as "women" and "men" as essential categories, nor is there a universal "breastfeeding mother." Otherwise, we risk creating an idealized mother who is able, through plentiful resources and support, to follow breastfeeding recommendations perfectly – to the detriment of those who are not afforded such opportunities.

Feminism is not an easy field to manage in relation to infant feeding research because, as Van Esterik (1995) and Tapias (2006) point out, for the most part, feminist anthropology, and indeed feminism in general, have avoided the topic of lactation and breastfeeding. Van Esterik (1995) argues that this is because breastfeeding is bound up with the reproductive aspect of women's bodies. Thus, it presents a dilemma for feminist theorists who seek to liberate women from the tyranny of reproduction. Yet she argues that "breastfeeding is a paradigmatic feminist issue for anthropologists because it requires rethinking some basic issues in anthropological theory, such as the sexual division of labour, the fit between women's productive and reproductive lives, and the role of physiological processes in defining gender ideology" (76). Van Esterik goes on to argue that breastfeeding should be considered a feminist issue because it is an issue of empowerment that challenges medical hegemony, the lack of integration between women's productive and reproductive activities, and views of the breast as primarily a sex object. Breastfeeding, moreover, requires structural changes in society to improve the position and condition of women, encourages solidarity and cooperation among women, and confirms a woman's power to control her own body (77).

The other theoretical framework I consider here is evolutionary theory. A consideration of evolutionary theory is relevant for two reasons. First, because lactation is a reproductive behaviour that influences human fertility and is sensitive to cultural ecology (Vitzthum 1994, 1997); second, because evolutionary theory offers an alternative to the biomedical view of breast-feeding (which privileges the health of the infant) by considering the mother-infant dyad, in which the benefits and trade-offs of infant feeding are considered for both mothers and infants (McDade and Worthman 1998; McDade 2001). While feminism and evolutionary theory seem to be odd bedfellows, there are examples of intersections: an evolutionary perspective need not be bound to biological determinism (cf. Waage and Adair Gowaty 1997; Stone 2016) and can be paired with a feminist agenda to highlight issues such as women's oppression and structural violence as issues relevant to breastfeeding.

Evolutionary biology and feminism both share the understanding of the maternal-infant dyad in terms of trade-offs. So often in the biomedical context, the infant/child is privileged over the mother; yet, in evolutionary terms, the mother's biology is always considered to be adapting to benefit her own survival as well as her offspring's. As an alternative to the public health or biomedical focus on infant health that treats women as passive feeding vessels, McDade and Worthman (1998) and McDade (2001) advance a model based on a life history approach from evolutionary biology. This model includes a maternal perspective that considers the costs and benefits of mothers' energetic, nutritional, reproductive, productive, and social norms, which are no doubt a part of the socioecological environment (McKerracher et al. 2017). This approach is more compatible with a feminist theoretical framework in that it includes mothers' constraints and agency in reproductive rights.

The concept of trade-offs between the mother and infant is also known as parent-offspring conflict theory (Trivers 1974). "Where the infant strives to be healthy as possible without draining the caregiver to a degree that she/he can no longer invest; the parent strives to raise healthy offspring that survive to reproduce at a minimal cost" (Tully and Ball 2013, 3). From an evolutionary perspective these are unconscious decisions on the part of the infant and parent players. Tully and Ball (2013), however, expand on this concept by creating a model of mother-infant breastfeeding trade-offs over time that incorporates parental or even family perceptions of potential costs to the mother and benefits to the infant that, presumably, would include both energetic and health costs to the mothers as well as costs in labour and psycho-social factors. Detailed research in both low-income and high-income countries surrounding the motivations, both conscious and unconscious, among families that drive breastfeeding practices is much needed to sort out how we can support mothers in breastfeeding to the degree that respects personal autonomy.

Going beyond the Maternal Focus

We must also consider why women are held responsible for the health of their children, even though there is overwhelming evidence of wider household, community, and global forces at work. Here again we can see that feminism can be brought to bear on this issue from different perspectives. In the same vein as supporting women's strengths in uniquely feminine traits and abilities like breastfeeding, Van Esterik argues that we should acknowledge women's very important role in feeding and nourishing children and other family members. By supporting women's "right to feed," it becomes apparent that there is an imperative to support women through all other social, economic, and political realms. This becomes bound up in the rhetoric around food security and can be extended to women as food producers and feeders. While this is an important activist position, it can lead to the slippery slope of blaming women when things go wrong with feeding, as has been pointed out by many authors writing critically about obesity research and attitudes taken up in the media and general public (Moffat 2010; Warin et al. 2012; Woolhouse 2017).

We can use a feminist position to interrogate the patriarchal structure of science to question why it focuses almost exclusively on the maternal child-feeding model. When female scientists look at these issues, they often come up with different ways of framing research questions. Researchers examining child feeding and care using evolutionary theory have shifted the frame of focus away from mothers. Kristen Hawkes (2003, 2004), for example, developed the grandmother hypothesis, which investigates grandmothers' roles as pivotal individuals in enhancing the survival of the next generation's offspring. According to Hawkes, in our evolutionary history of *Homo sapiens*, human grandmothers, who have finished reproducing and caring for their own children but, unlike other primates, continue to live for many years beyond menopause, play an important role in feeding young children, particularly in digging up foods like tubers (also known as underground storage organs) that would be challenging for young children to acquire. This would thus free up time and energy for mothers who are busy reproducing and caring for new infants. Sarah Blaffer Hrdy (2009) extends this model to include a variety of multiple caretakers, or allomothers, who performed a cooperative breeding strategy that permitted our hominin

Baby Steps

ancestors to produce slow-maturing, costly infants at shorter intervals. These allomothers could be grandmothers, but they could also be older siblings, aunts, uncles, and unrelated group members. Indeed, Blaffer Hrdy argues that we have evolved as a species to be a "cooperative breeder," and from this has flowed many other human traits, such as language and the ability to understand one another's minds to cooperate better than any other ape. These theories help us to decentre the "mother as the natural caregiver and feeder" and to question common scientific and media portrayals that assume that the responsibility for a child's nutritional well-being starts and ends with the child's mother.

If we extend this concept to "it takes a village to raise a child," we can go further in considering where the responsibility to feed children lies. While the family is a primary source of food and nutrition, both in the material form of food and in teaching and modelling how to produce, prepare, and consume food, we can and should go beyond the family into the larger community: neighbourhoods, daycare centres, schools, community centres. We can also look to governments to create policy that can guide and support families as well as monitor our food supply, food advertising, and how children receive food outside of the family home, when they are in childcare, school, and so on. It is at this point that, to support the argument that so much more than primary caregivers influence what and how children eat, I turn to examining children's food more generally.

2

Biocultural Variation in Child Feeding and Eating

Feeding and nourishing children is fundamental to the reproduction of the human species. Like other aspects of food and nutrition, the ways that adults feed children and how children feed themselves are shaped by biological and sociocultural factors. In this chapter, I investigate these factors using cross-cultural ethnographic examples. While there is a strong body of research on infant and young child feeding, as reviewed in Chapter 1, there is much less known about older child feeding and eating, demarcated from about four years of age (when breastfeeding usually has ended) to the end of adolescence (around eighteen years of age) with the transition to self-feeding. I begin with an overview of children's growth and development and then proceed to cross-cultural case studies of children's feeding. While there are biological constraints on child feeding, due to child growth and development, there is considerable cross-cultural variation in child feeding and caregiver-child feeding relationships. I focus on the variation in caregiver-child feeding relationships and children's food and eating with ethnographic examples from twentieth-century hunter-gatherer groups as well as from low-income and postindustrial countries. I then critically evaluate some of the so-called universals of child eating behaviour. Specifically, I consider evolutionary and developmental aspects of young children's eating habits with a discussion of the evolution of food preferences, tastes, and food neophobia (fear of new foods). This is distinguished from what is often in contemporary societies called "picky eating." Here I explore whether there is indeed any relationship between children's food preferences, taste, and picky eating. I conclude that picky eating is more socially and culturally constructed than innate, though an understanding of the biological basis of children's tastes and preferences is useful in trying to prevent children from becoming picky eaters.

Child Growth and Development and the Evolution of Childhood

In *Patterns of Human Growth*, biological anthropologist Barry Bogin (1999) describes how humans are unique as mammals and primates for having three biologically defined periods in our lifecourse prior to full adulthood and maturity: childhood (or early childhood), juvenile (or middle childhood), and adolescence. Early childhood lasts from approximately three to seven years of age and is defined by a moderate growth rate, dependency for feeding, a mid-growth spurt, the eruption of the first permanent molar and incisor, and the end of brain growth; middle childhood (what Bogin calls the juvenile stage) lasts from age seven to ten for girls or twelve for boys and is characterized by a slower growth rate, the ability to feed oneself, and cognitive transition leading to adult skills. Finally, adolescence extends from five to eight years after the onset of puberty and is accompanied by the adolescent growth spurt, the completion of permanent tooth eruption, the development of secondary sexual characteristics, and the intensification and practise of adult activities (55). Early childhood is marked by dependency on adults for survival; this is in part because of small body size but also because of an undeveloped cognitive capacity and motor development, both of which are needed to produce/acquire or prepare food, as well as certain limiting physical features such as immature dentition and digestive systems. The deciduous teeth, known as the "baby" or "milk teeth," cannot fully chew an adult diet, and thus some foods, at least in the early years, must be cooked or cut up into smaller pieces by adults. As well, since the digestive tract is smaller, a lower volume of food can be digested. Even at low volume, however, food dense in energy, lipids (fats), and protein is needed to support the very large and active human brain that is still growing during the early childhood years (75).

While these stages are biologically determined for *Homo sapiens* and the pattern of children's growth and development is universal, it varies in both amount and tempo, according to the environmental conditions that children experience. This variation has been demonstrated through studies of growth and development done by bioarchaeologists who use skeletal and dental remains from past populations in such locations as ancient Rome and medieval and post-medieval Europe (Lewis 2002; Prowse et al. 2010; Cardoso and Garcia 2009). Growth is a reflection of the environments in which children develop, with lower attained linear growth (height), called "stunted growth," and underweight usually due to lower quantity and quality of nutrient and energy intake as well as high infectious disease loads that impair growth. Similar growth patterns are also seen today in many low-income countries around the world (Prendergrast and Humphrey 2014), though researchers should be cautious about assuming that growth is affected by the same life conditions in both the past and present or in different geographical regions (Vercellotti et al. 2014).

Quantitative differences in growth affect the chronological timing of the stages of childhood. For example, populations living with low energy intake, high energy expenditure, and immune challenges from a high infectious disease load will experience puberty at a later age (Ellison et al. 2012). This contrasts with the earlier average age of puberty (marked most clearly by menarche in girls) in postindustrial countries (Reiches 2019). But despite variation in the timing of stages, humans universally have long childhood periods, much longer than all other primates and longer than our closest living non-human primate relatives, chimpanzees (Jones and Marlowe 2002). There are multiple theories as to why this is the case. One idea is that it is simply an artefact of having a long lifespan: mammals with long lifespans, like elephants, for example, have longer juvenile periods (Bock and Sellen 2002). But human childhood is even longer than that of those mammals with long lifespans and it has more complex stages, as described by Bogin (1999) above. Those trying to understand this unique human phenomenon look to evolutionary explanations from the study of life history.

One hypothesis, called "practice theory," proposes that the long juvenile period is a result of the need for an extended period of learning for humans in which acquisition of cultural knowledge is so crucial for individual and species survival. But further testing of this hypothesis reveals that a longer practice of foraging does not improve efficiency or survival capabilities, which for children is probably more limited by body size than by skill (Bock and Sellen 2002). Another hypothesis that has recently been supported by experimental data is based on brain growth. Human brains are very large relative to our body size, and large brains are metabolically needy, particularly during early development and growth. Energy, in the form of glucose, is diverted from the rest of the body that would be otherwise used for body growth, rendering a protracted period of body growth to adult maturity. Kuzawa and colleagues (2014) call this theory the "brain-body metabolic trade-off" and tested it with existing PET and MRI scans of children's brains to measure glucose uptake by age in comparison to body growth velocity. What they found is that, at the time of peak brain growth, when the brain requires maximal glucose levels, children's body growth is slowest, corresponding to the early childhood period of slow growth. Once the brain has reached maximum growth, around age seven, body growth begins again, exhibited in the mid-growth spurt that occurs from six to eight years and marking the end of early childhood (Bogin 1999).

No matter the reason for the long human childhood period, it entails high energy and nutrient demands, meaning that caregivers – mostly parents but not exclusively – are required to provision their young with high-quality food. Clearly, there can be no discussion about child feeding and eating without an examination of the caregivers and their relationship with children.

The Child-Caregiver Feeding Relationship

In academic and popular literature there is indeed a clear focus on caregivers, particularly mothers, who are often the primary caregivers and nourishers. These studies focus on parental feeding style as an important determinant of child nutrition. Anthropologist Katherine Dettwyler (1989, 696, emphasis in original) argues that "the degree and type of parental/caretaker control of food consumption *may be as important* as food availability, household socioeconomic status, or maternal workload in determining nutritional status in infants and young children." In her review of ethnographic evidence of parental feeding styles, Dettwyler states that styles range from "those that sanction maximum control by caretakers to those that allow almost complete autonomy for infants" and that "the degree of control exerted varies intraculturally as well, according to characteristics of the caretaker (e.g. age, sex, ethnicity, level of education, socioeconomic status) and/or characteristics of the children (e.g. age, sex, health, temperament)" (697). In Dettwyler's (1986) own study of families living in a peri-urban community in Mali, she describes a laissez-faire feeding approach, whereby mothers seldom put food directly into their children's mouths and those of all ages and genders are expected to feed themselves and determine how much and what they want to eat.

The emphasis on maternal feeding is a major focus of many nutritional studies in low-income countries, where there is a high proportion of children suffering from childhood malnutrition. A review of research studies of what the authors call "responsive feeding" (RF) sets out to determine how much RF influences child undernutrition and growth faltering in low- and middle-income countries. The authors define RF as a reciprocal relationship between caregiver and child, whereby the child signals food requests and the caregiver responds with food and emotional support that is a predictable experience for the child (Bentley, Wasser and Creed-Kanashiro 2011). A review of twenty-one published studies that included RF exposure and child nutrition outcomes yielded mixed results, which the authors attribute to the variety of measures and methodologies used. They suggest that more research effort be put into investigating this issue. I discuss in more detail the state of child undernutrition in low-income countries in Chapter 5, which addresses socioeconomic inequalities and food insecurity. Suffice it to say for now, however, that I would argue for an alternative position: that we should not give parental feeding style so much emphasis in a world of uneven access to resources. All things being equal, parental feeding style may indeed be an issue of concern, but all things are not equal, especially with regard to low-income nations.

In high-income countries parental feeding style is also of concern, but it is as much if not more an issue of overnutrition or overfeeding as it is of undernutrition. In Ellyn Satter's (1986) seminal article, "The Feeding Relationship," based on her own practice in eating and feeding therapy, she outlines how to develop a healthy feeding relationship with children that steers away from parental over controlling of food regulation in order to allow children to develop the ability to self-regulate their eating. In an age of concern about childhood obesity, she argues children who are deprived of food in an effort to keep them slim, what she calls "restrained eating," actually become more preoccupied with food and eating. With extreme parental control, the child's eating experience may become emotionally charged, which in the long run may put the child at higher risk for obesity and eating disorders. To summarize Satter's approach: "The parent is responsible for what is presented to the child to eat, as well as the physical and emotional setting. The child is responsible for how much is eaten or even whether anything is eaten" (355). While this is sage advice, the reality of feeding children, and families in general, is imbued with family and gender politics that sometimes make what is seemingly a simple task very complex.

In a fascinating study of Canadian women and their relationship with food and food work, Kate Cairns and Josée Johnston (2015) devote a chapter of their book, *Food and Femininity*, to a discussion of "maternal foodwork," which they subtitle "The Emotional Ties That Bind." Indeed, what is often not acknowledged in discussions of children's health and nutrition is how caregivers express love and feel guilt, or even anger and resentment, when feeding children. Cairns and Johnston conducted interviews with 129 food-oriented consumers, most of whom identified as women of diverse socioeconomic status and ethnic backgrounds living in Toronto. Of their sample a subset had children and spoke of their experiences in feeding them not only with a mix of joy and pride but also with fear of making mistakes or not shielding them from the dangers of a toxic world. In describing their role in feeding their children some mothers considered themselves to be "guardians of health and taste" (71). The authors give examples of mothers who say they secretly put vegetables and quinoa into macaroni and cheese: "creative efforts to 'trick' children into healthy eating" (72), as well as mothers who express pride and love in their maternal foodwork while they watch their children eat healthily and adventurously. Others divulge guilt about what they view as poor outcomes of not so healthy diets, such as one mother who believed she had fed her daughter too much chicken, the hormones in the meat allegedly resulting in the onset of her daughter's early menstruation.

The section of the chapter titled "Raising the Organic Child" distills many mothers' agendas, often in spite of financial constraints, to feed their children nutritious and "pure" food, mostly for health reasons but also to socialize their children into a world of ethical consumption and food justice. Cairns and Johnston (2015) describe this project as the "calibration" of both protecting the child and not being too "extreme" in their feeding practices. As one participant said: "Having a toddler things can get really intense … If he's like 'BANANAA!' and I can't get to an organic shop … and he's having a meltdown, then I'll go and get him a banana. And it won't be organic" (78). Many described the food they fed their children as "risk management" – as one thing in their environment, unlike the air we breathe or what's in the water, that they could control (80). Those who were living on fixed or lower incomes expressed frustration at the inability to buy organic food for their children. As Cairns and Johnston point out: "The continued attachment to the organic child ideal is rooted, in part, in the way that mothers are held *individually* responsible for protecting children's purity and socializing ethical consumers. Thus, this maternal food femininity is sustained by neoliberal conceptions of personal responsibility that are embedded within contemporary consumer culture" (83). I would add that this perspective follows in a long tradition of mother blaming and the perpetuation of the trope of the mother as solely responsible for her children's health (Moffat and Herring 1999). This is a point I take up more fully in the next three chapters.

Needless to say, it is important to note that mothers alone are not the only member of a family feeding children: many fathers shop, cook meals, and feed their children, as do extended family members, like grandparents and sometimes older siblings. As humans one of our hallmarks, although not unique in the animal world, is food sharing – that is, eating together as a kin group. Children rarely eat alone and usually eat with at least the primary caregiver if not multiple caregivers and other family members, including fathers, grandparents, and aunts/uncles as well as other siblings. Much has been made by the media and food writers like Michael Pollan about the disappearing family meal in contemporary society and why it's crucial for family, even civilization (Johnson 2013). Dietitians and child experts alike argue that it is an important site of food socialization that includes both nutritional and psychological benefits (Hammons and Fiese 2011). Ethnographic analysis of Canadian households with children demonstrate a relationship between screens and food provisioning behaviour that includes children eating individually through snacks more so than through family food-sharing (Kline 2016). A meta-analysis of studies of family meals and nutritional outcomes concludes: "children and adolescents who share family meals three or more times per week are more likely to be within a normal weight range and have healthier dietary and eating patterns than those who share less than three meals together" (Hammons and Fiese 2011, 1565).

The flipside of this, however, is that family meals can also become sites of power struggles and conflict. Anthropologist Richard Wilk (2010) questions the American idealism of the family meal as a US national political agenda. He argues that, even in so-called traditional small-scale societies, families do not always eat altogether in one spot; he describes his own fieldwork among Maya farmers in Belize: "Related men and older boys would sit on benches or squat at one end of the house where they were usually served their food by women, while women and younger children squatted on the floor around the hearth at the other end of the house" (430). As Wilk found out in his interviews with twelve American families who self-identified as having children who were "picky eaters," meals can be sites of power and gender struggles and are not always "happy meals."

Wilk's point is supported by a comprehensive survey of 107 parents of eight- to ten-year-olds living in Minneapolis conducted by Fulkerson, Story, and Neumark-Sztainerl (2008), who reported on barriers and benefits of eating home-cooked family meals. The authors found that, while more than 75 percent of most of these families ate home-cooked family meals together at least five times per week, 25 percent reported purchasing fast food at least once per week and a similar percentage reported buying takeout as frequently. Conflict about eating was reported on some days by 35.5 percent of parents and on most/every day by 4.7 percent of the sample. The most frequently reported aspects of meals that parents wanted to see change was the labour of preparing and cleaning up meals, followed by more time to plan and eat, a reduction in their children's pickiness, quicker and healthier meal planning, and less conflict. It should be noted, though, that parents also reported some benefits. The two most frequently reported enjoyable aspects of the meals were the "social nature," which included conversation and togetherness, and "aspects of relaxing and laughing as a family unit." Interestingly, only 23 percent of parents reported the benefit of nutritious home-cooked meals, which may be because of the high proportion of food prepared outside of the home or the challenges of cooking healthy meals within a busy lifestyle (Fulkerson et al. 2008). The authors did not report on the household incomes of the families in the study, but they do state that 85 percent of participants were college-educated and that 96 percent were white. These findings then may well be different among families with different socioeconomic or ethnic characteristics.

Immigrants' views about their feeding relationship with their children reveal different concerns, such as the effort to balance parental desires to maintain their foodways with their children's desires to fit into their host country's peer culture. In focus groups we conducted in Hamilton, Ontario, for a study called "Changing Homes, Changing Food," we spoke with immigrants and refugees, many of whom had raised children in Canada or were still raising children at the time of the interview (Moffat, Mohammed, and Newbold 2017). Parents spoke of their struggle in Canada to continue to feed children their own traditional food. Those with adolescent children said their children wanted to eat fast food with their friends. One participant described a compromise whereby children would eat caregiver-prepared food at home during weekdays and go out for fast food with friends on the weekends. Parents with younger children said they would often ask for

"Canadian food," which was usually described as pizza, pasta, sandwiches, and fast food. One woman from India with young children explained:

> Before, I don't know about lasagna or like pizza how to make. Now, I know the thing I make for them. They're happy ... My kids are happy now ... Before, ohhh ... still when I make my own food, they don't like. They don't like. They like Canadian food.

Compromises include making home-made pizza, which one mother from China described as "healthier" than the store-bought kind. This has also been documented by Helen Vallianatos and Kim Raine (2008) in their study of Arabic and South Asian immigrant women living in Canada who cook "Indian pizza," which adheres to dietary proscriptions such as dough made without eggs and toppings, and sauces and spices that are more palatable to the whole family's tastes but that satisfy children's desire for "Canadian" food.

New Canadian parents of school-aged children also report on how challenging it is to pack school lunches for them. This was for two reasons. First, there was concern about banned foods at school due to allergies. This concern has been documented more extensively in a study of newcomer parents living in Mississauga, Ontario, who display heightened concern about food allergies because they have not had much experience with allergies in their home country and because they believe that, as part of their civic duty as new Canadians, they should be vigilant about not sending allergenic food like peanuts to school (Harrington et al. 2015). Second, in our study in Hamilton some parents said that their children were embarrassed about bringing "traditional" foods to school and wanted to eat the kinds of foods that they saw other children eating. A Somali participant recounted her experience with packing school lunches for her children.

> I don't even give the children traditional food. One time, when we were new, I made them pasta and sauce and all the traditional food in it. After a few times, the kids were being looked at and the kids did not feel comfortable. So, they brought the food back. They didn't want it anymore, so I didn't want to give them traditional food for lunch anymore after that. The kids don't know what's good for them. If they are being looked at weirdly, they are going to bring back that food and not show it to their class.

But other Somali participants in that same focus group said that their children had the opposite experience: "My daughter took Somali rice one time and her friend, who is Canadian, tried it, ate it, and she liked it. And she said, 'Can your mom make that again?'" Thus, there appear to be variable responses to non-normative lunches brought to school. This could, in part, be due to schools' different demographic profiles: schools with more heterogeneous and multicultural student bodies may have more tolerant attitudes towards global foods.

Self-Feeding

The degree to which young children procure and prepare their own food and self-feed is related to the caregiver-child relationship in that it marks the absence of a central role of the caregiver in providing for children. Self-feeding, in addition to independent food procurement and preparation, has been a focus of anthropologists interested in life history questions about the evolution of childhood. While nonhuman primate juveniles acquire almost all their food after weaning, human primates depend more on adults to get large proportions of their food (Hawkes, O'Connell, and Blurton Jones 1995). Much of the research into this has focused on small foraging societies was been conducted mostly in the mid- to late twentieth century, some of it occurring before many of these hunter-gatherer societies were forced onto marginalized land where they were no longer able to maintain their hunter-gatherer subsistence patterns. Two of the most studied hunter-gatherer societies are the !Kung San of the Kalahari Desert in Botswana (Konner 2005) and the Hadza in north-central Tanzania, living around Lake Eyasi in the central Rift Valley (Hawkes, O'Connell, and Blurton Jones 1995). It's important to recognize that these societies do not represent "living fossils," and we cannot assume that they are models of our hominin ancestors, though their subsistence patterns are more similar to our ancestors' than are those living in agricultural and industrial/postindustrial societies. Hunter-gatherers, moreover, live in very diverse settings, ranging from the arctic to desert and tropical ecozones, and their economic, political, and ecological characteristics also vary widely. As Hewlett and Lamb (2005, 6) point out in the introduction to *Hunter-Gatherer Childhoods*, this is the reason they use "childhood" in the plural form.

It was thought previously that hunter-gatherer children were completely dependent on adults for their sustenance. This is in part because many gathered foods are difficult to extract, particularly tubers (also known as USOs or underground storage organs]) that do take some skill to locate and dig out (Tucker and Young 2005). As well, hunting can be dangerous and is a skill that takes years of practice and training, so hunting for bigger game is done by adults (Bird and Bliege Bird 2005). This conclusion was also based on the !Kung San ethnographic data, which indicated that children spent most of their time in play, though some of this play consisted of practising subsistence activities (Konner 2005). Kristin Hawkes and colleagues, however, challenge this notion by describing the intensive foraging activities of Hadza youngsters (Hawkes, O'Connell, and Blurton Jones 1995). Frank Marlowe, in his ethnography of the Hadza, states that by the age of four or five children are already getting much of their food from foraging. He calculates that girls of four to eight years old forage food that amounts to 361 daily kcals, about 25 percent of their requirements, and boys of the same age forage 277 daily kcals. Boys practise hunting in early childhood, and by five or six years of age can kill small birds and rodents (Marlowe 2010, 157). Child foragers often do not bring back food to camp but, rather, eat it as they forage. A lovely quote from a Martu forager child in the northwest section of Australia's Western Desert reported by Bird and Bliege Bird (2005, 129) describes how, when children get hungry, they go "hunting for little lizard, get him and cook it and eat him up. Me little bit big now, I go hunting myself, tracking goanna (monitor lizard) and kill him." It is clear from this quote that much of what at least some hunter-gatherer children eat is independently procured and prepared by themselves.

Tucker and Young (2005) speculate that variability in hunter-gatherer children's foraging may be influenced by travel distance to food sources and the dangers to children (or lack thereof) in the immediate environment. The !Kung, for example, live in a dangerous desert environment, so children stay closer to camp; however, even though !Kung children do not forage, they do contribute to food production by staying at camp to crack mongongo nuts, one of the important foods in the !Kung diet (Hawkes, O'Connell, and Blurton Jones 1995).

Despite the strong contribution of children to the group's subsistence, a review of a range of foraging societies still concludes that young people's consumption of food always exceeds what they contribute (Kaplan and Robson 2002, cited in Bird and Bliege Bird 2005, 130). This highlights the intergenerational food sharing that occurs in foraging societies. As Marlowe (2010, 158) puts it: "We tend to think of people being able to feed themselves when they reach adulthood, and it is true that by age 18 years, males and females acquire and bring back to camp as many daily kilocalories as they need to sustain themselves. However, no one ever really stops getting food from others among the Hadza. Parents are still giving food to their children into their fifties, and also receiving food from their children."

Adolescents: Transitioning from Caregiver Feeding to Self-Feeding

Some of the struggles that caregivers experience with feeding children often become more acute during the teen years. Adolescence is a time of transition. Biologically it is marked by the beginning of the pubertal growth spurt, one of the most intensive times of growth and development after prenatal and infant growth. It is also a time when pubertal maturation is occurring, when bodies are transforming from energy being allocated to growth and development to reproduction and maintenance (Reiches 2019). In addition to the biological changes, there are, of course, social changes happening as well. Though the timing can vary cross-culturally, all adolescents begin to gain more independence and agency in their lives, including more responsibility for feeding themselves. It is also characterized as a time in the lifecourse when individuals may be more influenced by their peers than their family and take more risks, which can be both beneficial and/or harmful to themselves and others around them. All these changes experienced during adolescence may negatively affect this group's eating patterns as well as its nutritional well-being.

Healthy food intake and attention to nutrition is important during adolescence. Apart from the fact that it is one of the most intensive growth periods, along with the prenatal and infant periods, which requires high energy and good nutrition (Bogin 1999), adolescent diets can set up patterns for lifelong eating that may decrease the risk of developing noncommunicable diseases (NCDs) later in life. A good example of one such disease is osteoporosis. Osteoporosis, characterized as low bone mass and deterioration of bone tissue, can lead to increased risk of fracture – usually of the hip, spine, wrist, and shoulder – and usually occurs later in life, after the age of fifty. Adequate calcium and vitamin D intake during childhood and adolescence is necessary to prevent osteoporosis because these nutrients are required for building bone, and individuals reach their peak bone mass and density – that is, when bones are strongest and hardest – near the end of adolescence. Thus, this is the time for optimal prevention of osteoporosis; yet most nutrition education campaigns for osteoporosis prevention target older adults, for whom it is effectively too late (Holland and Moffat 2017).

A decline in nutrition during adolescence may well be related to the fact that many adolescents have their own money and independence and want or need to eat many of their meals away from home. As well, they may skip meals, opting for high-energy but nutrient-poor snacks. This may be an issue in some populations more than others. A cross-cultural comparison of dietary habits among adolescents in São Paulo, Brazil, and Minneapolis–Saint Paul, USA, found that adolescents in São Paulo were more likely to regularly eat breakfast and lunch meals during the week and were much *less* likely to eat fast food more than five times per week (3 percent for Brazilian versus 21 percent for American youth). Participants from São Paulo were also *more* likely to report eating fruits and vegetables usually/always. Conversely, São Paulo youth reported eating *more* chocolate or other candy and soda pop at home compared to those from Minneapolis–Saint Paul (Estima et al. 2014), so food from home may not always be nutritious food.

In her ethnographic study of Irish low-income adolescents living in Belfast, Northern Ireland, Jennifer Williams (2016, 66–67) makes the point that adolescent food consumption can be described as a "model of autonomy and constraint since they can move freely within certain environmental spaces such as neighborhood stores and restaurants but must negotiate restrictions placed upon them by parents, teachers, and other adults in their schools, homes, and communities." Williams describes the youth clubs in Ireland, where there is a tension between serving both healthy and unhealthy foods such as sugary drinks and snacks. Youth clubs are positive places for teens to congregate, places where they can engage in sports and other activities and stay out of trouble. Because of the voluntary nature of the clubs, however, youth club leaders are obliged to offer some unhealthy foods in addition to healthy ones to avoid having youth leave to purchase food elsewhere. This epitomizes the challenge that many adolescent caregivers encounter: they may have some influence and control over feeding, but not as much as they did in children's earlier years.

Even young adults (those in their late teens and into their twenties) may be transitional in terms of feeding themselves: many are living at home or attending postsecondary educational institutions and may be dependent financially on their caregivers and even regularly receiving food and meals from them. Even though, at this point in their lives, many young adults may be more aware than adolescents of the importance of good nutrition and healthy eating, they may not consider that they are at risk for nutritional inadequacy – when in fact they may be. A study of the dietary intake of calcium and vitamin D and perceptions of nutritional adequacy among sixty young adults (age seventeen to thirty years) living in Hamilton, Ontario, uncovered that dietary intake and perceived intake often don't match. Based on a food frequency survey, 55 percent and 61 percent of the total sample were deemed to have inadequate intakes of calcium and vitamin D, respectively. Of those individuals, however, when asked if they thought they consumed enough of those micronutrients, 57 percent said yes for calcium and 78 percent said yes for vitamin D. The disconnect between actual and perceived micronutrient intake is problematic since only those who believe they are at risk for deficiencies will take steps to improve their diet (Holland and Moffat 2017). Interviews with this sample of young adults regarding the best way to educate them about nutritional prevention of osteoporosis revealed that young adults are most concerned about food (rather than nutrition per se) as well as fitness and weight loss. The prevention of diseases that occur later in life was not on their radar. Thus, nutrition education must be tailored in such a way that it is relevant to adolescents and young adults and matches their life views and interests (Holland 2020).

Child Eating Habits: The Biocultural Basis

Many people who work with, raise, or simply observe children eating will notice that there are some characteristics of their eating behaviour that appear to be universal. Let's begin with what is often considered a truism, that children are "picky eaters." To understand the phenomenon of picky eating is to realize that, when children are being fussy at mealtime, refusing to eat this or that, it may not be only because they want to torture their parents (though I'm sure there is a bit of that at play) but also because they are programmed through evolutionary history as a species to be discerning about food. *Homo sapiens*, as an omnivorous species – a species that eats both animal and vegetable foods and has very generalized dentition and digestive systems – eat a variety of foods from their local environment. In discovering what is edible lurks danger since some foods can be toxic (Rozin and Vollmecke 1986). Thus, we have "the omnivore's dilemma" – the ability and need to eat diverse foods but also the need to be discerning – a concept popularized by Michael Pollan (2006) in his book of that title. As part of this discerning palate, we have innate tastes, like a preference for sweet and a distrust of bitter: the sweet is a cue for foods with high energy and nutrients and the bitter a signal for possible toxic substances. In addition to innate tastes, we develop our preferences based on our experiences with food, so if we eat something that makes us ill, we usually develop an aversion to it (Rozin and Vollmecke 1986).

Children tend to be more conservative eaters than most adults, on average, but there is still variation along the pickiness continuum among children and there are even some adults who are also picky/fussy eaters (Kauer et al. 2015). There is good evidence to show that, between six and eleven months of age, while they are still completely dependent on their caregivers, children do not discriminate much in their eating (Birch 1999), although there is still a preference for sweet over bitter foods (Ventura and Worobey 2013). However, after twelve months and up to six years of age children become quite discerning. The fear of new foods may well be a built-in survival mechanism; as children become mobile and able to put things in their mouths at will, they must learn to distinguish between edible and inedible and that behaviour spills over to mealtime. It is thought that neophobia – literally the fear of new foods – is at its height in early childhood and then decreases through childhood into adolescence and adulthood. This is because with more experience with food there will be a decrease in novel foods, and, in keeping with the evolutionary argument, continuation of neophobia would be maladaptive for survival and reproduction of *Homo sapiens* as an omnivorous species with diverse nutritional needs (Dovey et al. 2008).

Researchers, however, consider picky/fussy eating to be "behaviourally and theoretically distinct from food neophobia" (Dovey et al. 2008, 187). Often neophobia and picky/fussy eating go hand in hand, but not always. Picky eating includes the rejection of novel or new foods but may go beyond just novel foods to the rejection of large categories of foods at different times, even familiar ones. Picky/fussy eaters usually eat inadequate amounts and types of foods that may be categorized by characteristics like colour or texture. (Dovey et al. 2008; van der Horst 2012). One of the main categories of foods that is often a target for picky eaters is vegetables, particularly those from the Brassicaceae family, also known as cruciferous vegetables (Brussels sprouts, broccoli, cabbage, cauliflower), which are bitter tasting. These foods are good sources of phytochemicals and have been shown to protect humans against cancers (Smolin, Grosvenor, and Gurfinkel 2012). There is, therefore, much interest in enticing children to get over their distaste for these and other types of vegetables so that they may acquire the beneficial nutrients. Again, it is important to make the distinction between neophobia and picky eating. Just because a child is neophobic about a food does not mean the child or the later adult will never eat it. It is now an oft-cited mantra that children may have to try a food up to fifteen times (that is, fifteen different experiences over time) before the food is routinely accepted (Dovey et al. 2008).

In addition to clear age-related patterns in neophobia, there is individual food preference variation in all age groups. In a frequently cited review of food preferences in the *Annual Review of Nutrition*, Leann Birch (1999) explains how genetic and environmental variables intersect. There is evidence, at least among adults, of individual differential sensitivity to the bitter substances 6-N-propylthiouracil (PROP) and phenylthiocarbamide (PTC) due to genetic variation: those who have the two recessive alleles being non-tasters and those who have one or both dominant alleles being tasters (Birch 1999). Some may remember doing these tests in high school or university genetics courses, where each student receives a slip of paper with PTC on it to determine whether or not they are tasters. This may explain why some people (tasters) will not under any circumstances eat vegetables from the Brassicaceae family – this discussion often arises at our holiday dinners, where Brussels sprouts are usually served. There is also some evidence that sweet taste preferences may be partially heritable (Keskitalo et al. 2007).

Genetic variation in taste, however, is only part of the story explaining food likes and dislikes. Individual personality traits may play a role: those who are sensation seekers or who need a high level of stimulation are often open to new food experiences, whereas those who overreact to tactile stimuli, "known as tactile defensive children," are more likely to refuse foods (Lafraire et al. 2016, 351). As Birch (1999) explains in her review of food preferences, contextual factors are also important. Parental influence on children's food tastes and eating styles can influence individual variation. Cues from what a mother eats during pregnancy and lactation are transferred through amniotic fluid and breast milk and can influence later preferences for flavours and food. As well, observation and modelling of both adults and peers eating a food like vegetables will encourage a child to try that food. The peer influence is often underestimated but is a phenomenon well known by any parent whose child has attended daycare: children who refuse to eat certain foods at home may eat them at daycare because their peers are eating them.

While there is a plethora of research on picky/fussy eating done in high-income, industrialized countries, mostly in Canada and the United States, there have only been a few studies to date in other parts of the world (Taylor et al. 2015). One study of school-aged (seven to twelve years) children living in urban and semi-urban locations in China found that 59 percent of the 814 children surveyed were characterized as "picky eaters" (Xue et al. 2015); this is comparable to similar studies of children in postindustrial Western countries, where rates are reported to be between 13 and 50 percent. By contrast, in studies done in rural areas of China only 17 percent of children were characterized by parents as picky eaters (Li et al. 2001). Another study from China focused on younger children (six to thirty-five months) across eight cities and found that 36 percent of preschoolers were deemed to be picky. Again, the authors comment that these are similar to levels found among children from Western postindustrial countries (Li et al. 2017). It is striking that, in rural China, the prevalence of picky eating is much lower. It is possible that picky eating is a behaviour associated with urban affluence or that it is low on the list of priorities of parents who may be struggling with poverty and food insecurity.

So, while neophobia may have biological and evolutionary roots, picky eating appears to be more influenced by sociocultural context. Indeed, one does not have to go outside of Western societies to see stark cross-cultural differences in the way children and caregivers approach child-feeding and eating. To wit the popularity of several popular books authored by North American women who spent years living in France, where they raised their young children. These authors counter the idea that picky eating among children is universal. Karen Le Billon's (2012) *French Kids Eat Everything (And Yours Can Too)* humorously documents, as stated in the subtitle of her book, "How Our Family Moved to France, Cured Picky Eating, Banned Snacking, and Discovered 10 Simple Rules for Raising Happy, Healthy Eaters." A similar book by Pamela Druckerman (2012), called *Bringing Up Bébé*, also documents cross-cultural differences between children's eating styles and parents' approaches to child-feeding in France versus North America. Both authors describe their initial culture shock and how they and their families adapted to the culture of eating in France, pointing out all the differences along the way. What they discover in France is a very different approach to child-feeding – children eat mostly what adults do and mostly like it too. Children in France are expected to try new foods, and they have very structured mealtimes: breakfast, lunch, goûter (afternoon snack), and supper. Meticulous thought and meal planning is put into meals served to children in *crèches* (daycares) and schools. Meals in daycares and schools include an entrée (usually vegetable), a main course that is a dish of meat and vegetables, or a vegetarian or fish dish – not burgers, chicken fingers, or French fries – followed by a cheese/yogurt/fruit course. Children's lunches

Biocultural Variation in Child Feeding and Eating

are accompanied by the obligatory baguette and water and sometimes wine, if you're a teacher (more about French school meals in Chapter 4). While these books are not meant to be scientific or scholarly studies of cross-cultural variation in children's eating habits, they do raise some interesting questions about whether North Americans are raising a generation of picky eaters instead of working, as do the French, to overcome those so-called natural tendencies in children.

As Druckerman (2012, 200) explains:

> Though French kids eat hamburgers and fries sometimes, I've never met a French child who ate just one type of food or a parent who allowed this. It's not that French kids are clamoring for more vegetables. Of course they like certain foods more than others. And there are plenty of finicky French three-year-olds. But these children don't get to exclude whole categories of textures, colors, and nutrients just because they want to. The extreme pickiness that's come to seem normal in America and Britain looks to French parents like a dangerous eating disorder or, at best, a wildly bad habit.

Why do we care about picky eating? Besides the fact that it's a nightmare for parents at mealtimes, a review of studies of food intakes of picky children concludes that children characterized as picky eaters consume fruits and vegetables less often, with less variety in their diets and lower intake of dietary fibre (Taylor et al. 2015). The multitude of studies out of the United States reflect the concern that American parents have about children who are picky eaters, offering strategies to reduce picky eating, such as reducing parental pressure that creates a negative eating environment and making cooking and eating fun. An extreme version of picky eating is called avoidant/restrictive food intake disorder (AFRID) and is listed in the American Psychiatric Association's *Diagnostic and Statistical Manual of Mental Disorders*, 5th edition (DSM-5). It would be interesting indeed to know the prevalence of picky eaters among children in France, something I could not find in the existing literature. It is not clear whether the lack of studies about picky eaters in France is due to the lack of a problem or just that the research has not yet been done.

It is clear, however, that the French care very deeply about educating their children concerning the joy and importance of food. In the past twenty years, the French National Farmers Union has countered agricultural technoscience and large-scale agriculture with an appeal to consumer taste and the promotion of the *techne*, or artisanal production of French foods

(Heller 2007). Teaching the taste and *techne* of food takes place with school children through extracurricular educational programs like La Semaine du Goût, an annual fall event during which they spend a week visiting food artisans, cooking and tasting different foods from local regions in France so as to appreciate French cuisine. Based on ethnographic fieldwork in the Loire Valley, Wendy Leynse (2006) describes "journeys of ingestible topography" to educate children to be "situated eaters" by experiencing localized French food production and consumption, also known as *terroir*. Leynse describes this educational movement as, in part, a reaction to distrust of the quality and safety of mass-produced foods and concern about "the perceived 'steam-roller' effect of American fast-food culture on French eating habits and tastes" (145). This I believe is what we have to learn from other food cultures like that of France, where children learn that eating and their foodways should be pleasurable and slow, and that they can and should partake in eating the food that adults eat. Persistence of picky eating among children, past the early pre-school years, becomes "pathological," as Pamela Druckerman (2012, 200) puts it. And the concern goes beyond poor dietary habits or malnutrition: it's about a rejection of valuable aspects of our food cultures, our connection to our environment, and our humanity.

Summary

The long period of life after infancy to maturity is unique for humans in terms of biological, developmental, and social changes. These developmental periods are accompanied by variable child feeding stages, which progress from complete dependency on caregivers through the transition to more autonomous self-feeding. Given the wide range of ecological and cultural patterns of human subsistence and food consumption, it is not surprising that children's eating and feeding varies from one population to another. Even among small-scale foraging societies there is variation in how much children procure and prepare food and self-feed.

Humans, more than any other animal, are dependent on caregivers for intensive feeding, and this may have a large impact on children's nutritional status. Poverty resulting in food insecurity for families or concerns about environmental toxins or ultra-processed foods – among other challenges in the global food system – may overwhelm parents' desires and ability to nourish and protect their children despite their best intentions. The child-caregiver relationship, especially in American and Canadian families, is complex and often fraught with gender and generational struggles.

Despite cross-cultural variation in timing, however, most children transition out of feeding dependency during adolescence and into adulthood, when individuals begin to feed themselves independently. The best hope for launching young adults into the world of food and eating is to support them in childhood to form healthy eating habits and relationships with food.

For *Homo sapiens*, as omnivores with a wide repertoire of food choices, it's not surprising that there are some evolutionary reasons young children experience taste preference/aversions and neophobia at specific developmental stages, particularly during toddler and preschool years, when children are more mobile and need to differentiate between safe and dangerous foods. Whether that neophobic stage morphs into picky eating, however, is a matter of cultural practices of child rearing and foodways that vary within some countries (e.g., urban versus rural China) or between countries (e.g., Canada/USA versus France). The French approach to child feeding is seen at both familial and institutional levels, where French children are expected by caregivers to eat food that is shared by the whole family and are educated to appreciate French food culture. It will be interesting to see, with an increasingly globalizing world, if these traditions continue in countries such as France.

3

Children's Food in the Age of the Industrial Diet

At the end of the twentieth century the social sciences began to recognize children and childhood as a serious topic of scholarship, as I discuss in the introduction. Allison James and Alan Prout's (1997, 3) edited volume *Constructing and Reconstructing Childhood* sets out "central tenets of the emergent paradigm" in childhood sociology, which begin with understanding the institution of childhood as a social construction. Though James and Prout acknowledge the biological immaturity of children as well as universal components of childhood in all societies, they assert that the form of the institution of childhood varies historically and cross-culturally. For example, while today in most societies it is illegal for children to work in the labour market – and in some postindustrial middle- and upper-class families many children do not even work informally in the home – historically, children have worked in agriculture and industry and continue to work in formal and informal sectors in low-income countries. A historical analysis of British conceptualizations of childhood from the eighteenth century until today indicate multiple constructions and reconstructions of childhood, including the romantic, wage-earning, schooled child, and the child of the welfare state (Hendrick 2015). These constructions of childhood continue to change as societies evolve.

In this chapter, I consider children's food as part of the institution of childhood and argue that it is a socially and culturally constructed category. Special dietary requirements are a physiological necessity for children, in the form of human milk/infant formula and weaning foods, as well as for their growing and developing bodies. But for the most part specialized children's food is a recently constructed phenomenon, a product of scientific nutritionism and the industrialization of the food system (Patico and Lozada 2019).

Food manufacturers have constructed, or perhaps responded to, the desire for specialized children's food items that are convenient, palatable, and fun, and often advertised as "healthier" or at least as nutritionally fortified. The twentieth century was declared the "century of the child" (James and Prout 1997, 1), a time when children's rights, health, and well-being were recognized and scrutinized by governmental and non-governmental bodies all over the world. In tandem with, or perhaps inspired by, the focus on the child, food manufacturers produced and marketed a whole range of specialized foods for children. These children's foods are marketed to both children and their caregivers. Many of the foods that North American children eat every day, like breakfast cereals, are a product of the industrial food system and have been normalized as benign and as a healthy part of a child's diet.

Many caregivers believe that, since they nurture children from before birth and through the early years, they can protect them from harmful foods and that their children will continue to have excellent nutritional health throughout their lives. Though this may be true for many, most children will be exposed in one way or another to influences beyond their parents' control through daycare, school, peers, and media. And in much of the world, even within the home, what individuals and families eat is influenced by our industrial food system and food culture. While many nutritionists focus on the individual and family as the locus of control and responsibility for nutritional well-being, Marion Nestle (2002), in her bold book *Food Politics*, exposes just how much of the food we eat, the food system, and food policy is controlled by multinational corporations and their commercial interests. Out of choice in some cases or often from necessity due to financial constraints, many families in North America are propelled to eat foods that are based on what Anthony Winson (2013) calls the "Industrial Diet."

This chapter focuses on the industrial food system, with its deep commercial interests in creating and shaping children's food and food products. I begin with a review of children's special nutritional needs and then move to the construction of children's food as an artefact of the industrial food system. I do this by reviewing in detail the history of three quintessential products that have been specifically marketed to children: fast food, breakfast cereals, and processed snack foods. These foods have one important ingredient in them that is also a central part of the industrial food system: sugar. I briefly review the history of sugar and then, through an exploration of Western children's food culture (e.g., Halloween trick-or-treating, birthday parties, Easter, etc.), discuss why children are attracted to sugar both biologically and socioculturally. I also review the transformation of sweetness from its form as cane sugar to high-fructose corn syrup and whether this highly processed sweetener is nutritionally worse than older versions, such as sucrose.

Finally, I address marketing and advertising to children and the impact that it has had on North American children's diets. Proponents of neoliberalism in Canada and the United States argue that there is no place for government regulation and policy that inhibits the free market – and that includes the unfettered promotion of selling food products to children. Many nations around the world, however, are beginning to doubt the wisdom of this approach once they see its deleterious effects over the past thirty years, with the rising prevalence of noncommunicable diseases (NCDs), otherwise known as "chronic" diseases such as type 2 diabetes and heart disease. At the end of this chapter, I explore some of the successes and challenges of policy in countries that regulate children's food marketing. A review of these policies shows that, while they are no panacea, they are a step in the right direction.

Special Nutritional Needs versus Special Food Needs

At no time in our life do we require so much high-quality food to maintain our nutritional well-being as when we are growing and developing from conception through to physical maturity (age of eighteen years for females and twenty years for males). During the first year of life (infancy) babies triple their weight and double their length, and after that the next highest period of growth velocity occurs during adolescence. In comparison to overall body growth, brain growth occurs more rapidly in early childhood, and by seven to eleven years of age the brain has almost completed (95 percent) its volumetric growth (Caviness et al. 1996), approximating adult size, though prefrontal cortex functions of the brain are not fully developed until well into the twenties (Giedd 2015). This rapid growth requires fuel (energy) in the form of fat and carbohydrates. Also necessary is protein, which is the building block of cartilage, muscles, and the nervous system, essential components of growth and development. These macronutrients – carbohydrates, fats, and protein – fuel growth, development, and maintenance and are required for growing children in larger amounts relative to body weight compared to adults, who, once mature, move into maintenance mode.

Similarly, the micronutrients, vitamins (organic) and minerals (inorganic), though named for the fact that they are required in much smaller amounts compared to macronutrients (Smolin, Grosvenor, and Gurfinkel 2012), are also needed in higher quantities for children's growth and development. Consider, for example, the mineral calcium. It is needed in more relative abundance during childhood compared to adulthood. Ninety-nine percent of calcium is stored in the bones and teeth, where it supports structure and function. The other 1 percent circulates in the blood to be used for essential metabolic functions such as vascular contraction and vasodilation, muscle function, nerve transmission, intracellular signalling, and hormonal secretion (Institute of Medicine 2011). Though bone is dynamic throughout the lifecourse and requires new calcium deposits with remodelling, the deposition of calcium is higher during the growth of the skeleton, peaking in adolescence as reflected in the higher recommended amounts of calcium in the recommended dietary allowances (RDAs) for children aged nine through eighteen years (Table 3.1).

So children have special nutritional needs, like more calcium, but does that translate into special food needs? One "special food" discussed by anthropologist Andrea Wiley is cow's milk. In North America and some other populations around the world, such as that in India, drinking

TABLE 3.1
Recommended dietary allowances (RDAs) for calcium

Age	Male	Female	Pregnant	Lactating
0–6 months*	200 mg	200 mg		
7–12 months*	260 mg	260 mg		
1–3 years	700 mg	700 mg		
4–8 years	1,000 mg	1,000 mg		
9–13 years	1,300 mg	1,300 mg		
14–18 years	1,300 mg	1,300 mg	1,300 mg	1,300 mg
19–50 years	1,000 mg	1,000 mg	1,000 mg	1,000 mg
51–70 years	1,000 mg	1,200 mg		
71+ years	1,200 mg	1,200 mg		

* Adequate intake (AI)

Source: National Institutes of Health. Office of Dietary Supplements. n.d.

milk throughout childhood – usually cow's milk – is considered important for children's growth and well-being. This is perhaps because infants drink mother's milk, so it is considered normal for them to continue drinking other animals' milk after weaning (Wiley 2016, 2019). In North America the promotion of cow's milk (henceforth milk) for children has been attributed in part to the high amount of calcium found in it (as explained above, calcium is a mineral necessary for bone growth and strength). However, as Wiley points out, milk does not contain only calcium: it has an abundance of nutrients, including protein, carbohydrates, and multiple minerals and vitamins, as well as saturated fat (which when sold commercially is customized in content) and a variety of immune factors and steroids (Wiley 2016, 11–12). But do children after infancy require milk? As seen in Table 3.1, children have high RDAs for calcium. Even though the RDA for children under eight years of age is lower than that for adults, children also have much lower body weights than adults, so per kilogram of body weight the requirement is still higher. The amount of calcium found in a serving of milk and other dairy products, like yogurt and cheese, is quite high compared to that of other foods that contain calcium. An eight-ounce glass of nonfat milk contains 30 percent of the daily value of calcium compared to 25 percent for tofu and 9 percent for kale. Foods providing 20 percent or more of its daily value are considered high sources of the nutrient (NIH n.d.). It would seem that drinking milk is a good way for children to obtain calcium, but then so is eating tofu.

As Wiley (2017) points out in her chapter "Cow's Milk as Children's Food: Insights from India and the United States," drinking fluid cow's milk (as opposed to other dairy products such as cheese or yogurt) has been normalized in many parts of the world. This is based in cultural beliefs about the need for milk to support child growth as well as in the history of milk as a required element in many school meal programs (see Chapter 4 for a discussion of milk in school meal programs.) The story of milk in our evolutionary history and modern food system is a long and complicated one, and it has been researched extensively and presented in fascinating detail by anthropologist Andrea Wiley (2016) in her book *Re-imagining Milk: Cultural and Biological Perspectives*. An important point that Wiley makes and that is relevant to the discussion of special children's foods is that, for many of the world's populations, fluid milk is not digestible after infancy. This is because for much of our species the gene that produces lactase in adulthood shuts down sometime after about one to two years of age.

Lactase is the enzyme that allows us to digest lactose, the sugar found in milk; without the ability to digest lactose, milk itself cannot be digested and often causes severe abdominal and gastric discomfort. Though the commonly used term for this condition is "lactose intolerance," Wiley prefers the term "lactase impersistence" as it underscores the underlying genetic mechanism behind the condition, and is a reminder that most mammals do not drink milk after they are weaned, and because most humans – particularly those with Asian, African, and Indigenous American ancestry – are lactase impersistent. Population genetic research on lactase persistence indicates that, through natural selection, some 35 percent of the world's population, particularly those with ancestry from Europe and northern South Asia, have mutations in a chromosomal region upstream from the lactase gene that cause it to stay active throughout life. In *Re-imagining Milk* Wiley addresses how, in North America, milk has come to hold such a special place as a children's food, and why the milk industry and the promotion of milk drinking has more recently spread into East Asia (China, Japan, and South Korea), despite the fact that many people in these countries are lactose impersistent. At this juncture, I refer you to Wiley's book to get the full story, but I point out here that, in its ties to the food industry and global capitalism, the promotion of milk as a children's food is related to other children's foods.

One further example before I move into a detailed discussion of ultra-processed foods marketed to children is that of the recent food product "toddler milk," or "growing up milk." This is a powdered drink that is designed for one- to three-year-old children and that is marketed as promoting healthy brain growth because it contains DHA (docosahexaenoic acid, a type of omega-3 fat). A study of US toddler milk and infant formula sales and marketing from 2006 to 2015 found that advertising spending on toddler milk increased fourfold and that sales increased 2.6 times precisely when advertising and sales of infant formula declined (Choi, Ludwig, and Harris 2020). In short, the creation and marketing of toddler milk happened at the moment that infant formula sales began to decrease. Toddler milk advertising preys on parents' fears that their children may not be consuming enough nutrients (Khazan 2020). Paradoxically, toddler milk may do more harm than good. Nutrition experts do not recommend toddler milk and argue that it undermines breastfeeding up to two years and beyond and can be detrimental because it is expensive and contains added sugar, possibly distracting toddlers from eating nutritious foods (WHO 2016b).

The Creation of Children's Food in the Era of Industrial Food

Apart from weaning foods, there is not much cross-cultural research on the topic of children's foods from a non-Western perspective. In an article titled "Does Child Food Exist for Rural Malays?" Elizabeth Elliott Cooper (2013) analyzes the perspectives of caregivers living in rural Sarawak on the island of Borneo, to determine whether they categorize certain foods specifically as children's foods. She concludes that there *is* such a thing as children's food, but it's a subset of primary adult foods and usually comprises those foods prepared differently, more simply, with less spice and milder flavours, often in a single pot. However, when Malay caregivers were asked to sort specific foods into either adult or children's foods, it is striking that the only foods, apart from milk and rice porridge, that were labelled specifically as children's foods were commercially produced items such as Nestum (Nestlé's commercial porridge), candy, ice cream, chocolate, crisps/chips, and sweetened condensed and powdered milk.

Similarly, in my research on children's food and nutrition in both urban and rural Nepal conducted in 1995 and 1998, I found, through twenty-four-hour dietary recall surveys of children's foods, that urban children living in Kathmandu were regularly fed commercial products such as Nestlé's Cerelac (instant weaning cereal) as well as sweet treats, primarily in the form of packaged biscuits and locally made puff pastries (Moffat and Finnis 2010). These commercially prepared foods were easily accessible in what might be thought of as "convenience stores," small shops set up in garages or shacks dotted along the roadsides, selling snacks and beverages along with cigarettes and other sundry items. The presence of these commercially produced "children's foods" was much less conspicuous in rural Nepali children's diets, though there was one convenience store in the hill village where I conducted research that sold packaged biscuits that appeared in some children's dietary recalls.

In China, Jun Jing (2000) explains in his introduction to his edited volume *Feeding China's Little Emperors* the term for children's food – *ertong shipin* – did not appear in a Chinese dictionary until after 1979. Jing speculates that there was an assumption by the dictionary compilers that, after weaning, children ate food that was much the same as that consumed by adults, and it was not until the 1980s, with major economic and agricultural reforms in China, that children's food became a part of popular Chinese culture, "a linguistic marker of social change" (10). That social change included a significant increase in Chinese children's influence on family spending. A 1995 survey estimated that children living in Beijing households shaped 70 percent of spending, nearly double that in American households (6–7). In summary, then, while there may be a perception that children eat foods in different ways with different modes of preparation, it appears that the concept that there are unique foods produced for and consumed by children only is an invention of the contemporary food industry that is now ubiquitous in many non-Western countries, at least in urban centres.

Arising in the industrialized food system, but increasingly spreading to global markets, are three categories of foods that have been specifically produced and marketed for children: fast foods, breakfast cereals, and snack foods. Before dealing with each of these in detail, let's review the history of the industrial food system, which began in the United States. According to Anthony Winson (2013) in *The Industrial Diet: The Degradation of Food and the Struggle for Healthy Eating*, the industrialization of food began around 1870 and intensified after 1945. It was initiated with the patenting of milled flours and companies like Coca-Cola and Kellogg, which began branding their products, and then it developed into the mainstream degradation of food. Industrialization has happened through three main processes: "the simplification of whole foods, the speed-up of the turnover time of capital employed in the food sector, and the growing use of macro-adulterants in producing edible commodities" (Winson 2013, 133). The macro-adulterants that Winson refers to are salt, sugar, and fat, used to produce what he has coined "pseudo foods" – that is, foods that do not contribute to healthy sustenance of the body and in fact do more harm than good. Not only do pseudo foods have macro-adulterants in them that make them incredibly appealing to consumers, but they also contain chemical additives that inexpensively but effectively transform their colour, texture, taste, and shelf life. The inexpensive production (chemical flavours cost much less than flavours made from real ingredients) and the long shelf life of pseudo foods renders these commodities very profitable. To wit, in 2016, the food and beverage industry was number seven on the list of the top ten industries that produce the most billionaires (Peterson-Withorn 2016). According to Oxfam's (2013) report *Behind the Brands,*

> 10 big food companies – Associated British Foods (ABF), Coca-Cola, Danone, General Mills, Kellogg, Mars, Mondelez International (previously Kraft Foods), Nestlé, PepsiCo and Unilever – collectively generate revenues of more than $1.1bn a day and employ millions of people directly and

indirectly in the growing, processing, distributing and selling of their products. Today, these companies are part of an industry valued at $7 trillion, larger than even the energy sector and representing roughly ten percent of the global economy.

In an article by Juliet Schor, author of *Born to Buy: The Commercialized Child and the New Consumer Culture* (Schor 2004), and co-author Margaret Ford, they discuss the commercialization of childhood as it relates to food purchases by children. Children are lucrative for the food industry not only because they have their own money that they spend on food but also because they influence their parents' purchases. Children are also huge consumers of media, in which they are exposed to junk food marketing (Schor and Ford 2007). I examine children's food product marketing later in this chapter, but first let's look at some of the main foods that have been specially developed for and marketed to children.

Fast Foods

In *Fast Food Nation*, Eric Schlosser (2002) argues that fast food was born of the 1940s car culture in the United States: the first successful fast-food restaurants were drive-ins (customers were served in their cars) located in Southern California, attracting Los Angeles adolescents. The McDonald brothers, Maurice and Richard, set up one of these drive-ins, but within the decade they had converted their business to a sit-in restaurant with a "speedee" self-service model, eliminating cutlery and dishes and replacing all sandwiches with burgers only. In this type of venue working-class families with young children could eat out, and it became the prototype for all fast-food restaurants thereafter. Ads like "give mom a night off" appealed to the stay-at-home mothers who worked diligently at home preparing meals for their families but needed a night with no cooking every once in a while (BBC n.d.). In the 1970s, with more mothers working outside of the home and the rise of advertising directed towards younger children, fast-food consumption continued to grow among the "family with young children" demographic. McDonald's was the first to develop meals specifically catering to young children. The "Happy Meal" contains smaller portions of food along with prize toys, which are included in each meal. Though McDonald's has a variety of means to attract children to its restaurants, such as character mascots like Ronald McDonald and indoor playgrounds, the key hook in its strategy is the toys. Toys found in Happy Meals tap into the latest kid craze, such as Pokémon, Tamogotchis, and movie characters, to name just a few of the popular themes (Schlosser 2002). As these are often collectibles, they are highly sought after and require repeat visits. Many fast-food chains have copied these marketing strategies, successfully attracting children. In the US alone, consumption of fast food by children went from 18 percent of children's total energy intake in the late 1970s to 32 percent in the mid-1990s (Guthrie, Lin, and Frazao 2002).

Over the past few decades fast food has become a more common consumer item around the world, where it is increasing annually. In China alone transnational food corporations (TFCs) such as McDonald's and Yum Foods (KFC, Pizza Hut, Taco Bell) have exploded with more and more of the population eating fast food on a regular basis – it is particularly alluring to Chinese children and adolescents, for whom fast food is associated with the trendiness of the West. Barry Popkin (2006) has written extensively on what he calls the "nutrition transition" that has happened globally over the past thirty years, producing diets that now contain significantly more meat, fats, and sugar. Popkin explores multiple drivers of the transition, three of which are increasing income, urbanization, and TFCs. These are also drivers of increasing consumption of fast foods. While in the US and Canada we often associate fast-food consumption with lower-income households, in low- and middle-income countries it is urbanization and the rise of income, particularly for middle and higher socioeconomic status families, that enable more families to afford to eat at fast-food restaurants (Kearney 2010). TFCs have been expanding rapidly into countries like China. According to IBISWorld, despite a weakened world economy and growing awareness of the health risks associated with fast food, the global fast-food industry will continue to grow thanks to international expansion (Couillard 2019).

Though TFCs are largely US-based and "uniformity" is a mainstay (Schlosser 2002, 5), when they move into countries outside of the US, they "localize" to the specific cultural context. In James Watson's (2006) edited volume *Golden Arches East*, he explores issues of globalization, or "glocalization," through case studies of five fast-food restaurants that moved into Asian countries. The theme that unites all these case studies is the way these restaurants slightly deviate menu items or marketing to appeal to local tastes and aesthetics. A prime example of this is seen through the story of KFC's move into China, as described by Eriberto P. Lozada, Jr. (2000). When KFC first arrived in Beijing in 1987, it introduced Colonel Sanders, the old man with a white beard. KFC in China, however, quickly ascertained that the Colonel, a reference to the originator of the restaurant and its Southern origins in the state of Kentucky, reminded people of their grandfathers and did not attract them to the restaurant. So the mascot was changed from the Colonel to "Chicky" (*Qiqi*). "Chicky is a white-feathered chicken dressed in big red sneakers, red-and-white striped pants, a red vest marked with the initials KFC, and a blue bow-tie. His blue baseball cap (also with KFC logo) is worn pulled to one side, as is the rage in hip-hop culture of the United States; Beijing children see such images in music videos regularly aired on local television" (Lozada 2000, 119). As Lozada explains, in addition to making the KFC restaurants very child-friendly, replete with smaller seating, lower hand-washing stations, play areas, and hostesses giving out toys, KFC promoted its restaurants by developing partnerships with educators and parents and by sponsoring sporting and school-based competitions.

No matter where in the world fast food is eaten, everyone can agree that it is contributing to declining nutritional health. A large national survey of 6,212 children and adolescents (aged four to nineteen) in the United States from 1994 to 1996, and again in 1998, indicated that, of those surveyed, 30.3 percent ate fast food on one of the two non-consecutive survey days (Bowman et al. 2004). Another study used this same national survey to examine the dietary intake of adults and children who reported eating fast food on the two non-consecutive survey days versus those who did not. The authors found that both adults and children who ate fast food more frequently had higher intake of energy, fat, saturated fat, sodium, and soft drinks, and lower intake of vitamins A and C, milk, fruits, and vegetables compared to those who did not (Paeratakul et al. 2003). Clearly, a significant proportion of the US population is eating fast food and that is detrimental to nutritional health.

If parents and even older children know that fast food is so unhealthy, why continue to eat it? In a survey of 605 adolescents and adults living in Minneapolis–St. Paul, Minnesota, who regularly eat at fast-food restaurants, the three most frequently cited reasons for eating fast food were: fast food is quick, restaurants are easy to get to, and the food tastes good (Rydell et al. 2008). It appears that most people know that fast food is not healthy, as only 21 percent of the US sample in Minneapolis/St. Paul agreed with the statement "They [fast-food restaurants] may have many nutritious foods to offer." A study on the broader topic of children's nutritional knowledge surveyed 354 children aged seven to thirteen years living in South Australia. The authors found that children's knowledge of nutrition had no impact on their desire to eat less healthy foods like fast foods. This was particularly seen among eleven- to thirteen-year-olds who possessed higher nutritional

Children's Food in the Age of the Industrial Diet   75

knowledge than the younger children in the sample but who were more likely to eat unhealthy foods because of their "hedonistic nature" (i.e., desire for pleasurable taste) and perceptions of favourable social acceptability (Tarabashkina, Quester, and Crouch 2016). It appears that great taste and convenience trump nutrition.

But given fast-food restaurants' attempts to offer some "healthy" menu items, there is a faint hope among the consuming public that the nutritional harm of fast foods may be mitigated by pairing the fast-food staple, like burgers and fries, with a healthier beverage or dessert option. Indeed, with the growing awareness about the rise of childhood obesity and concern about the effects of fast food on children's health, some fast-food restaurants have attempted to make their children's meals healthier. McDonald's Happy Meal now has meal options such as salads and fruit bags. These are thinly veiled tactics to lull parents and children into thinking that fast food is not "too unhealthy," though I wonder how many children choose the salad or fruit bag option.

While fast food is a lucrative children's food product, it is not (or is mostly not) consumed daily. I now move on to foods that are frequently found in many North American families' grocery carts and pantries and may be consumed on an almost daily basis.

Breakfast Cereals

Breakfast cereals are made-in-America products that were created at the end of the nineteenth century as "health foods." Granola, a breakfast cereal that can be home-made or bought commercially through numerous large and small food companies, is still considered to be synonymous with "health food." One of the original and most enduring breakfast cereals, cornflakes, was created in Battle Creek, Michigan, in the late nineteenth century by John Harvey Kellogg, a surgeon and Seventh Day Adventist who ran a health spa, where he served the cornflakes. Later, his younger brother, Will Keith Kellogg, mass marketed the cereal as Kellogg's Corn Flakes. There were other types of health-food breakfast cereals to follow, such as C.W. Post's Grape-Nuts, and the Quaker Oats Company's Puffed Rice/ Wheat (Bellis 2019).

It was not until after the Second World War and with the beginning of the baby boom that food companies began to produce breakfast cereals marketed to the youth demographic (Gitlin and Ellis 2012). At this time, the United States was still in the thralls of what food historian Harvey

Levenstein (2013) calls "Vitamania," the relentless fear of vitamin deficiencies, especially among children. Because breakfast cereals are heavily fortified, food producers were easily able to advertise them as a complete source of vitamins and minerals, thereby absolving the companies and parents of feeling guilt about any of the less healthful ingredients. To appeal to children, many of the cereals, which previously had been made with very few adulterants, were radically changed by the addition of sweeteners, artificial colouring, and branding that was directly marketed to children in the form of cartoon characters. Some of the iconic characters that still exist today are Kellogg's Tony the Tiger and Snap, Crackle and Pop, along with General Mills's Lucky Charms Leprechaun singing "They're magically delicious!" Another marketing ploy was to include coupons on the cardboard of the cereal that typically couldn't be cut out and mailed in to redeem the prize until the cereal was eaten (though as a child I often carefully removed the plastic sleeve full of cereal, cut out the cardboard coupon, and then returned the box contents without too much damage).

The appealing aspects and marketing of children's foods are directed not just at children but also at their caregivers. Children are typically dependent on adult caregivers to provide them with food, though in many hunter-gatherer societies, like the Hadza in Tanzania (see Chapter 2), children are surprisingly adept at foraging for their own foods, sometimes at as early as four years of age (Hawkes, O'Connell, and Blurton Jones 1995; Marlowe 2010). In postindustrialized societies children are much less independent, but there are children who, from an early age, do prepare food for themselves, particularly within busy households. Breakfast cereals are one such item that is conducive to children's "foraging," especially on weekend mornings, when parents may wish to sleep in. Cooking can be dangerous for a young child, so what could be more convenient than pouring breakfast cereal and some milk in a bowl? One of the most iconic breakfast cereal television advertisements ever created, which ran on TV from 1971 to 1984, showed two older brothers with their younger brother, Mikey, at a table discussing a new breakfast cereal called Life. Though children were featured in the ad, Quaker Mills Company was not marketing the cereal directly to children at all – what child would want to eat something called Life with basic packaging and no cartoon characters on it? What the commercial showed was children assessing the food as delicious and eventually feeding themselves without any parent in sight. What more could a parent ask for?

During my perusal of a local supermarket, part of a major Canadian supermarket chain near my home, I eyeballed the aisle devoted to breakfast cereals and estimated that about one-third of it comprised of cereals specifically marketed to children. These include four major companies: Kellogg, General Mills, Post, and the joint cereal partner Nestlé-General Mills. There are approximately sixteen major types of cereals made by these companies, with multiple variations of some of them. An example of one line of the more long-standing and famous children's cereals that is high on the pseudo food scale is Post's Monster cereals, the most famous example of which is Count Chocula. Other newer cereals of the same ilk are based on popular Hollywood children's movies such as *Cars* and *Despicable Me*. Yet other cereals are modelled on children's confectionary goods, like Reeses Puffs, Cookie Crisp, and Nestlé's Nesquik. It's hard to see how these crossover cereals can be considered breakfast food, except that they have some cereal grain in them – Cookie Crisp even advertises that it is made with whole grain and that it is fortified with vitamins and minerals. In three-quarters of a cup of Cookie Crisp with half a cup of milk there are 190 calories, 210 milligrams of sodium, and a whopping seventeen grams of sugar. That is equal to drinking almost half of a twelve-ounce can of Coke (containing thirty-nine grams of sugar), and if the child eats more than three-quarters of a cup of the cereal, which wouldn't be hard to do, then the serving of cereal approaches the amount of sugar found in a full can of soda pop. Compare this to the American Heart Association's recent recommendation that children over two years of age should consume no more than six teaspoons or twenty-five grams of added sugar each day (Vos et al. 2017). With a bowl of Cookie Crisp cereal for breakfast the child will have already maxed out their daily sugar limit with their first meal of the day.

My supermarket scan and nutritional assessment of children's cereal is supported by a Canadian study of the nutritional content and healthfulness of "child-targeted" and "not child-targeted" breakfast cereals (Potvin Kent, Rudnicki, and Usher 2017). In an analysis of 262 unique breakfast cereals the authors found that child-targeted cereals were *lower* in fibre, protein, and fats and significantly *higher* in sodium and sugar. They were also *less* likely to be classified as healthier cereals and there were none that were sugar-free, with the majority having two to three different sugars added. If we go back to the original intent of breakfast cereal as a health food, we can see how breakfast cereals marketed specifically to children were a stroke of genius: they offer "health" in the form of a food fortified in vitamins and minerals that appeals to children, and they simultaneously serve parents' needs because they promote children's self-feeding. As we see in the next section,

Children's Snack Foods

As discussed above, children have high nutrient needs, but they also have small stomachs and cannot always eat the whole amount of food that they require for their nutritional well-being in three structured meals. It is recommended that for young children a meal or snack should be offered every two to three hours, with a consistent daily pattern. These snacks in between meals, however, should be nutritious, focused on vegetables and fruit, grain products, milk and alternatives, and meat and alternatives (Smolin, Grosvenor, and Gurfinkel 2012). Unfortunately, snacks in North America have become synonymous with high-energy, high-fat and/or high-sugar and high-sodium foods. In a study of trends in snacking in the US based on national surveys of food consumption, Piernas and Popkin (2010) found large increases in snacking between 1989 and 2006. Children were moving towards three snacks per day, with more than 27 percent of their daily calories coming from snacks. The largest increases were in salty snacks and candy, but desserts and sweetened beverages remained the major sources of calories from snacks.

It's hard to know whether food companies are responding to the increase in snacking and thus creating and marketing snacks specific to children or whether they have actually precipitated the increase in snack consumption by offering up a larger range of children's snack items. Another quick study at my local supermarket produced the following inventory of snacks that are specifically marketed to children. This is a narrow range of snack items, since there are many more snacks, such as chocolate bars, potato chips, pretzels, and so on, that are not specifically marketed to children but that children still eat. However, in the interest of understanding the industry's response and creation of "special" children's food, I wanted to investigate what kind and how many snacks are *specifically* marketed to children. Like breakfast cereals, it appears, as seen in the inventory (Table 3.2), that many of the snacks are created to serve multiple purposes: satisfying some nutritional needs of children, making the food convenient for parents and accessible to be independently eaten by small children, and providing foods that children will find appealing and fun.

Charlene Elliott (2010) calls this snack food branding and marketing "eatertainment." The "fun" element of these snack foods is communicated through

TABLE 3.2

Inventory of snack foods specifically marketed to children found in one Canadian supermarket

Type of food/ beverage	Product (marketing theme)	Company (brand)
Fruit snacks	Fruit by the Foot (*Despicable Me*) & Fruit Roll-Ups (*PAW Patrol*)	General Mills (Betty Crocker)
	Fruit Snacks & Fruit Crushers	Kellogg
	FunBites & Fruit To Go	SunRype
	Zoo Animals	President's Choice (No Name)
	GoGo squeeZ	Materne
	Fruitsations Fruit Rockets	Mott's
Sweet snacks and snack bars	Cinnamon Toast Crunch Treats (*Cars, Star Wars*)	General Mills (Betty Crocker)
	Dunkaroos	General Mills (Betty Crocker)
	Golden Grahams S'mores & Lucky Charms Treats	General Mills
	Nutella & Go	Nutella
	Pop-Tarts	Kellogg
	Lunchbox granola bars	Nature Valley
Cookies and crackers	Snak Paks (*Emoji Movie*), Animal Crackers, Teddy Grahams, Mini Oreos, & Mini Chips Ahoy!	Christie
	Bear Paws	Dare
	Goldfish	Campbell Soup Co. (Pepperidge Farm)
	Honey Crunchy Cubs Graham Cookies, Zookies	President's Choice
Yogurts	Yop, Minigo, Tubes	Yoplait
	Danino yogurt drinks	Danone
	Nanö Drinkable Yogurt Yogurt Tubes	Iögo
Cheese	Cheese Strings Ficello	Black Diamond
	aMOOZa Cheese Twists	Kraft Canada
Frozen treats	Popsicle (*SpongeBob SquarePants*)	Good Humor-Breyers (Popsicle)
	Popz	Nestlé
	Li'l Treats	Chapman's
	Eggo Minis	Kellogg (Eggo)
	Toaster Strudel	General Mills (Pillsbury)
Beverages	Juice Boxes (featuring cartoon bears made of fruit)	Coca-Cola (Minute Maid)
	Fruit Punch	Dr. Pepper (Hawaiian Punch)
	Kool-Aid Jammers	Kraft (Kool-Aid)
	FruitZoo Juice Xoxes (*Cars*)	Lassonde (Oasis)

the use of cartoon characters and children's celebrities and extra-bright packaging as well as the food itself, which is often meant to played with – for example, squirtable apple sauce and yogurt tubes or fruit rollups. Elliott argues that part of the reason caregivers go for this type of food is that it taps into modern, Western cultural ideas about childhood, whereby childhood is synonymous with fun and play. She states, moreover, that "eatertainment" distracts modern children from their occupation of isolated and lonely spaces in households due to the decrease in the number of siblings in families and the increase in parents' work time. This phenomenon has also transpired in Japanese society, though for different reasons. Anne Allison (1991) documents the labour of Japanese mothers who prepare *obentōs* (boxed lunches) for their nursery school children. These *obentōs* consist of small pieces of food cut and arranged into elaborate scenes displaying cute animals, toys, or nature. Purportedly, this is done to assist children in adjusting to school and as a sign of the mother's commitment to her child and to being a mother.

In North America the issue of snack food convenience for parents is something that even young children recognize as important. In the early 2000s, I conducted focus groups about healthy eating and nutrition with young children in elementary schools in Hamilton, Ontario. We showed them photos of various kids' foods. One of the pictures was of a Lunchable, not a snack food per se as it is marketed as a meal, but in the same territory. When asked whether that would be a food they would like to eat, students aged seven to eleven years cited a variety of reasons they would choose Lunchables. Some of the reasons, with motivations categorized in brackets, were: "because I like it" (preference); "because I don't usually get them for lunch" (novelty); "because in the hot dog ones there's special treats in them" (fun); "cuz most of them are healthy" (perceived as healthy); "because it's already made for you and your parents don't need to make it" (convenience). Lunchables high in fat and sodium are a nutritionist's worst nightmare, and yet, as pseudo foods, children consider them to be at least somewhat healthy and also, according to one child at least, to make their parents' lives easier. Energy-dense snacks have even become embedded in the economy of schools. This is demonstrated in Deborah Crooks's (2003) study of the sale of high-sugar and high-fat snack foods in an elementary school in a poor district in eastern Kentucky, which demonstrates that these snacks are sold to fund activities and programs that are on par with those in schools in richer districts.

As seen in Table 3.2 there is some nutritional value in some snack food items (e.g., yogurts and cheese strings), but most have only the illusion of being nutritious as they contain empty calories. A nutritional profile of 367 food products targeted at children as "fun food" in a Canadian supermarket found that 89 percent of the foods could be classified as of poor nutritional quality (Elliott 2008). The snack category that is perhaps most egregious in its attempt to masquerade as a healthy children's food is "fruit" snacks. I put "fruit" in quotation marks since they are made with minimal fruit and maximum sweetener. Witness the ingredient list for Fruit Roll Ups: corn syrup, concentrated pear puree, corn syrup solids, sugar and/or golden sugar, modified palm oil, citric acid, sodium citrate, pectin, monoglycerides, malic acid, ascorbic acid, acetylated monoglycerides, colour (contains tartrazine), and sulphites. The Center for Science in the Public Interest actually sued General Mills in 2011 on the grounds that its packaging and claims were misleading: General Mills claimed that Fruit Roll Ups were "fruit-filled and healthy," despite having the same nutritional profile as candy. The suit was settled out of court with General Mills, and in 2014 the company stopped claiming that the product was made with real fruit (Hughlett 2013).

Snacks specifically marketed to children are not exclusive to the United States and Canada. An article on the top twenty snacks that any child raised in Hong Kong would know include the following: (1) egg puff waffles paired with ice cream or filled with custard, chocolate, or matcha cream; (2) deep-fried curry fish balls; (3) *put chai ko* a soft pudding cake made from sugar and adzuki beans and skewered on a bamboo stick to look like a lollipop (Li, n.d.). Though these may sound slightly healthier than those found in North America, with fish and beans as ingredients in two of the snacks, the list goes on with many more straight-up candy/cookies (like Pocky) and salty snacks (like Pretz). Children's snacks, whether they are commercially produced or made by small vendors and sold as street food, are all good business. As Bernadine Chee (2000) describes in her ethnographic study of eleven-year-old students living in Beijing, there is strong peer pressure among urban school children to try the latest expensive and fad snack foods, and many parents of single-child Chinese families willingly give out pocket money so that children can consume these snack-food symbols of modernity to cultivate social relationships.

Sweet Child o' Mine

One of the common ingredients in most of these children's foods is sugar. Sidney Mintz, in his seminal anthropological analysis of the political-economic and cultural history of sugar in *Sweetness and Power: The Place of Sugar in Modern History* (1985) and "Time, Sugar, and Sweetness" (1979), illuminates just how novel and habituated the use of sugar has become in contemporary culture. As Mintz explains, prior to the production of sugar from sugarcane, humans were exposed to sweet taste only through fruit and honey. Europeans' first use of sugar, produced from sugarcane that was grown in the Middle East and the Mediterranean, was in small amounts and usually for medicinal purposes. In medieval Europe it was dispensed through apothecaries and was used regularly by royalty only. In the following centuries, though, it became more commonly used for preserving fruits and meats and in alcoholic beverages like wine and rum. Beginning in the seventeenth century, sugarcane, a plant native to Asia, was exported to the Caribbean Islands along with African slaves who worked on the plantations, producing it cheaply with great profit for the owners. In the late seventeenth century and into the eighteenth, sugar was mass produced from sugarcane and, later, beets, making it accessible to the masses. Mintz (1979, 1985) describes sugar as a "drug-food" and argues that, with the rise in industrialism in the nineteenth century, sugar became a necessity of the proletariat: a quick and cheap energy source, an appetite suppressant, and a necessary item in the day of a factory worker taking breaks to drink tea or coffee sweetened with sugar.

There is a debate in the scientific literature about whether sugar is in fact addictive. Certainly, there is a "hedonic" aspect to sweetness. As Mennella, Bobowski, and Reed (2016, 172) explain:

> Sweetness as a sensation starts on the tongue. When sweet-tasting (nutritive and non-nutritive) ligands stimulate a receptor on taste cells, the resulting signal is conducted via G proteins which activate pleasure-generating brain circuitry, where sweet taste perception and hedonics arise. The hedonic "liking" and motivation "wanting" signals for a sweet taste are distinctly modulated through brain mesocorticolimbic circuitry involving the nucleus accumbens and ventral pallidum.

These authors go on to explain that the sweet taste receptor and the proteins that are involved with intracellular sweet signalling are encoded by genes that are under-expressed in some people due to genetic variation, explaining differences in sweet taste sensitivity and preferences. Sweet taste receptors are also connected to the production and secretion of hormones, most notably dopamine. This has been demonstrated mostly in animal models,

Children's Food in the Age of the Industrial Diet   83

mice and rats, but since there are similarities between the rodent and primate taste systems, this is likely the case for humans. This may be suggestive of a similar neurobiological set-up, like that of addiction to cocaine or heroin (which are also dopamine inducers), in that addiction-like behaviours can be caused by sucrose. A review of the science behind sugar addiction, however, problematizes the current research, and given the important fact that sugar is rarely eaten on its own, encompasses more issues, such as the desire for palatable foods, which may also contain fat, and therefore may be related to a more general food addiction. As the authors state, perhaps the most important question, and one relevant to a discussion about children, is whether or not sweetened foods produce addiction-like behaviours such as cravings that may lead to habitual consumption (Westwater, Fletcher, and Ziauddeen 2016).

Research devoted to children's food choices and taste has been linked to discussions about child obesity and the bid to get children to eat healthier foods, in particular vegetables. Children's predilection for sweet tastes is linked to the evolutionary development of high recognition of tastes that signal non-toxic foods such as fruits that are high in energy from carbohydrates. This is true for all humans (and maybe mammals) but is perhaps more highly sensitized for children, who have taste receptors that are more acute than those of adults. Studies of babies indicate that they always respond more positively to sweet foods, and children have a higher preference for sweet taste, which remains heightened through childhood and declines during mid-adolescence to adult levels. This preference may be linked to our evolved taste signalling that sweeter foods are high in energy and correspond to higher energy needs during growth and development (Mennella, Bobowski, and Reed 2016). It is no wonder, then, that Michael Moss (2013), in *Salt Sugar Fat: How the Food Giants Hooked Us*, titles the first chapter of his book "Exploiting the Biology of the Child."

But tastes can be acquired as well through early life exposure and habituation. Although we crave fat and sugar, we are not necessarily programmed to eat it in the quantities that we do today in the era of industrial food. While heightened desire for sweetness during childhood may be biologically driven, and sweet taste preferences are partly genetically determined (Keskitalo et al. 2007), genetic predispositions do interact with the eating environment in the development of food preferences (Birch 1999). The appropriate level of sweetness in varying foods is learned during childhood. One experimental study of children aged six to eleven years showed increased preference for a sweet drink with repeated exposure over eight days; interestingly, this was not the case for a sour drink given to a control group (Liem and de Graaf 2004). Given that habitual consumption of sugar-sweetened beverages and sweets begins early in childhood in many industrialized societies – sometimes in high amounts even starting from six months of age, as found in Finland (Laitala, Vehkalahti, and Virtanen 2018) – it is not surprising that children today have even more heightened taste and preference for sweet taste in their foods than did children of earlier generations.

Indeed, it is this biocultural interaction between innate craving for certain foods and cultural patterns of child feeding that we need to examine. While the heightened desire for sweet taste among children may be biologically universal, the amount of sugar we feed children varies through time and space. Prior to the mass production of sugar, as described above, sugar was either not available or was not affordable for most people. Once sugar was readily available, it was not limited either geographically (except maybe in the case of remote communities) or by income. And since the development of high-fructose corn syrup – a cheaper and more easily manufactured sweetener used in processed foods from the late 1970s on and now the primary sweetener in processed foods – sweeteners have become more ubiquitous than ever.

We have come to expect that children will want, demand, and eat sugar; however, cultural associations between children and sweetness predate the industrial food system. Think about the nineteenth-century Grimm's Fairy Tales, such as "Hansel and Gretel," which features a cannibalistic witch who lures children into her oven with a house made of gingerbread, cakes, and candy (Lang 1965). Or how about the nursery rhyme "What Are Little Boys Made Of?" (Opie and Opie 1997, 100–1)? Though the boys are made of nasty things like snips and snails and puppy-dogs' tails, the second verse contrasts this with a description of sweet girls:

What are little girls made of?
What are little girls made of?
Sugar and spice
And everything nice [or "all things nice"]
That's what little girls are made of

Gender stereotypes aside, this nursery rhyme associates all goodness with sweetness. And this trend continues into modern children's literature. Goldman and Descartes's (2016) analysis of Scholastic Publishers' "100 favorite books for preschoolers" found that sixty-nine of the books depicted food.

Of these, 26 depicted sweetened baked items; 12 sweeteners such as honey, sugar, jam, and so on; 10 sweetened drinks; 8 candy; and 7 ice cream. With further analysis of the centrality of the food item and the affect associated with it, the authors found that sweetened baked items had high centrality and positive affect (80 percent of books featuring them); in contrast, fruits, and particularly vegetables, were less likely than sweetened items to be portrayed centrally or with positive affect. Though I have not seen a comparable analysis of books for older children, my experience of reading these books with my children indicates that, if this analysis were to be done, there would be similar findings. *Charlie and the Chocolate Factory* by Roald Dahl (1964) stands out as a classic example of sweetened food being portrayed as both central to the plot and associated with positive affect.

As I write this chapter my son is downstairs sorting the copious Halloween candy items he just acquired from trick-or-treating. As I gave out my own fair share of candy to the kids who came to the door (not wanting to be the one on the block who gives out toothbrushes!), I pondered why almost every kids' cultural event – think birthday parties, Easter, candy canes at Christmas – in the Western (mainly Christian) tradition is associated with sweet treats. Though some of these celebrations come from long-standing traditions, what's different today is the magnification of the amount of sweets at each event. Sugar consumption, moreover, has become quotidian; where it was once an occasional and special treat, sweet foods are now ubiquitous and added sweeteners are found in almost every processed food, even foods we think of as savoury such as bread and pasta sauces.

The Health Effects of Sugar

Should we worry about sugar? Indeed, that is a reasonable question considering that there are many other "bad" foods to be concerned about, like those high in saturated fat and salt. North Americans for many decades saw sugar as rather delightful or at least benign, and, since the mid-twentieth century, we have been brought up on the fear of fat and the association between high-fat diets (particularly those high in saturated fat) and heart disease. As Harvey Levenstein (2013) explains in *Fear of Food: A History of Why We Worry about What We Eat*, the promotion of the low-fat diet and what Levenstein calls "lipophobia" was instigated in the 1950s by an American physiologist named Ancel Keys, who, after vacationing in Naples, Italy, and conducting some rather unscientific studies of cholesterol levels in Madrid and Naples, determined that the Mediterranean diet, a diet generally low in dietary fat, was responsible for lower levels of coronary heart disease in these populations compared to those in the US. This was followed by a relentless campaign by Keys and others, with endorsements from *Time* magazine and the American Heart Association, along with commercial interests from food manufacture. Soon sales of whole milk and butter nosed-dived and manufacture of vegetable oil and margarines escalated. In 1960, food manufacturers figured out how to produce partially hydrogenated oils with less saturated fat than butter. Ironically, these partially hydrogenated fats (aka artificial trans fats) were later determined, with overwhelming evidence, to raise levels of low-density lipoprotein (LDL) cholesterol, or "bad cholesterol," while reducing levels of high-density lipoprotein (HDL) cholesterol, and were banned for sale in Canada in September 2018 (Canadian Food Inspection Agency 2019). As Levenstein points out, one of the unintended consequences of the "war on fat," aside from the unrestricted use of partially hydrogenated vegetable oils (trans fats) in processed foods, was the replacement of fats by sugar. A quick perusal of the nutritional labels of many of the low-fat products – previously endorsed as "heart healthy" by the American Heart Association and the Heart and Stroke Foundation of Canada – indicates that sugar is the main ingredient. Indeed, a systematic, empirical study of sugar content of regular versus low-fat or nonfat comparable food items proves that processed food that is lower in fat is higher in sugar (Nguyen, Lin, and Heidenreich 2016).

In 2009, the American Heart Association published a scientific statement in the journal *Circulation* warning about the detrimental effects of dietary sugars on blood pressure, lipids, and inflammation and obesity (Johnson et al. 2009). The Heart and Stroke Foundation of Canada (2014) also published a position paper, stating: "Excess sugar consumption is associated with adverse health effects including heart disease, stroke, obesity, diabetes, high blood cholesterol, cancer, and dental caries (cavities)." Further, it states: "Individuals who consume greater than or equal to 10 percent but less than 25 percent of total energy (calories) from added sugar have a 30 percent higher risk of death from heart disease or stroke when compared to those who consume less than 10 percent. For those who consume 25 percent or more calories from added sugar, the risk is nearly tripled" (1). In 2015, the World Health Organization (WHO) published a report to go along with its new guidelines for sugar intake for adults and children, which limit free sugars to less than 10 percent of total energy intake. Free sugars "include monosaccharides and disaccharides added to food and beverages by the manufacturer, cook or consumer, and sugars naturally present in honey, syrups, fruit juices and fruit juice concentrates" (WHO 2015, 4). The authors of the report conducted a systematic review of the evidence, mainly randomized controlled trials (RCTs) and cohort studies (longitudinal), and focused on two main health effects: body weight and dental caries. For body weight the overall conclusion is that the relationship to changes in body weight for both reducing and decreasing free sugars was moderate for both children and adults. For dental caries, a systematic review of non-randomized intervention trials and observational (cross-sectional) studies indicates positive associations between the amount of free sugars and dental caries in both children and adults (WHO 2015).

One of the newest sweeteners on the scene, as mentioned above, is high-fructose corn syrup (HFCS). It is a fructose-glucose liquid sweetener alternative to sucrose (table sugar) first used in the food and beverage industry in the 1970s. It now accounts for about one-half of the sweeteners used in the US; countries that follow the US with the highest percentage of HFCS used as a national sweetener are South Korea, Japan, and Canada. It is popular in the food industry due to its chemical stability, ease of use, and price stability since it is made from North American corn, which is grown abundantly in the US (White 2008). In 2004, Bray and colleagues hypothesized that HCFS may be responsible for the rise in obesity that occurred between 1960 and 2000 around the same time that HCFS was growing in use as a sweetener in processed foods. They argue that the digestive and absorptive processes and metabolic effects of glucose and fructose are different. They note that there is a low insulin concentration after consumption of fructose that is associated with a lower average leptin concentration. Leptin is a hormone that regulates our appetites; the lower the leptin, the lower the signalling to our bodies that we are satiated. They link the high use of HCFS in soft drinks in the US with the dramatic rise in obesity (Bray, Nielsen, and Popkin 2004). Debate abounds about Bray and colleagues' hypothesis. More recent RCT studies that include different groups consuming sucrose versus HFCS, or HFCS versus glucose, or straight-up fructose have found no differences in the production of inflammation associated with type 2 diabetes and cardiovascular disease (Kuzma et al. 2016), lipid profiles, weight gain (Lowndes et al. 2014), and nonalcoholic fatty liver disease (Chung et al. 2014). Whether or not HCFS is more culpable in increasing obesity on a metabolic level is still debatable, but the fact that it's cheaper and easier to use in food manufacturing surely implicates it for making the use of sweetener in processed foods even more ubiquitous.

While we need to be careful about fearing the latest food and running from one nutrition warning to the next, some of the emerging data on the harmful health effects of sugar should make us pause – especially when humans are now beginning to consume sugar earlier in the lifecourse and in greater quantities. Though there has been concern about the increase in the use of HFCS, particularly in North America, where it is ubiquitously used in processed beverages and foods, thus far there is no good evidence to indicate that it is any worse than other sweeteners. In short, sugar is sugar in no matter what form.

Commercial Food Products and the Colonization of Children's Minds

I use the word "colonization" in this subhead to be provocative, but even a brief review of children's food advertising invokes this metaphor. Junk food marketing, or what is called "noncore" food advertising by the authors of a comparative study of children's television food advertising in thirteen countries across five continents, is highly pervasive on a global level. Their analysis of television programming content indicates high levels in all the countries sampled, with the highest proportion of noncore foods in children's advertising found in programing in Germany, the United States, and Canada (Kelly et al. 2010). Many nations, including Denmark, Sweden, the United Kingdom, Belgium, Greece, and Norway, along with the province of Quebec in Canada, ban advertising specifically targeted at children. The bans all differ slightly in terms of age restrictions or certain types of programming (e.g., specifically during children's programming only). Why have these governments chosen to legislate this? As I show in the first part of this chapter, children's food products – part of a lucrative billion-dollar food industry – are very high in free sugars, fats, and salt, and are implicated in contributing to a higher risk for a number of NCDs such as heart disease, obesity, type 2 diabetes, and dental caries. While certainly children and their caregivers are implicated in consuming these products, the food industry works hard to increase the consumption of these products through marketing and distribution. I first review the current understanding of advertising food to children and some of the potentially negative outcomes before returning to the question of whether banning children's food product advertising could aid in decreasing the consumption of unhealthy foods.

From a developmental perspective, young children are the proverbial "sitting ducks" when it comes to advertising because cognitive reasoning, which would enable them to understand the purpose and motivation behind advertising, does not develop fully until late childhood. A review of developmental psychologists' studies of children's cognition in relation to advertising indicates that, somewhere around the age of eight, children begin to understand the perspective of advertisers and their motivation to sell products; it is not, however, until later childhood (ten to twelve years old) that children are skilled at conceiving of multiple points of view and thus of the motivations behind advertising (Young 2003). Even for older children, however, advertising can sometimes be misleading or confusing. Harris and colleagues (2017, 2) investigate an advertising phenomenon that they call "health halo" ads, whereby a nutrient-poor food product is advertised in the context of healthy lifestyle messages, "such as depicting children engaging in sports and then going out for fast food to celebrate, or an ad for sugary cereals that also shows fruit and milk on the table." The authors studied the impact of health halo television commercials on children's ratings of the foods and found that children aged seven to eleven years were more likely to rate nutrient-poor foods as "healthy" if they were advertised in health halo commercials. These findings did not differ by gender, age, or TV viewing habits.

While we know that advertising can acutely influence children, the next empirical question is whether junk food advertising directed at children actually influences their behaviour and their health outcomes – that is, are they more likely to eat more nutrient-poor food and have poorer nutritional outcomes? A survey of Grade 5 and 6 students in Melbourne, Australia, demonstrates that heavier TV use, particularly commercial TV viewing, is associated with more positive attitudes towards junk food and higher reported junk food consumption. The authors argue that junk food advertising contributes to normalizing unhealthy eating (Dixon et al. 2007). A similar study of elementary school children (aged four to twelve) in the Netherlands found a strong association between exposure to advertising and consumption of unhealthy foods. They, too, argue that this goes beyond specific brand consumption to generic consumption of unhealthy foods, supporting what they call the "spillover effect" (Buijzen, Schuurman, and Bomhof 2008).

In examining the question of whether food advertising influences health outcomes, most studies measure the association between TV watching, exposure to children's advertising, and obesity. One of the first landmark studies to measure this relationship was conducted by Steven Gortmaker and colleagues (1996). They documented a dose-response relationship between the prevalence of overweight and the number of hours watching

TV in ten- to fifteen-year-old children. In other words, the more TV the children watched, the higher their risk of being overweight. This study, however, could not differentiate the cause of weight gain associated with television viewing: Was exposure to food advertising directed at children increasing energy intake or was the television viewing decreasing energy expenditure (i.e., replacing physical activity with sedentary TV viewing)? Studies that have looked more directly at the effects of television advertising on obesity, however, do find some direct nutritional effects. For example, a study of the relationship between the numbers of ads for sweet and fatty foods per hour on children's television and estimates of prevalence of child overweight in the United States, Australia, and eight European countries showed a significant and positive association between the two variables. The authors found that advertising could explain up to half of the variation in child overweight among these countries (Lobstein and Dibb 2005). As Stephen Kline (2016) points out in a discussion of the effects of children's advertising on their nutritional health, food advertising may be most detrimental by influencing the cultural habits or lifestyle practices of children and their families rather than through product or brand promotion. In an analysis of culture and eating in Canadian children's food ads, Kline (2016, 283) notes a dearth of references to family meals and the promotion of four eating occasions: eating out (fast food), eating convenience foods, snacking, and eating on the run.

In addition to understanding how junk food advertising affects children's diets, it is important to consider how we can limit it. As mentioned above, there are many countries that have legislated bans on advertising to children. The UK introduced its ban in 2007 and is the most recent addition to the group. There are surprisingly few studies that have evaluated the effectiveness of these bans. One study done in Quebec, where a ban on children's advertising has been in place since 1980, evaluated the impact of the ban on fast-food consumption. The authors very cleverly designed a natural experiment by using household-level expenditure survey data to estimate the number of meals purchased at fast-food restaurants. Their "treatment" group was francophone households in Quebec – they limited it to French-speaking households since they primarily watch Quebec-based stations, where the ban applies, as opposed to English media from outside of the province. Their "control" groups were both anglophone households living in Quebec and anglophone and francophone households living in neighbouring Ontario, and within those treatment groups they included households both with and without children. The authors deliberately

Children's Food in the Age of the Industrial Diet 91

included Ontario households in order to control for cultural differences influencing fast-food consumption between anglophones and francophones living in Quebec. The findings showed that francophone households with children in Quebec (those subject to the children's advertising ban) bought less fast food and that this was associated with a statistically significant effect at the household level. The authors estimate that this effect amounts to an annual drop of $27 million in fast-food sales due to the ban (Dhar and Baylis 2011).

While the findings from Quebec are impressive, it is worth mentioning the complexity inherent in establishing children's advertising bans. A study published in 2011 evaluated the effectiveness of the ban in the UK four years after legislation was introduced in 2007. The UK ban restricts ads for foods high in fat, salt, and sugar (HFSS) on all children's channels and on non-children's channels during or around programs typically watched by four- to fifteen-year-olds. The authors monitored ads broadcast in one region of the UK over one week during periods six months before and six months after regulations were implemented, and they compared these data to viewing data on four- to fifteen-year-olds. While HFSS food advertising was absent from the broadcast slots designated in the ban, children were still exposed to these ads in other viewing periods. The authors state: "Perversely, we found that exposure to HFSS food advertising, as a proportion of both all advertising and all food advertising seen, increased for all viewers following introduction of the scheduling restrictions" (Adams et al. 2012, 5). Adams and colleagues did not analyze these data according to the age of the child, but it is probable that older children were more likely to be exposed to these ads than younger children, who would more likely view younger, child-specific programming and, therefore, have less exposure to ads during other television programming slots. Nevertheless, it underscores the pervasiveness of and difficulty in reducing exposure to HFSS food advertising altogether, particularly for older children and adolescents.

Another difficulty in restricting advertising to children occurs in countries like Sweden, where Swedish-language, state-run television bans advertising directed at children under thirteen years old, but many households have access to satellite television channels that have no such ban. Some countries, like the US, have established initiatives to decrease children's advertising through self-regulatory mechanisms. In 2006, the United States launched the Children's Food and Beverage Advertising Initiative to "encourage healthier dietary choices in advertising directed to children under 12 years of age." Monitoring of ads viewed by children over subsequent years demonstrates that by 2015 children saw just 3 percent fewer food television ads and 86 percent of ads still promoted HFSS foods (Boyland and Harris 2017, 761).

While I'm a fan of intervention policy, my hunch, based on my in-house observations of my teen children, is that these television advertising regulations that are already somewhat ineffective will soon become moot. Children are watching less traditional cable and satellite TV and are viewing more online streaming and internet, including YouTube and social media, where ads are more subliminal and harder to police. Many media watchdogs are extremely worried about the incursion of advertising into children's online programming. Take, for example, the Children's YouTube channel that, while family friendly with educational programming like *Reading Rainbow*, also mixes advertisements with content so that "boundaries are blurred" (Greenberg 2015). As Julia Greenberg explains, the Federal Communications Commission in the US has strict rules about how network and cable channels can advertise to kids, including time limits on the number of ads allowed per hour during children's programming and a ban on TV characters' selling products; however, no such regulations apply to online programming.

Should we give up and throw in the towel? No, absolutely not. A policy position paper by Kim Raine and colleagues (2013) states unequivocally that Canada needs to act to effectively legislate a ban on children's advertising that features unhealthy food. In Canada there is only self-regulation (except for Quebec) through the Broadcast Code for Advertising to Children and the industry-initiated Children's Food and Beverage Advertising Initiative. These initiatives are obviously ineffective, given that Canada is one of the top countries in the world when it comes to advertising unhealthy foods to children, as reported above (Kelly et al. 2010). As Raine and colleagues point out, though, the challenges with new and emerging media are significant. As well, much of the Canadian media comes from the US, and it is difficult to regulate cross-border media. They advocate for "a Canadian (federal) government-led national regulatory system prohibiting all commercial marketing of foods and beverages to children under 18 years of age, with exceptions for 'approved public health campaigns promoting healthy diets'" (Raine et al. 2013, 247). And they specifically define marketing as pertaining to "all media through which children are or can be targeted," including product placement, websites, text messages, point-of-purchase,

Children's Food in the Age of the Industrial Diet   93

and so on (ibid.). Their list of media is extensive though probably not exhaustive.

Summary

Children's food as a special category of food items is a creation of the industrial food system in the United States that has spread globally from the end of the nineteenth century and continuing into the twenty-first. Though these processed food products for children are thinly veiled as having enhanced nutritional properties – they are often fortified with vitamins and minerals – they are mainly convenience products that are marketed to children through the use of appealing media characters and packaging. Fast-food restaurants have also created child-specific menu items that are usually associated with characters and/or toys.

Most children's foods are highly sweetened to make them palatable and tasty. Children are more attracted to and have a higher desire for sweet taste than do other age groups. This is due to biological factors such as the need for high energy intake during growth and evolutionary-derived survival mechanisms that favour avoidance of bitter taste to prevent ingestion of toxic substances. Prior to the sixteenth century, however, for most people sweet tastes were only garnered through fruit and honey, making the consumption of sugars rare. Though there is debate about whether sugar is truly addictive, there is no doubt that the taste for sugar can become habitual, and this starts very early in life with regular consumption of sugars from a young age. There is now mounting evidence that the consumption of high amounts of free sugars is harmful to human health. Due to epidemiological evidence that links high sugar consumption with heart disease, stroke, obesity, diabetes, high blood cholesterol, and dental caries, the World Health Organization, the American Heart Association, and the Heart and Stroke Foundation of Canada have all issued guidelines on the daily maximum limit on free sugars.

There are many references and practices in Western culture that associate sweet taste and sugar with children, all of which may be readily seen in children's literature and common children's celebration events. The consumption of sweetened food by children continues to be normalized through media advertisements directly marketed to children. Due to global concerns about child obesity, the discussion about controlling or restricting advertising of children's food products has stepped up. A handful of nations have implemented legislation that restricts food advertising (or advertising of all products) to children on television; other nations are discussing it, but given the new and emerging media (e.g., the internet and social media) and the globalization of media in general, we will have to become more creative and vigilant moving forward.

4

It Takes a Village
School Feeding Programs

"It takes a village to raise a child." This oft-repeated and much clichéd proverb – most recently the title of one of Hillary Rodham Clinton's books – is said to have originated in Africa. National Public Radio attempted to research the origins of this proverb and concluded it may be from a Swahili term, with others citing Native American origins. As one commenter, Lawrence Mbogoni, an African studies professor at William Paterson University, interpreted the proverb:

> [It] reflects a social reality some of us who grew up in rural areas of Africa can easily relate to. As a child, my conduct was a concern of everybody, not just my parents, especially if it involved misconduct. Any adult had the right to rebuke and discipline me and would make my mischief known to my parents who in turn would also mete their own "punishment." The concern of course was the moral well-being of the community. (Goldberg 2016)

I use this proverb to make the point that feeding children from birth to adulthood is of considerable importance to the future health and well-being of our species as a whole and, thus, is the responsibility of all of us, not just immediate caregivers. Although feeding children is often constructed as mainly the responsibility of primary caregivers, usually parents – and usually mothers – the reality is that children obtain their food from many different people. Humans are "cooperative breeders," meaning we rely on alloparents, or other caregivers, to successfully raise our offspring (Blaffer Hrdy 2009). Thus, in the context of postindustrial societies around the world, I extend the "village" as a metaphor for larger units such as the local community, municipality, and state levels of society and governance. In other words, it does not matter whether we procreate our own children or not: we are all responsible for the well-being of the next generation.

Though aspirational, in modern times this philosophy has not been upheld since the 1980s, when neoliberal governments placed more responsibility for raising children on individual families, with an accompanying reduction of welfare provisions (de Benedictis 2012). Within this neoliberal framework, parents – and especially mothers – are blamed for their children's poor nutritional outcomes (e.g., child obesity) (Power 2016). Paradoxically, the economic cuts that save money in the short term cost society more in the long term through increases in diet-related NCDs, such as type 2 diabetes and cardiovascular disease, that are expensive for health care systems. This is another reason to strengthen community and institutional structures that support children's nutrition.

In this chapter I examine institutional and societal influences on feeding children, with a focus on schools. School is a daily part of children's lives around the world, and it is one of the locations where children obtain food on a regular basis. Not only do schools provide food for children but the people within schools – educators and peers – greatly influence what children eat. Though schools are quite similar globally, they also differ in significant ways through time and space. Thus, it is important to examine school feeding from historical and cross-cultural perspectives because it allows us to question our own assumptions and practices, to think about alternative perspectives, and to consider how we can improve the way we feed children.

I begin with an overview and history of school meal programs and then focus on research I have done in partnership with Danielle Gendron on school nutrition in France and Japan. I examine case studies from these two countries,[1] and then I contrast them with North American lunch programs, highlighting the lack of school feeding programs in Canadian schools.

The History of School Food

Providing children with food at school goes back to the late nineteenth and early twentieth centuries in some parts of North America, Europe, and Asia, where lunches were offered on a school-by-school basis in response to widespread hunger and poverty. As school became mandatory, school meals

It Takes a Village

were seen as essential and also as incentive for poor families to send their children to attend school and to leave family labour on farms or in factories. This is still the case today in many rural areas in low-income countries (WFP 2013). School meal programs in the US became formalized by government funding in the early twentieth century. As Susan Levine (2008) describes in *School Lunch Politics*, the political support for a national school lunch program was grounded in a concern for the well-being of children living in poverty through the Great Depression of the 1930s, but it also served to help the agricultural sector, which was floundering at that time, due to the downturn in demand for food and the drop in agricultural prices. Thus, surplus food, like potatoes and milk, that farmers could not get to market were bought by the US Department of Agriculture to provision the large amount of food required for the school lunch program. The US government, under Roosevelt, was able to satisfy the needs of both farmers and children. To this day the National School Lunch Program (NSLP) continues to be overseen by the US Department of Agriculture (USDA) (Levine 2008; Poppendieck 2010).

The ongoing political support for the NSLP after the Depression was fuelled by the need for a reserve of well-nourished men to send to the Second World War, known as "defence nutrition": there was concern about the high rates of malnutrition among children in the US and reports of young men failing draft physical examinations (Poppendieck 2010, 50). The school food programs were also viewed by school lunch reformers, using the emerging science of nutrition as a way to thwart "mental dullness and its attendant evils" (Ziegelman and Coe 2016, 78). The NSLP was solidified in 1946 as an act in Congress. Despite the establishment of the act, throughout the twentieth century there were battles to keep it adequately funded. During the 1960s, there was increasing criticism of the USDA's inability to provide free lunches to the poorest of children in the US, and the program increasingly became caught up in President Johnson's "War on Poverty" and civil rights activism. This activism helped to undergird the political will to continue to expand the NSLP to this day (Fitchen 1988; Levine 2008).

School Meals in Global Perspective: Case Studies from France and Japan

The World Food Programme (WFP), in *State of School Feeding Worldwide* (2013), reports that school meal programs are established in low-, middle- and high-income countries, with an estimated 368 million children worldwide receiving meals at school. In 2010, China, as part of the project to address intergenerational poverty, implemented a pilot school feeding program that was scaled up in 2011 to serve an estimated 38 million children (WFP 2013, 33). India, with the largest school feeding program in the world (113.6 million primary school children receive a daily mid-day meal), adopted a rights-based approach with universal school meal programs. The WFP points out, however, that universal rights do not always translate into universal practice in India, and disparities remain due to financial constraints at state level (30).

The WFP argues that, beyond the obvious benefits of improving student nutrition and learning, school meal programs can operate as a food-based social safety net for vulnerable families and children. As well, school meal programs can support local agricultural production and thus contribute to the economic welfare of families and communities. This approach has been outlined in *The School Food Revolution*, which highlights case studies from New York, London, and Rome, where school meal programs have been developed with local food procurement systems (Morgan and Sonnino 2008). The WFP (2013) report concludes that school meal programs must be made more efficient and that there is a need to strengthen the evidence base for their benefits and to share knowledge about them around the world.

To date, with the exception of the documentation of model school lunch programs in Italy, Finland, Brazil and Colombia (Ashe and Sonnino 2013; Morgan and Sonnino 2008; Raulio, Roos, and Prättälä 2010; Sidaner, Balaban, and Burlandy 2013), most studies have focused on the poor nutritional quality of school meal programs in the US and the UK and on how to improve them (e.g., Clark and Fox 2009; Nelson et al. 2007). Much less attention has been paid to successful school meal programs located in Europe – with the exception of Italy and Finland (citations above) – and in Asia. In 2013, Danielle Gendron (previously Thrasher) and I researched school meal programs in Japan and France, respectively (Moffat and Thrasher 2016; Moffat and Gendron 2019). Despite geographic and cultural differences, these meal programs have some commonalities. Though there is a long history of school meal programs in France and Japan, within the past two decades, both nations have targeted their meal programs as sites of intervention for improving child nutrition and preventing obesity. As part of this, Japan and France introduced legislation to enforce strict nutritional guidelines for meal programs. Both these high-income nations, moreover, invest sustainably in social programs such as education and health care, and have cultural and economic interests in food and food production. We argue that these

It Takes a Village

meal programs are excellent models for potential programs for other nations that either do not have them at all – for example, Canada, one of the few G8 nations that lacks a government-funded school meal program (Hernandez et al. 2018) – or for countries, like the US, that do have government-funded school meal programs but have been heavily criticized for their nutritional and social failings (Poppendieck 2010).

Case studies from high-, middle-, and low-income countries focused on the systematic use of local food in school meal programs demonstrate the considerable impact that school food procurement can have on the development of local agriculture, thus leading to a more sustainable public food system (Morgan and Sonnino 2008). In France, a number of large food-producing companies make either the ingredients or whole meals delivered to schools. With government mandates to include a certain percentage of local and/or organic foods, these companies must adapt their procurement strategies. In Japan, many schools have relationships with local farmers to buy food directly. This happens in France as well, where some school districts will buy, for example, whole organically raised cows for the production of meals in school kitchens.

One of the key findings from interviews we did with parents and educators in France and Japan was that school meals are viewed as an essential way to educate children about healthy eating and food literacy. Children's eating habits and future dietary habits are influenced during infancy and early childhood by parental role modelling (Scaglioni, Salvioni, and Galimberti 2008). If that parental role model is absent or not ideal, then school meals can provide an alternative. Moreover, as children grow older, they develop what Hill (2002, 264) terms "nutritional autonomy," whereby peer role models become more influential in their lives. Also, as discussed in Chapter 3, as children age, they are exposed to more food advertising. Since much of the peer interaction takes place at school, it makes sense that children share healthy eating experiences together. In its position statement, the Academy of Nutrition and Dietetics recommends that intervention programs "integrate education with supportive environmental change. In school and child-care settings the most successful interventions at achieving behavior change coupled educational messages with institutional change, so that children are taught about healthy eating and physical activity while provided healthy foods and more opportunities for physical activity" (Hoelscher et al. 2013, 1380). At this point, more evaluation of the influence of school meal programs on dietary habits is required. In France, one national study of dietary and physical activity behaviours of children who participated in school lunch programs versus those who did not found that those who participated had less sedentary behaviour and higher dietary diversity. Though the authors admit that this is not necessarily a causal relationship (Dubuisson et al. 2012), the results are promising.

Close-Up on School Meal Programs in France and Japan

Beginning in the 1880s and through the twentieth century, *restauration scolaire* (student restaurants) in France, informally called "the canteen," and *gakkō kyūshoku* (school lunch programs) in Japan became more formalized and increasingly overseen by the national French and Japanese governments (Agliano Sanborn 2013; Téchouyeres 2003). In France, *restauration scolaire* is administered at the level of the municipality, and, in the case of Paris, within each of the twenty *arrondissements* (administrative districts). Each municipality or district within Paris has its own mayor and *caisse-des-écoles* – a public establishment that administers school funds and oversees meal programs. Though the overall structure of school restaurants is similar across municipalities and districts, there is variation in the management by each *caisse-des-écoles*. In France, approximately 66 percent of students eat lunch at school at least once a week (Bertin et al. 2012), and in Paris, where there are many dual working parent families, participation is estimated to be even higher.

France deliberately and proactively subsidizes its payment scheme so that no student is unable to afford school lunch. In France a *quotient familiale* (family index) is calculated yearly, based on household income and living expenses, and the family is charged accordingly. In a wealthier district of Paris, the government pays for 50 percent of the program; in less wealthy districts, parent funding can drop to 35 percent. Families of the lowest income level pay as little as eighteen cents (USD) per day. It should be noted that the same meal is served regardless of amount paid. Since all payments are made monthly by parents, no one at the school knows whether a child receives a subsidized meal or not.

In contrast to France, the consumption of school meals is compulsory in Japan, even for teachers. In Japan, although all meals are available at low cost – between three to five US dollars per meal – there is no overt recognition that some families may be unable to afford them. The municipal government subsidizes meals by paying for the upkeep and maintenance of school lunch facilities, equipment, and staff; families pay the costs only for the food. Individual schools determine the cost per meal, and it varies by

It Takes a Village 101

grade level; younger students eat less, so the cost per meal is less. Students receive meals regardless of their payment status because lunch is part of the curriculum. Where Danielle Gendron did her fieldwork in Utsunomiya, Japan, there was a reported 4 to 5 percent non-payment rate for school lunches. Teachers explained that they are responsible for collecting outstanding lunch payments from parents by calling and writing letters, though students continue to receive lunches regardless of whether payment was made or not. As Anne Allison (1991, 199) notes in her study of *obentō* boxes in preschools, teachers in Japan hold legal authority and possess the ability to affect students' future successes. For instance, reports written by teachers may impede a student's entrance into high school. This, in part, explains why the lunch non-payment rate is so low in schools. A school nutritionist explained to Danielle: "[If a student hasn't paid] for like a month, we don't care because we have so many students so we can cover it, but if so many parents don't pay the money, like every month, then there will be so many problems." Though not explicitly stated, throughout multiple interviews it was inferred that it is at the teacher's discretion whether families should be pursued for payment.

The following vignettes of school meals in Paris and Utsunomiya are based on field note excerpts from our visits to primary school lunchrooms in these cities.

Lunchtime in Paris

School meals in a primary school located on the outskirts of Paris are eaten in the canteen in one of two thirty-minute shifts to accommodate all students. At one of my visits to observe a school lunch in Paris children entered the canteen noisily and washed their hands. Lunch consisted of an entrée, salad or fruit/vegetable, a main course (cereal/grain, meat or meat alternative, and a vegetable), followed by a cheese/yogurt and fruit course. Children chose their own places at tables and ate with enthusiasm – boisterous but relaxed.

At another school, children grabbed trays and served themselves cabbage and lettuce or cucumber salads to start, followed by a main course of beef with green beans and carrots, and finished with sliced, canned peaches and yogurt or fresh cheese. Children drank water poured from pitchers and helped themselves to baguette bread from bowls distributed around the room. I chatted with children and they told me they really liked the school food; it appears they were telling me the truth as I observed that not much was left on their plates at the end of the meal. In this multi-ethnic classroom, children appeared to be enjoying their meal in harmony.

In another school situated on the outskirts of Paris, a canteen staff person generously served tofu ravioli. She tried to serve students salad to which many shouted "pas de salade," but she managed to put a few leaves on their plates anyway. Teachers barked orders while canteen staff kept up a friendly rapport, singing songs, asking the children how they were doing.

At several schools there were lunch *animateurs*, adult supervisors who encourage eating and sociable lunch behaviours, though at another school observed there was much less interaction between staff and students. At the end of the meal in all the schools I observed, students took their dishes to a washing station, where they disposed of leftover food, sorted dishes, and then ran out into the school court-yard for recess break.

Lunchtime in Utsunomiya

In a fourth-grade classroom, students were quietly chatting and gig-gling as they rearranged the rows of desks into two tables of ten. Three students assigned as the *tōban* (lunch work group) put on their white aprons, hats, and sanitary face masks in order to retrieve lunch from the school kitchen. The *tōban* returned and unloaded pots of food, dishes, and utensils onto a table at the back of the class-room. The students formed a line to receive their lunches; I was invited to follow them. I picked up a tray, and then a *tōban* student served pan-fried mackerel on one side of the plate and mixed steamed vegetables with ham on the other before placing it on my tray. Next a bowl of rice was placed on the bottom left of my tray, followed by a bowl of miso soup on the bottom right. Finally, the teacher directed that I place chopsticks on my tray between the rice and the miso, and milk at the top right. The utmost care and atten-tion was paid to the proper serving of food and the correct place-ment of dishes on each tray.

It Takes a Village

Once everyone was served, the class gave thanks for the meal, and *itadakimasu* (I humbly receive) was said in unison, as it is said before all meals eaten in Japan. Although students chatted with one another, the main focus was on eating; students helped themselves to more food once they finished their first serving. A game of *janken* (rock/paper/scissors) broke out between five students to determine who would receive the last three pieces of mackerel.

I found that the appearance of the food was better than its taste. Far from bad, it was, however, bland: the vegetables were overcooked, the pan-fried mackerel soggy. The miso was the standout feature, and, as expected, the rice was cooked to perfection. Despite some shortcomings, this meal was nevertheless far superior to any school food I had ever eaten. Meals vary in quality between schools, belying how kitchen staff budget food ingredient costs while being aware of the affordability for local families. Some meals seem what would be considered more authentically Japanese (by both outsiders and Japanese people themselves) than others.

After everyone was finished eating, about twenty minutes, students said *gochisōsamadeshita* (it was a feast), as is said at the end of every meal in Japan. Students then performed lunch clean up: desks were wiped clean and placed back into rows, dishes and utensils were packed back onto the cart and returned to the kitchen, and floors were swept.

School Lunches in the New Millennium: Focus on Nutrition

Since the year 2000, many countries have sought to improve their school meal programs in light of concerns about public health issues like obesity as well as newer concerns about the promotion of food sovereignty and local agriculture (Morgan and Sonino 2008). Probably no one has done more for the cause of school lunches than celebrity chef Jamie Oliver. His documentary series, *Jamie's School Dinners*, features Oliver attempting to improve the quality of school dinners in the UK. Politicians paid attention to what Oliver was saying, and this resulted in new school food policy in the UK, reducing fried foods and banning soft drinks. As a result of Oliver's attention to school meals, over three years Tony Blair's government injected another £208 million into school meals in the UK (Garner 2009).

With less fanfare, France and Japan also overhauled their public nutrition programs. In 2005, *Shokuiku Kihon Hō*, the food education law, was legislated nationwide in Japan. The purpose of the law, translated as "nurturing through food," is to mandate that all public institutions, including schools, educate individuals on the importance of eating habits (Mah 2010). This law is incorporated into school programs, as described by Utsunomiya's Board of Education coordinator: "*Gakkō kyūshoku* (the school meal program) focuses on food education in order to ensure both physically and mentally healthy lives for children, but not only to provide daily nutritional requirements; *gakkō kyūshoku* also means, 'to eat happily.'" These laws have been instituted as part of a reaction to the rise in obesity that is connected to – in the minds of many public health practitioners in Japan – the rise of fast foods. A school nutritionist in Utsunomiya voiced this concern:

We have to stop people from getting fat. The problem is, if a child doesn't know how to eat then they won't know how to eat as an adult ... Say a child likes sugar and when they grow up, they still will eat sugar and soda pop and they don't want to eat vegetables, and they don't eat meat and then they will be unhealthy, they will have glucose problems. We have to stop this. We have to teach students about how to eat and that is to learn about being healthy. (Moffat and Thrasher 2016, 139)

In 2001, France launched the *Programme National Nutrition-Santé*, the National Nutrition and Health Program – with the mandate to deal with the nutritional needs of youth, taste, and food safety and to stop child overweight and obesity. It was at this point that more serious attention was paid to the quality of food served in school restaurants (Hercberg, Chat-Yung, and Chauliac 2008; Salanave et al. 2009; Téchouyeres 2003). Monthly menus are posted at each school and on school websites, and only one meal is offered. Menus are colour-coded by food group to indicate which foods are organic and/or locally procured. This is considered a convenience to parents so that they can plan evening meals in accordance with what children eat during the day. It also makes explicit the efforts to serve nutritious and well-balanced meals that include organic and locally produced foods.

Nutrition lessons in France, unlike the more explicitly didactic approach taken in Japan, are taught through experiential learning – that is, children are taught "how to eat" in a healthy and structured manner. The structure of

It Takes a Village 105

this healthy eating is distinctively a French style of eating as described by one parent of a five-year-old child living in Paris:

> I believe that the canteen helps because it shows you that you have an entrée with vegetables, that you have fish or meat, plus either veg plus rice, pasta, it's usually both of them, and then you have a milky product, cheese or whatever, and then a fruit. So in their day-to-day life kids can experience that, they see that there's always fruit and veg at a meal. (Moffat and Thrasher 2016, 139)

In summary, school meal programs in France and Japan are excellent models of school-based obesity prevention and nutrition interventions (Moffat and Thrasher 2016). This approach is two-pronged: (1) through public or social responsibility that ensures nutrition security for all children, regardless of income level, and (2) through education about nutrition, food, and eating based on experiential modelling of school meals served on a daily basis.

Making Gastro-Citizens

Beyond the concern for improving eating habits and the nutritional well-being of children, both Japan and France invest in school meals because food is very dear to the national culture and heritage of these nations. Both nations promote regional cuisine and local food production, which they have applied to their school meal programs. This trend is connected to larger national interests in the value of local food and gastronomic heritage. French cuisine and Japanese traditional cuisine (*washoku*) have been added to UNESCO's Intangible Cultural Heritage of humanity list (UNESCO 2010, 2013). Both nations are concerned about the encroachment through globalization of American foods, particularly fast food. In Europe the rise of the Slow Food Movement has been a very direct and organized reaction to this (Pietrykowski 2004).

Coupled with the fear of fast food is the desire to strengthen food sovereignty. In 2008, Japan passed *Chisan Chishō*, the Local Production for Local Consumption Act (LPLC), which promotes local agriculture throughout Japan. Its implementation in school meal programs requires that 30 percent or more of the school lunch menu be sourced locally (Agliano Sanborn 2013, 49). As Assman (2015, 180) argues, this law is connected to "culinary nationalism," a reaction to recent globalization (read "Western encroachment") that is changing Japanese food culture. In addition to concerns about preserving Japanese cuisine, the LPLC is imbued with appeals to a healthy national body and food safety and quality through the use of domestically grown fruit and vegetables that are promoted as "'delicious' and 'healthy' Japanese ingredients" (Takeda 2008, 23).[2]

School meals emphasize the "Japanese element," and teachers incorporate lessons on agriculture into their curricula (Takeda 2008). In addition to the provision of meals, children are explicitly educated about food: nutrition and eating are part of the daily curriculum. This was observed by Danielle Gendron in Japan, where students learn about food and eating through lessons, and information about the food is delivered as embellishments to the actual meals. Before, during, or after meals a teacher or nutritionist tells students about the ingredients used in the meal and talks about their health and nutritional benefits. Special emphasis is placed upon the local foods served; often ingredients come from farmers living close to the school, so that naming a farmer tells students the exact location of the produce. Even foreign assistant language teachers working in the schools were cognizant of the lessons being taught to children, as the following quote below indicates:

> I think that if you were to ask students to give you certain foods that are high in iron or protein or calcium or whatever, I think they would be able to do it ... I think that it would be partly down to the fact that they are told during their lunches ... When they are taught that the food comes from certain places, I think that that sticks with them, they do know what their areas are capable of doing, capable of producing, what sorts of foods come from their local areas. (Assistant language teacher)

School lunch provides a venue for students to learn about the significance and history of dishes that originate in local regions and to ensure that the consumption of such meals and local food traditions continue to be practised. The vice-principal of an elementary school articulated: "We [Japanese] are very traditional, and it [i.e., school lunch] provides delicious traditional food. That is something that school lunch can do, carry on local traditions in order to foster a love and appreciation for their [i.e., students'] own region."

Gakkō kyūshoku also places importance on teaching normalized mealtime behaviours. Teachers and nutritionists demonstrate how food should be properly presented, as emphasized in the serving of lunch each day in a particular formation. How food should appear, be arranged, and eaten are lessons embodied in these school meals. One important part of eating in Japan concerns the correct use of chopsticks. Mastering the use of chopsticks is a marker of being Japanese and is part of the formative enculturation of Japanese children (Allison 1991, 207). Thus, special emphasis is placed on the younger children to ensure that they understand the placement of food on the plate and how to use chopsticks.

Like the Japanese, the French are also concerned about the rise of fast food as well as industrial agriculture and the agrofoods industry. As discussed in Chapter 2, in France the focus on nutrition education is accompanied by an equal emphasis on explicitly teaching children about French food and culture. This was clearly articulated by a school board official I interviewed in Paris: "We try to educate taste. We consider having one mission that is at the crossroads – we are getting deep into French matters – we consider that the school lunch program is at the crossroads of several of the Republic's missions: a mission of educating and a mission of promoting public health" (Moffat and Gendron 2019, 70). This quote perfectly encapsulates and makes explicit the blending of teaching "taste," both in the sense of food and more broadly in the sense of class-based or national taste distinction as conceptualized by Bourdieu (1984). It amounts to what we have coined "gastro-citizenship," the emphasis on learning and embodying culinary heritage as part of children's education, becoming good citizens through the consumption of particular foods. School meal programs in Japan and France are part of the larger national project to produce gastro-citizens (Moffat and Gendron 2019).

Despite the rhetoric around connecting *gakkō kyūshoku* to Japanese and local cuisine, Gendron observed that school meals were of variable quality and of variable adherence to traditional cuisine, with some meals including of white bread instead of rice.[3] The obligatory addition of milk to school lunch in Japan is also not in keeping with traditional Japanese cuisine but, rather, is part of the rise of milk drinking and the milk industry in East Asia (see Wiley 2016). In Paris, where in some arrondissements there was considerable time and effort spent in producing very high-quality "cooked-from-scratch" meals, other school districts outsource school food to multinational food production companies, with meals being delivered to schools in the morning and reheated at lunchtime. In my interviews with school meal organizers, I found that those opposed to this system thought it was preferable for the food ingredients to be sourced directly by the *caisses-des-écoles* and cooked in school kitchens. As evident in the varying quality and authenticity of school food in Japan and France, some of the promotion of school meals as a representation of national cuisine is in the imaginations of the school administrators and educators rather than in the reality of the food served. Though we participated in some school lunches and ate with children, we did not sample a large proportion of the food, nor did we interview children about their perspectives on school meals. We realize this is a shortcoming of the research. While many of the adults in both Utsunomiya and Paris were very proud of their school meal programs and spoke very highly of them, we don't really know what the children thought of them. This speaks to the need for more research to be done with children in general (raised in the Introduction) and, more specifically, concerning their thoughts on school food.

School Food Challenges

It is important not to romanticize school meals as a panacea for all the problems related to food insecurity and poor dietary habits. School food can be of poor quality and can sometimes exacerbate inequalities among children. For example, in *Free for All: Fixing School Food in America*, Janet Poppendieck (2010) discusses how minimal the dietary guidelines are for school meals in the US. There is also the problem of what are called "competitive," or à la carte, foods that children can buy to replace the meals on offer. As Poppendieck explains, in order to subsidize the NSLP, for which some children qualify because they live in a low-income household and are thus eligible to obtain reduced-price or free lunches, à la carte foods are sold to increase profits. These à la carte foods are usually high-fat and sugary items that are not subject to the NSLP dietary guidelines and thus contribute to the portrayal of US school food as unhealthy. In addition to nutritional concerns the whole system can fail those children who need it most. First, parents have to apply, be certified, and then verified for the free or reduced-price school lunches, proving that their income is low enough to qualify, and parents don't always follow through on this procedure. Then there is the problem of stigma because students who get free meals are identified with their tickets or swipe cards. This becomes even more obvious as there are often two lines, one for the school meals that are subsidized and another for the à la carte items that are not (Poppendieck 2010). The poor quality of school food in the US was highlighted by Jamie Oliver's reality television series *Food Revolution*, which spent its first season inside schools in West Virginia, oftentimes berating low-level school administrators and cafeteria staff for the poor quality of the school food. This made for great reality TV, but, unfortunately, fed into stereotypes of poor, working-class families and did not address the reality of underfunding, which is part of neoliberal agendas to place the responsibility for feeding children solely on families instead of on the state. One can refer back to historical concerns that tie into school meal programs and nationalism (discussed above), where school meal programs were built on concerns about building bodies for military purposes (Levine 2008). In more modern contexts, as seen in France and Japan, feeding programs are designed to grow nutritionally healthy and fit citizens. It appears that in the US, particularly in poor school districts, this vision is lacking, at least for those citizens who are envisioned as having unhealthy and unfit bodies.

The French and Japanese models are much more equitable as, in the case of France, children do not know whose lunch is being subsidized, and, in the case of Japan, they all pay one very low price. In both France and Japan meals are all the same for everyone, so there is no stigma or shame involved in eating school meals. Though these programs are laudable for their social inclusion, however, there is potential for social exclusion. In both countries school meals are limited in their accommodation of students' dietary restrictions, which may be for medical (in the case of food allergies/sensitivities) or cultural/religious reasons. Students who wish or need to participate in these programs are forced to submit their food requirements and needs to the greater good of these states' mandates to feed every child equally. In 2013, when I was researching school lunches in France, though vegetarian meals were served randomly throughout the month, there were no vegetarian alternatives served daily. This meant that students who did not eat meat, or ate only halal meat, were not able to fully participate. Though there was an alternative offered on days when pork was on the menu, educators and nutritionists who were interviewed considered it impossible to serve halal meat and said that they could not accommodate religious food restrictions, both for logistical reasons and, as phrased by a primary school principal, because the "Republic's school should remain everyone's school" (Moffat and Thrasher 2016, 138). This principal worked at a school just outside of Paris, in a poorer, working-class area with a high proportion of immigrants in residence. The principal insisted that there should be no attempts to cater to religious food restrictions, though they conceded that alternatives to pork were reasonable.

France has a history of operationalizing state secularism, *laïcité*, through its refusal to accommodate religious requirements in food or dress in national institutions. In 2005, the "pork affair" erupted in an elementary school in a Paris suburb, where a teacher allegedly forced three-year-old students to eat pork in their school meals. Muslim parents protested with legal representation, demanding that they have the right to school lunches without pork. The event was settled out of court, with the agreement that students could opt out of certain menu items and that all ingredients would be clearly posted on school meal menus (Selby 2011). School meals were politicized again when National Front leader Marine LePen declared that non-pork alternatives for Muslim students would be banned as "contrary to France's secular values" in the eleven municipalities where her party was contending (Daily Mail Reporter 2014). This ban was in fact enacted in 2015 in a town near Paris governed by Mayor Jean-Paul Beneytou, where non-pork alternatives are no longer an option on the school lunch menu (Chrisafis 2015). On the other side of this debate are those who have called for standard vegetarian alternatives to be compulsory in all schools, as proposed in 2015 by a member of the French National Assembly, Yves Jego (BBC News 2015). To date this issue has not been resolved.

School Food in Canada

Despite the fact that there are challenges in many national school meal programs, Canada stands out like a sore thumb as the only country in the G8 that does not have a government-funded and -managed school meal program (Hernandez et al. 2018). After the Second World War there was intense debate in Canada about whether a national school lunch program should be developed, but the federal government decided to take an individualist approach and to supplement family wages with income assistance rather than to fund a universal school meal program that would collectively be responsible for children's nutritional well-being (Carbone, Power, and Holland 2020). Today we are in much the same situation. In a UNICEF report on youth well-being across Sustainable Development Goals for forty-one high-income nations, Canada was ranked thirty-seven out of forty-one in working towards Zero Hunger for children. In other words, Canada ranked better only than Malta, Turkey, Mexico, and Bulgaria; the United States, though only ranked at thirty-six, was above Canada (UNICEF Canada 2017). For a nation that prides itself on social programs in the area of health and publicly funded health care, Canada is doing appallingly poorly in the area of child nutrition, a determinant of health that is critical to preventing illness and promoting health and well-being.

In the majority of publicly funded elementary schools in Canada students bring packed lunches to school. Frequently, there are home and school fundraisers that sell pizza or sub sandwiches to students once a week to raise funds for school events and equipment. But most days children bring their own lunch to school. Though it would be nice to think that lunches coming from home are lovingly prepared by parents following Canada's Food Guide and that children are dutifully eating these nutritious lunches at school, the lived reality is much different. Harassed single- or dual-parent working families throw together lunches for their children in the morning (or the night before if they're really organized), using many of the processed snack foods, cheese strings, fruit rollups, and so on discussed in Chapter 3 (see Table 3.2). Parents often resort to these snack foods due to lack of time or to pressure from kids: "that's what my classmates get," or so they say. Once kids are at school, in the twenty minutes or so they have to eat, they often eat the treat or snack and throw out the apple or whatever else might contain more nutritional value. Indeed, studies of food brought from home in primary schools in Canada (where packed lunches are the norm and there is no real comparison) and the US and UK (where they are not the norm and can be compared to school meals) demonstrate that packed lunches are of low dietary quality and do not meet school meal standards (Evans et al. 2010; Hubbard et al. 2014; Tugault-Lafleur, Black, and Barr 2017).

That's the good scenario if you come from a middle-class family that can afford, in terms of finances and time, to pack a lunch. The more deplorable reality in Canada is that one in six Canadian children under the age of eighteen are affected by household food insecurity (Tarasuk and Mitchell 2020). In these households there isn't always enough food to pack a nutritious lunch, and many students go hungry. There are no school nutrition programs in Canada that are completely funded by government. For example, breakfast programs receive an amalgamation of funding from provincial and municipal governments, parents, corporate donations, and non-governmental organizations (Godin et. al 2017). Breakfast Clubs Canada supports an army of volunteers who serve children breakfast before the start of the school day. While these volunteer groups are aided by some financial resources, they still rely on food donations that may not be of optimal nutritional value. These programs are also precarious because they rely ultimately on the goodwill of volunteer workers. This is not a sustainable way to feed children. It also does not address the need for children to eat more than breakfast during the day.

Publicly funded high schools in Canada usually have cafeterias that sell a limited selection of food, such as sandwiches, soups, salads, burgers, and fries, with a variety of daily specials. These cafeterias are run by third-party companies contracted by school boards (Winson 2008). With regulations about school food, like the School Food and Beverage Policy, which came into place in 2011 in Ontario, many companies pulled out of schools because they claimed that, without being able to sell "junk food" like French fries, the cafeterias were no longer profitable, as cited in a media report (Cross 2013). Outspoken Dr. Yoni Freedhoff of Ottawa's Bariatric Medical Institute was quoted as saying: "The fact that kids are going across the street to buy crap is not an argument to sell crap in the schools. They can buy tobacco in the stores as well, but I don't think that would be a good thing to sell in the schools even if it made schools a profit" (CTV News 2011). Despite Freedhoff's logical argument, the fact is that high school students can and will leave campus to seek food at other venues. The foodscapes around schools challenge attempts to encourage healthy eating at school: one study from Montreal even indicated that there appears to be a gradient whereby schools in more socioeconomically deprived areas have foodscapes with higher densities of fast-food outlets, making children living these areas even more at risk for diet-related diseases (Kestens and Daniel 2010).

Despite these challenges, there are ways forward. First, many adolescents do want to eat healthy food but will tell you that, when the food sold at their cafeteria is unappealing and unhealthy, they will go elsewhere or will not eat at all. Second, even if adolescents might go astray in their eating habits, we should ensure that younger students, those as young as three or four who stay at school all day where they eat at least 30 percent of their daily food requirements, have access to high-quality and nutritionally optimal meals. As mentioned above, food habits start early, and healthy, enjoyable eating must be modelled experientially to children.

There is a growing movement in Canada in support of establishing school meal programs. One of the most organized and convincing advocates of a national school food program is the Coalition for Healthy School Food, part of Food Secure Canada. It seeks investment from the federal government to mount a cost-shared universal healthy school food program (Food Secure Canada n.d.). In its position paper it cites a number of health- and wellness-related reasons to support its call for the program: school food programs can increase the consumption of fruits and vegetables; they can assist in student learning and success by improving concentration and mental

It Takes a Village

health; and school food programs can create jobs and support local economies (Coalition for Healthy School Food n.d.). These calls for a national school food program are getting attention from different sectors, including the Canadian Medical Association (Collier 2015), public health nutritionists (Hernandez et al. 2018), and the mainstream media (CBC News 2017b).

There are a few schools and organizations in Canada that have independently forged ahead to improve the state of school food. For example, Inuksuk High School in Iqaluit has established a healthy free lunch program three days a week, where students volunteer or are even hired part-time to make and serve lunches to other students. They have taken the "farm-to-table" into their own hands by creating and using greens from their own school hydroponic towers, where they source most of their kale, lettuce, and herbs (Frizzell 2018). FoodShare has been pioneering in its Good Food Café project, which it runs in Toronto schools: it has taken over cafeterias in some schools and brings in lunches to others. With student input it has introduced a variety of healthy meals to expose children to meals that include fruits and vegetables. These innovations are important to examine as models of what could be done more widely in Canada (DiFelice 2015). Finally, former premier Rachel Notley's NDP government in the province of Alberta made the most significant gains by piloting a government-funded school meal program. It began in 2016 with an allocation of $250,000 CAD to each of fourteen publicly funded kindergarten to Grade 6 schools in Alberta. The schools designed their own combination of breakfast, nutritious snack, and lunch meals. The preliminary evaluation of the program was so favourable that the government forged ahead to expand it in the remaining elementary schools in Alberta (Alberta Government 2017). Finally, in 2019, Justin Trudeau's federal Liberal government announced its long-awaited National Food Policy, which included a federal commitment to work with the provinces and territories to develop a national school food program to deliver healthy food to Canadian children before and during school (Hui 2019). So far, this is only a theoretical commitment, but it's a start.

Summary

Schools can and should be more than just institutions where children are warehoused for six hours per day. Educators, especially those in elementary schools, are caregivers and role models and, like families, should nourish children in both mind and body. School food should be included in this nurturing approach, and it must be of the best quality and served in the most inclusive and enjoyable settings possible. As Danielle Gendron and I have concluded from our research on programs in France and Japan, school meals should be part of national public health programs and should be used as a tool to prevent noncommunicable, dietary-related diseases (Moffat and Thrasher 2016). Since the beginning of the twenty-first century a number of school-based interventions have been implemented that are grounded in behavioural and short-term interventions. A review of these programs concludes that the effects overall are modest (Katz 2010). A large randomized-control trial of a school obesity intervention in primary schools in the UK found that, in schools where the intervention took place as opposed to those in which it did not, there was no significant difference in child obesity after thirty months of the program. The intervention consisted mostly of increasing physical activity at school, but there was also a healthy-eating component that included education-related activities such as healthy cooking classes aimed at both students and their families. This school intervention program, while probably quite positive, was ultimately considered a failure because there was no change in obese and overweight children's body mass index scores after thirty months. A news article in the *Guardian* emphasized this failure in its headline: "Schools are not the answer to childhood obesity epidemic, study shows" (Boseley 2018). In Chapter 6, I discuss more about the framing of childhood obesity as an epidemic and how that promotes short-term, non-systemic, and ultimately futile approaches to preventing obesity. But suffice it to say, improving school meal programs requires more than short-term fixes for weight loss; it requires systemic changes that establish dietary habits for life – and modelling good food and ways to eat that do not include shovelling processed food into one's mouth as fast as possible, which is what occurs in many schools throughout Canada and the US.

School food can also serve as a way to create change in the whole food system while simultaneously educating the next generation. As was done in the 1930s by the US government when it gave farmers a helping hand by buying food for school meals (Levine 2008), school food procurement can support local farmers and educate children about the value and environmental sustainability of eating local, fresh, and nutritious food. There are examples of this all over the world, in Asia, Europe, South America, and some school districts in New York State (Morgan and Sonnino 2008). Canada is very far behind these places as it has no formalized structure or government oversight of school food programs. Now is the time to change the program, to learn from other countries' accomplishments and mistakes to make a uniquely Canadian school meal program.

It Takes a Village

Like so many other aspects of our social and economic structures, the COVID-19 pandemic is shining a light on the institutional importance of school food. School closures throughout the world resulted in children missing out on their school meals, which had a devastating impact on their nutritional well-being, particularly so for those living in food-insecure households (Rundle et al. 2020; Van Lancker and Parolin 2020). One can only hope that the demonstration of the effects of their absence will strengthen our resolve to expand and improve school meals in the future.

5

Global Malnutrition and Children's Food (In)security

No social or economic problem facing the world today is more urgent than that of hunger. While this distressing state of affairs is not new, its persistence in spite of the remarkable technological and productive advances of the twentieth century is nothing short of scandalous.
– DRÈZE AND SEN, *HUNGER AND PUBLIC ACTION*

The outrage expressed by Jean Drèze and his co-author, Nobel Prize–winning economist Amartya Sen, in the preceding epigram (Drèze and Sen 1989, v) is no less valid in the twenty-first century than it was in the twentieth. One in three children under five years of age suffers from malnutrition and at least one in two under five suffers from nutrient deficiencies (UNICEF 2019).

While the news about child hunger and malnutrition is dire, there has been some positive change in the new millennium. Between 2000 and 2016 there was a global decline in stunting (a measure of chronic growth retardation, discussed in further detail below) of children under five years of age, from 32.7 to 22.9 percent. In other words, there was a global decrease from one in three to one in four, or from 198 million to 155 million, stunted children. Despite this positive trend, local conditions that give rise to chronic growth failure in certain parts of the world, such in West and Central Africa, remain stubbornly persistent, where the number of stunted children has increased over the same time period from 23 million to 28 million (Development Initiatives 2018).

The manifestation of malnutrition, defined by the WHO (2016a) "as deficiency, excess or imbalance in a person's intake of energy and/or specific nutrients in relation to their requirements" has also changed in the new millennium: malnutrition is increasingly associated with overweight, prevalence rates of which are now reported in global statistics on child malnutrition. In 2016, 41 million, or 6 percent, of children under five around the world were overweight. While this prevalence plateaued for many regions, Eastern Europe and Central Asia had a statistically significant increase in the number of overweight children between 2000 and 2016 (Development Initiatives 2018). There is also a phenomenon in low- and middle-income countries called the "double burden of malnutrition" that is hitting Southeast Asian countries hard, as well as some sub-Saharan African and Central and Southern American nations. The double burden of malnutrition refers to the occurrence of both undernutrition (micronutrient deficiencies, underweight, and stunting and wasting) and overweight and obesity in the same population, households, and even individuals (Popkin, Corvalan, and Grummer-Strawn 2020). The coexistence of both undernutrition and overweight/obesity is paradoxically related to both poverty and systemic flaws in the global food system, a central premise of Raj Patel's (2012) aptly titled book, *Stuffed and Starved*.

I begin this chapter with a discussion of malnutrition in low-income countries, using my own research in Nepal as a case study to illustrate the experience of child malnutrition in one local context. Here I argue that malnutrition in low-income regions is not just about food or the lack thereof but, rather, has to do with a complex interplay among multiple factors that include a polluted environment, household poverty, and lack of investment in health care and infrastructure at both national and international levels. I then move on to an overview of food insecurity, its definitions and measurement, and its ramifications for physical, sociocultural, and psychological well-being – with specific reference to children. This is followed by discussions of child malnutrition and food insecurity as they are manifest and patterned in high-income countries, with a focus on Canada and the United States. Though children in these high-income countries do not generally experience malnutrition in the form of underweight, they do suffer from malnutrition in the form of micronutrient deficiencies and overweight/obesity in addition to related poor health outcomes. I then examine policy as it relates to children's food insecurity in high-income countries, with a focus on Canadian versus American approaches. I conclude with a reference back to Raj Patel's thesis that child malnutrition is the product of a global food system that is inadequately serving children and future generations.

Malnutrition in Low-Income Countries

Undernourishment of a child may begin before they are even born. The most common measure of prenatal malnutrition or inadequate foetal growth is low birthweight (LBW), which is marked by a newborn weight of less than 2,500 grams (5.5 pounds). In 2013, an estimated 16 percent (or 22 million) of babies were born with LBW. This is no doubt an underestimate since many children in low-income countries are not weighed at birth (Development Initiatives 2018). There is a strong association between neonatal (first twenty-eight days postpartum) mortality and LBW (Bogin 1999). Those babies who survive are more likely to experience impaired immune function and infectious disease, reduced muscle strength, and lower cognitive abilities (Martorell 1999). LBW due to inadequate foetal growth is related to the mother's condition. While many environmental factors, such as smoking, alcohol, environmental toxins (Bogin 1999), and infections such as malaria (Ramakrishnan 2004), can increase the risk for LBW, approximately half of LBW babies are the direct result of the undernutrition of mothers. Studies done in low-income countries show that pre-pregnancy size is a well-known determinant of LBW, indicating that this is an intergenerational problem from mother to daughter and so on (Ramakrishnan 2004). South Asia currently has the highest prevalence of LBW (28 percent), twice as high as sub-Saharan Africa (13 percent) (Development Initiatives 2018).

Even if an infant is not born with LBW, malnutrition can quickly become a problem for children, and the onset of this is usually in the first three months of life. It is manifest by slow infant growth in both weight gain and length; this is usually precipitated by inadequate infant and young child feeding, as discussed in Chapter 1. In low-income countries malnutrition in infancy is associated with a higher prevalence of infant mortality due to infectious diseases such as diarrheal diseases and pneumonia (Walson and Berkley 2018).

Malnutrition in low-income countries is sometimes a result of catastrophic events, either natural disasters or political disasters – for example, droughts, earthquakes, or war. This is manifested in sudden weight loss and dehydration among children, usually occurring in sub-Saharan Africa, where most of today's famines occur. However, for the most part, malnutrition is a slow, relentless, and chronic phenomenon that reveals itself in frequent illness, learning challenges, and shorter attained stature, with accompanied lower muscle mass and physical work capacity.

This type of malnutrition, known as "chronic malnutrition," is measured through attained height and weight of children relative to their chronological

Global Malnutrition and Children's Food (In)security   119

age. Height-for-age and weight-for-age indices are standardized by comparing them to a population reference, most commonly the WHO growth reference (de Onis et al. 2007), and then converted to a percentile of the reference median. Two cross-sectional indicators of poor child growth are "stunting" and "wasting." Stunting is indicated by low height-for-age and wasting by low weight-for-height. Stunting is the pathological end result of low linear growth (height), whereas wasting marks current, acute malnutrition (Waterlow 1973). The cut-off points for stunting and wasting are scores below the third percentile of the growth reference, where the fiftieth percentile is the median of the normal distribution of growth, relative to the WHO's normal growth reference (Gibson 1990). As with LBW, South Asia continues to have the highest prevalence of stunting and wasting among children under five; in 2018, the prevalence of stunting in this region was 34 percent and the prevalence of wasting was 15 percent. While there is also a high prevalence of stunting in sub-Saharan Africa (33 percent), the prevalence of wasting is lower, ranging from 6 percent in Eastern and Southern Africa to a high of 9 percent in West and Central Africa (FAO 2019).

A common misunderstanding about malnutrition among children in low-income countries is that it is due solely to low energy (calories) and/or protein intake. While this is frequently the case, even with adequate amounts of energy and protein, children may suffer from micronutrient deficiencies. Micronutrient deficiencies can cause a wide range of physical and cognitive impairments in children, including growth failure (Milward 2017). An example of a micronutrient deficiency that is still widespread in low-income regions of the world is vitamin A deficiency – once again this has the highest occurrence among children aged six to fifty-nine months in South Asia and sub-Saharan Africa (Development Initiatives 2018). It is the leading cause of preventable childhood blindness (xeropthalmia) and is associated with impairment of immune function leading to childhood illness such as diarrhea (Stevens et al. 2015). Unlike overall undernutrition, micronutrient deficiencies can be addressed to some degree with supplementation; targeted programs in many regions of the world have been successful, though this requires a strong public health care system (Development Initiatives 2018).

A Case Study from Nepal

I use Nepal as a case study here not only because it is where I conducted research on infant and young children's nutritional health and well-being in the 1990s but also because it is a low-income nation. More specifically, it is a low-income nation in the region of South Asia, which, as stated above, has the highest prevalence of child malnutrition in the world. This stubbornly high prevalence of malnutrition has been coined the "Asian enigma" (Headey and Hoddinott 2015) since malnutrition persists there despite the fact that many of the economies in this region have been growing rapidly for at least a decade. In the 1990s, when I was doing my doctoral research in Kathmandu, Nepal, the infant mortality rate and under-five mortality rate were 99 and 142 per one thousand, respectively; a whopping 60 percent of children under five years were stunted, many of them severely so (Headey and Hoddinott 2015). Nepal was at that time, and continues to be, a poor nation by global standards, ranking twenty-eight out of the thirty poorest nations in the world (Tasch 2017). Apart from a ten-year Maoist revolution that occurred from 1996 to 2006, Nepal has been a relatively peaceful nation with, at this point, a more-or-less functioning democracy and the strong presence of a number of international government development agencies as well as many international and domestic NGOs that are working on poverty alleviation and the improvement of children's nutritional status.

The focus of my study was the Tibeto-Nepali carpet-making industry in Kathmandu. In 1995, it was a magnet for Nepali young adults who were leaving their villages to work as carpet weavers and spinners, and, as they frequently told me, to make a better life for their children – mainly to gain access to health care and schools, all of which were (and are) wholly inadequate in rural regions. Wages for weavers and spinners were low – the field was dominated by women who earned less money than their male counterparts – though many of the larger factories provided subsidized lodging. Families with young children under five years of age working in the carpet-making industry were the participants in my study. My research questions were as follows: How do women negotiate their productive and reproductive roles and what impact does that have on their children's health? How does the urban environment affect children's health? What do young children eat and how does their diet affect their growth and development? These were the questions with which I entered the field, with an overall view of attempting to understand the biocultural determinants of young children's health and nutritional status.

At a descriptive level it was clear that a large proportion of the 283 children under five years of age that I measured at least once during the course of a year's fieldwork were stunted and underweight, though not so much wasted. Stunting and underweight was highest in children from one to five years of age, and lowest among the infants. A comparison of the average stature in centimetres for the Nepali boys and girls relative to the World

Global Malnutrition and Children's Food (In)security

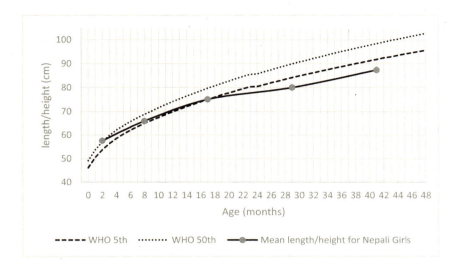

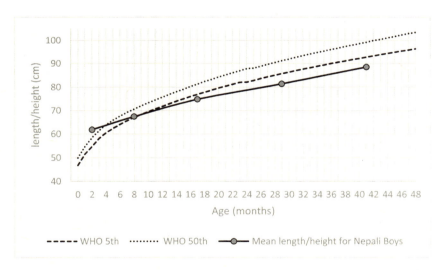

FIGURE 5.1 Linear growth rate of Nepali children from birth to five years compared to the WHO 50th and WHO 5th growth references. | Courtesy of author.

Health Organization growth reference shows that these Nepali babies began, on average, at the WHO 50th percentile; however, by eight months of age their mean length was at the WHO 5th percentile, and, by eighteen months of age, it had dropped below the WHO 5th percentile, where it continued to track into the fourth year of life (Figure 5.1).

The growth faltering these children experienced early in their lives was indeed a form of chronic malnutrition, but what were its specific determinants? I investigated young children's diets by conducting twenty-four-hour food frequency recalls that were done with parents at every measuring session. A profile of a typical weaning diet (from four to six months up to the end of breastfeeding, which lasted on average to 2.5 to three years of age) consisted of daily rice flour pabulum (called *litho*) for infants, and, as they became older, rice and *dal* (lentil soup). Only about a third of the children ate meat and less than 20 percent ate eggs on a regular basis. Milk tea (with sugar) was a daily beverage for young children, and "sweets," mostly in the form of sweet digestive-type biscuits or commercially sold puff pastries, were a ubiquitous feature of children's diets. Seven out of forty-four children in the twelve- to eighteen-month-old category were reported by parents to have eaten very little – a piece of bread or a snack – on the food-recall survey day. Many mothers cited illness as the reason. Some mothers said that after one year of age, children ate whatever the rest of the family was eating, so there were no special meals prepared for them – a form of the "laissez-faire" approach to early child feeding as discussed in Chapter 2. What is clear is that these families, on an extremely tight budget, had a limited diet that extended to the weaning diet of young children.

In addition to diet, I looked at factors beyond what they were eating and at the children's environment and its impact on their nutritional health. The range of illnesses that young children experienced, as reported by parents, indicated that these children suffered from a wide array of infections. Most common were gastrointestinal (GI) diseases, as indicated by symptoms of vomiting and diarrhea or "worms" that were self-diagnosed by parents through observation of bloated stomachs or worms found in the stools. Approximately one-third, or 34.6 percent, of the sample suffered from a GI illness within the previous two weeks of the survey. From this larger sample of children, I had a smaller sub-sample of seventy-one stools analyzed for indications of parasites. Thirty out of seventy-one individuals (42 percent) had evidence of either a helminthic (worm) or protozoan (such as an amoeba) infection in their stool. In other words, these children were suffering from chronic parasitism, due to polluted water and food, consistent with the very high prevalence of reported GI infections. More children over one year of age than under one were reported by parents to be suffering from parasitic infections, most likely because, as they got older, their diets diversified and they were more mobile and thus more likely to interact with a polluted environment (Moffat 2003).

The impact of disease on child growth has been well documented. Studies in a variety of low-income countries have indicated that the presence of infectious disease significantly reduces child weight gain (Becker, Black, and Brown 1991) as well as length/height gain (Black, Brown, and Becker 1984). Recent research based in Nicaragua and conducted by Barbara Piperata and colleagues (2019) indicates that common enteric pathogens found in children's stools, like *Salmonella* and *Campylobacter*, can adversely affect the gut microbiota of children, which could have long-term implications for children's nutritional health and well-being. Diarrheal diseases have been a major focus of interest in child health studies, although in some cases respiratory diseases – specifically lower respiratory tract diseases like pneumonia and measles – are also implicated in growth retardation. It is important to note, as Cole (1989) points out, that the impact of an infectious disease will vary with the specific environment, which includes the prevalence of the disease, the level of health care, and the socioeconomic conditions in that community. Diarrheal diseases have been most closely scrutinized because of their known biological means of causing malnutrition (Chen 1983). Diarrhea can be an appetite depressant, leading to statistically significantly reduced food intake among children (Martorell et al. 1980), but acute diarrhea can also cause malabsorption and loss of important nutrients such as protein, nitrogen, and fat (Mann, Hill, and Bowie 1990). My survey findings were corroborated by parents' thoughts on this issue. When I asked parents whose children were assessed as stunted and/or underweight if they thought their children were small – and, if so, why – 59 percent of them cited illness as the reason, and an additional 10 percent specifically cited GI problems. Only 4 percent cited not enough or bad food, and a further 8 percent said they had no or low-quality breast milk (Moffat 2000).

What were the biocultural determinants of malnutrition that these children in my study experienced? I argue that they were intimately related to their urban biophysical environment. Within the environment there were a variety of factors at the community level, including many people living in a small area that was lacking adequate water, toilet facilities, and sewage treatment, combined with inadequate housing and low-quality food. This environment led to a high pathogen load for children that was synergistically exacerbated by poverty from low wages that were stretched to buy food, clothing, school fees for children, and health care, among other basic needs.

The good news is that, according to Nepal's Demographic Health Surveys conducted in 2001, 2006, and 2011, there has been an impressive and rapid reduction in malnutrition since 2001. The national prevalence of stunting declined from 56.6 to 40.6 from 2001 to 2011 – the most rapid decline in child stunting in the world (Headey and Hoddinott 2015). Studies of the drivers of this reduction conclude that the following five factors explain reduced stunting prevalence: (1) increases in average birthweight, indicative of improvements in maternal nutrition; (2) asset accumulation for households, meaning rapid growth in household income; (3) educational improvements and, specifically, maternal education; (4) increased access to health care, including prenatal, neonatal, and postnatal care; and (5) sizeable improvements in sanitation, specifically in the reduction of open defecation and more toilet use (Headey and Hoddinott 2015; Cunningham et al. 2017). All these improvements are linked with social, economic, and policy changes at both community and national levels and on multiple fronts (Cunningham et al. 2017), emphasizing that there are profound links between the political economy, the biophysical environment, and child health. Regrettably, there is still an unacceptably high proportion of children in Nepal who continue to experience growth stunting, and Headey and Hoddinott (2015) note that progress in improving access to clean water has been very slow. Access to clean water, to higher wages and employment, and to higher-quality food for young children must increase to see further progress in children's nutritional health.

With these conclusions, I emphasize that most malnutrition in low-income regions of the world occurs because of poverty and lack of resources at the household, community, and national levels. Families for the most part know how to feed their children and are well intentioned in their desire to see their children grow and prosper. A systematic review study of international evidence for the impact of intervention programs on improving complementary feeding of children aged six to twenty-four months through maternal education indicates that these programs have little effect on improving children's nutritional outcomes (Dewey and Adu-Afarwuah 2008). This is a final point that ties together lessons from my fieldwork case study and the more recent studies that have examined the drivers of success in improving nutritional status in Nepal (Headey and Hoddinott 2015; Cunningham et al. 2017). Improving children's nutrition "requires the contributions of a diverse array of sectors" (Cunningham et al. 2017, 36) that must focus on decreasing poverty and improving the infrastructure, resources, and the biophysical environment in both households and local communities.

~

In the spring of 2019 I visited Kathmandu again, twenty-one years after doing postdoctoral research there in 1998. As an epilogue to this case study of Nepal's changing child growth indicators, I noticed, with my eyes popping out of my head, the frequency with which I saw, through visual observation only, overweight and obese children. This was not something I ever saw in the Kathmandu Valley in the 1990s. These are clearly children living in affluent households whose families are able to afford a plentiful supply of food that no doubt includes the large two-litre plastic containers of Coca-Cola I witnessed in Nepali households (only small glass bottles of Indian and Nepali brands of soda were commonly consumed in the 1990s, and only on special occasions). The emerging multinational fast-food chains, such as KFC and Baskin-Robbins, were both conspicuous in downtown Kathmandu. Affluent and urbanized children's celebrations are now connected with Western cultural rituals that focus on sweets. For example, I witnessed a child's birthday party hosted at the hotel where I was staying: it included a birthday cake and many sweets that were given to the guests as part of the celebration. Birthday parties are not part of the traditional suite of Nepali celebrations and festivals. Living in Nepal in the 1990s, I never witnessed any child or adult celebrating a birthday party or eating a birthday cake.

There are a few studies that have documented the recent rise of child obesity in Nepal. One study of children attending a private school in Kathmandu surveyed 986 children aged six to thirteen years and found that 14.6 percent were overweight and 11.3 percent were obese (Koirala et al. 2015). Another study discusses the overall prevalence of adult obesity in Nepal in the context of the global emergence of obesity in low- and middle-income countries, particularly in South Asia (Vaidya, Shakya, and Krettek 2010). As discussed above, this is part of the "double or dual burden of malnutrition" seen in many low- and middle-income countries around the world that is related to the global increase in diet-related NCDs such as type 2 diabetes and heart disease (WHO 2017). This double burden is connected to what Jonathan Wells (2012b) describes in his analysis of the role of capitalism in global obesity, whereby emerging food markets dominated by multinational food corporations infiltrate countries that were formerly impoverished by colonial and postcolonial food systems that reduced their capacity to control their own food production and markets. In these low-income countries a person can be born with a low birthweight, grow up stunted, and then have an enhanced metabolic susceptibility to obesity with the rapid nutrition transition within their lifetime and exposure to obesogenic foods like sugar-sweetened beverages. This phenomenon is mirrored, though not as dramatically, among people living with food insecurity in high-income countries.

Food (In)security and Malnutrition in High-Income Countries

While hunger continues to be a widespread problem for humanity, it is one part of the more encompassing phenomenon called "food insecurity." The most common and, I would say, most useful definition of food security comes from the Food and Agriculture Organization: "*Food security* exists when all people, at all times, have physical, social and economic access to sufficient, safe and nutritious food which meets their dietary needs and food preferences for an active and healthy life." Added to this definition is a refinement to specify the level of analysis at the household: "*Household food security* is the application of this concept to the household or family, with individuals within households as the focus of concern" (FAO 2003, section 2.2, emphasis added). This is an important addition when considering children, as most children (though not all, of course) are dependents in households. In measuring food insecurity at the household level, children are counted separately in the measurement process. The tool for measuring food (in)security in the US and Canada is a questionnaire called the Household Food Security Survey Module (HFSSM), adapted from the one developed by the United States Department of Agriculture in 1995 and employed with some modifications in the Canadian Community Health Survey.[1] The HFSSM focuses on self-reports of uncertain, insufficient, or inadequate food access, availability, and utilization due to limited financial resources, and on the compromised eating patterns and food consumption that may result. It is a standardized set of questions that focuses on households, with a subset specifically for households with children (Government of Canada 2012).

The Food and Agriculture Organization (FAO 2008) has conceptually divided food security into four dimensions: physical *availability* of food; economic and physical *access* to food; food *utilization*; and *stability* of the other three dimensions over time. These dimensions are useful because they allow us to unpack the variety of reasons and levels at which individuals, households, and communities can experience food insecurity. In high-income nations of the world, physical food *availability* is not usually a problem, as it can be in low-income nations, especially during times of political instability (such as war) or natural disasters (such as earthquakes). Even in nations like Canada, however, food availability may be a problem in northern and circumpolar communities, where transportation of food from the south is often dependent on air transportation, and where food is exorbitantly expensive and not properly subsidized by the Canadian government (Galloway 2014, 2017). Northern Indigenous communities also must contend with the lack of availability of "country foods" – foods that are hunted or fished, such as seal or caribou – due to declines in animal populations as a result of disturbances from mining, deforestation, environmental contaminants, and climate change (Power 2008).

Food *access* is undoubtedly the largest impediment to household food security in high-income nations, stemming from insufficient income to buy both the necessary quantity and, more often, the necessary *quality* of food that people require to support their physical, social, and cultural needs. This is particularly acute when it comes to children who are growing and developing. Sadly, food insecurity affects and is more prevalent among households with children under the age of eighteen. In the US in 2017, 15.7 percent of households with children were living with food insecurity compared to the overall prevalence of 11.8 percent for all households (Coleman-Jensen et al. 2018). In Canada, the prevalence of food insecurity among households with children is also higher than the national prevalence. As reported in Tarasuk and Mitchell (2020), overall 17.3 percent of households with children under the age of eighteen in Canada are affected by food insecurity. Food insecurity among children, however, is not evenly distributed across the country: it is especially acute in the Far North, where a full 78.7 percent of children living in Nunavut live in food-insecure households. This has been described by Valerie Tarasuk as "a national tragedy" (CBC News 2017a).

In reviewing the sociodemographic profile of households with children experiencing food insecurity, one key factor pops out: lone parent families are overrepresented. In the US, 30.3 percent of food-insecure households were headed by single women and 19.7 percent by men (Coleman-Jensen et al. 2018). Of the Canadian households reporting food insecurity in 2017–18, 26.1 percent were headed by males and 33.1 percent by females. As well, households in Canada where the respondent identifies as Indigenous or Black are disproportionately affected by food insecurity (Tarasuk and Mitchell 2020).

With the exception of the Far North, where food prices are exorbitantly high, food insecurity in the US and Canada is, for the most part, not about the high cost of food per se; rather, it is more related to low income and the high cost of other living expenses, such as rent, utilities, and medications, to name some of the essentials that substantially deplete the household income before food is purchased. Food is considered essential but is an elastic commodity, having some cost flexibility when households try to reduce their monthly expenses (Power 2014). As a way of illustrating the reality of these struggles, local health units in Canada create the Nutritious Food Basket, which is a calculation of expenses for a variety of families living in different circumstances and purchasing food accordingly. The basket includes approximately sixty foods that represent a nutritious diet for individuals in various age and gender groups. The City of Toronto, for example, reports the living expenses for a household of four people who are receiving Ontario Works (provincial income support program). At the end of the month, after the family has spent $914.41 in food to match the Nutritious Food Basket items (this does not include any treats or the ability to invite anyone for a meal), it would have $44.59 left over to pay for telephone/internet, transportation, childcare, household and personal items, clothing, school supplies, and so on (City of Toronto 2019). It is obvious that something has to give in this scenario, and it might very likely be the quality and even the quantity of purchased food. Clearly, social assistance funding is not sufficient; but, indeed, as Tarasuk demonstrates, of those in Canada who report experiencing household food insecurity, 65 percent of these households report their main source of income is from wages and salaries (Tarasuk and Mitchell 2020). So even improving social assistance funding would not be sufficient to eradicate food insecurity in Canada, though it would go a long way to improving it.

How do families with low income reduce their food costs? Some will rely on food banks, some on extended family and friends, and some parents, particularly mothers, will skip meals or eat less to buffer their children from hunger (McIntyre, Officer, and Robinson 2003; Olson 2005). The outcome of protecting children from the nutritional effects of food insecurity is demonstrated by Sharon Kirkpatrick and Valerie Tarasuk's findings from a study of the prevalence of nutrient deficiencies as measured by twenty-four-hour dietary recalls conducted in the Canadian Community Health Survey among children, adolescents, and adults. The authors found that higher estimates of inadequacies in protein and some vitamins and minerals manifested in adults and, to some degree, in adolescents in food-insecure households but not in children (Kirkpatrick and Tarasuk 2008). Elaine Power's ethnographic study of lone mothers in Atlantic Canada and Janet Fitchen's of rural families in New York State show clear evidence that

Global Malnutrition and Children's Food (In)security   129

mothers regularly sacrifice their needs for the sake of their children (Fitchen 1988; Power 2005).

While the quantity of food for children living in food-secure households may not always decline, the quality of their food may suffer. Empirical studies demonstrate that energy-dense foods containing refined grains, high in sugar and fat, are the lowest-cost options for consumers; fruits and vegetables that have more nutrients, but lower energy, pack less bang for the buck – they're less palatable and don't provide satiety to hungry people (Drewnowski and Specter 2004). "Poverty diets" in the US, as described by Janet Fitchen, are excessive in fats, sugars, and starches, and deficient in protein and vegetables, with cycles of plenty and dearth depending on paycheques or social assistance payments. This may result in times when access to money results in eating less nutritious food.

> For all poor people, the constraints of having to feed a family on an inadequate budget are exacerbated by the fact that hunger is cognitive as well as metabolic. The necessity of keeping children reasonably satisfied despite the shortage of money may take its toll on nutritious eating. In one common management strategy a mother responds to her children's complaints about being hungry by giving them a food item that is not only filling but also desired and liked. A package of frosting-covered cupcakes (high in desirability, sugar, and cost, but low in needed nutrients) may quickly pacify a child, thereby addressing the perceived and expressed hunger of the moment and allowing the mother to turn to other demands on her time and attention. Repeated reliance on this strategy, however, may lead to long-term nutritional deficit for the child. But the child's fussing now is more pressing and immediate and cannot be ignored; malnourishment, on the other hand, is delayed, is not so readily apparent, and has a less clear cause. (Fitchen 1988, 322)

Obtaining food may also be a geographic problem, where lack of physical proximity to food outlets also relates to the "access" part of food insecurity. The study of "food deserts" – a term first coined in the UK by Cummins and Macintyre (2002) – is defined as urban areas with low access to healthy and affordable food. This definition is also relevant in Canada and the US, where many supermarkets relocate to suburban areas or lose customers to superstores that outcompete grocery stores in downtown neighbourhoods (Larsen and Gilliland 2008; Walker, Keane, and Burke 2010). Those living with low income may not own or have access to an automobile, making it much harder to get to these superstores. Parents with young children in tow may want to but cannot physically haul large bags of groceries with heavy fresh produce and may have to rely on convenience stores that don't sell fresh produce or on more energy-concentrated processed foods in smaller packages. Several studies indicate that low-income urban neighbourhoods in Canada and the US tend to have more "convenience, variety, or corner stores" that stock limited fresh produce and more processed foods, leading to unhealthier diets (Latham and Moffat 2007; Walker, Keane and Burke 2010).

Food *utilization* can refer to the body's biological ability to use the food that is consumed. This may be impaired for physiological reasons in the case of gastrointestinal parasites that are common in low-income countries with poor water and sanitation infrastructure. A more common reason in the case of high-income countries is a disease that impairs the digestive system, such as celiac disease. More generally relevant in the category of food utilization in North America is "food use" – that is, a household's ability to buy, cook, and safely prepare nutritious food (Barrett 2010; FAO 2008). While many people know how to cook nutritious and safe food, there may be cases where some support is needed. For example, some newcomers, when they first arrive in their host country, may be challenged by navigating supermarkets with new and strange products, reading ingredient and nutrition labels, and cooking with novel methods and foods (Moffat, Mohammed, and Newbold 2017). There are also youth and families who are homeless or living with precarious housing who are without kitchens and appliances and are unable to prepare meals for themselves and their families (Smith and Richards 2008). Or there are deficits in time in this increasingly fast-paced lifestyle: many families are working multiple jobs with precarious employment, and lack the time to cook, so that purchased fast food becomes the norm (Szabo 2011; Slater et al. 2012). Finally, some members of the younger generation may lack what is often referred to as "food literacy": those who are not food literate have not learned any culinary skills, have little knowledge of healthy eating, and end up relying on purchased, ready-made processed foods that are of lower nutritional quality than those prepared from fresh ingredients (Vaitkeviciute, Ball, and Harris 2015). All these situations related to poor food use would fit into the Food and Agriculture Organization definition of food insecurity.

The Health Effects of Food Insecurity

While there are clear associations between household food insecurity and child malnutrition in low-income countries, the relationship is less consistent in high-income countries (Hadley and Crooks 2012). Although frank malnutrition is not often seen among children in high-income countries, the effects of household food insecurity on children and their families in these countries are not benign. There is a growing literature that documents the association between food insecurity and the physical health of children. A large retrospective study out of the US, for example, documents an increased risk of food-insecure infants and toddlers being reported by caregivers as in "fair or poor health," and the odds of being hospitalized since birth for food-insecure families is almost a third larger than it is for those who are not food insecure (Cook et al. 2004). Another large retrospective study of the health effects of hunger, an extreme manifestation of food insecurity, based on the Canadian National Longitudinal Survey of Children and Youth from 1994 to 2004–05, found that children and youth who reported ever being hungry and multiple episodes of hunger were likely to have poorer general health, though this was not found for chronic conditions or asthma (Kirkpatrick, McIntyre, and Potestio 2010). These health effects can reverberate throughout the child's life and into adulthood, with long-term health effects later in the lifecourse. There is a clear link between food insecurity and chronic nutrition-related diseases such as hypertension and type 2 diabetes (Seligman, Laraia and Kushel 2009; Tarasuk et al. 2013). These are diseases that are set in motion from preconception (as per the earlier discussion of the developmental origins of health and disease), leading to intergenerational continuity of the effects of food insecurity on individuals and their descendants. Food insecurity has also been associated with low calcium intake and low bone mass among eight- to eleven-year-old boys, which can have long-term implications for chronic diseases (such as osteoporosis) in later adult life (Eicher-Miller et al. 2011).

There is some association between food insecurity and a higher risk of developing obesity. In North America the association is stronger for women compared to men and children. This ultimately, however, can have some bearing on children since there is growing evidence of a strong positive relationship between obesity before and during pregnancy and the risk of developing NCDs like type 2 diabetes and cardiovascular disease in future generations (Laraia 2013). The association between food insecurity and overweight and obesity among children is complicated: severe food insecurity can result in underweight children, and moderate and mild food insecurity can be associated with a higher prevalence of obesity, though the evidence is equivocal (Eisenmann et al. 2011). The mechanisms underlying the association between food insecurity and malnutrition are multifactorial. Part of the problem may be the lack of access to fruits, vegetables, lean meats, and generally fresher and more expensive foods, as described above. There may also be metabolic disturbances (such as visceral fat and insulin resistance) associated with the stress of living with food insecurity and poverty more generally, as well as regular cycles of food scarcity followed by abundance, leading to binge eating behaviours (Laraia 2013).

There is also a strong association between food insecurity and mental health. This is well documented in low-income countries like sub-Saharan Africa (Decaro, Mangyama, and Wilson 2016; Hadley and Patil 2006), but it is also indicated in North America. A large survey out of the US found that mothers are more at risk for major depressive episodes and generalized anxiety disorders when food insecure. This is accompanied by behaviour problems among their preschool-aged children (Whitaker, Philips, and Orzol 2006). A prospective cohort study in Quebec, in which children's mental health was assessed at 4.5, 5, 6, and 8 years of age, showed a clear and statistically significant association between food insecurity and hyperactivity/inattention in boys and girls (Melchior et al. 2012). Another longitudinal study out of the UK found that food insecurity was associated with children's emotional problems (Belsky et al. 2010). One of the few studies to examine the impact of food insecurity directly on children from their own viewpoints was undertaken in Mississippi, using qualitative interviews with thirty-two children aged eleven to sixteen years who were likely to have experienced food insecurity. Not only did these children talk about eating less and eating "cheap" foods, but they also said they experienced shame due to being labelled as poor as well as anxiety, worry, and sadness due to not having enough food and the consequent limitations on their social activities (Connell et al. 2005). Again, these issues continue to affect children into their adulthood and may have profound impacts later in life, even if they move out of food-insecure households.

Policies and Programs to Address Food Insecurity among Children

Clearly, we require policies and programs to address food insecurity among children and their families, both for their physical and mental health as well as for the future well-being of communities and nations. A growing group of scholars of food and nutrition in Canada has repeatedly emphasized the need to increase household incomes to reduce food insecurity (Collins, Power, and Little 2014; Kirkpatrick and Tarasuk 2009). Valerie Tarasuk (2001, 496) states: "It may well be that the most effective responses to

Global Malnutrition and Children's Food (In)security 133

household food insecurity are not those that focus on food and food-related behaviors but rather those that lessen economic constraints on poor households." Social assistance and welfare benefits have not kept pace with inflation in either Canada or the US and thus have not been sufficient to reduce household food insecurity (Power, Little, and Collins 2014). It is instructive to note, however, that Canada has, with the guaranteed annual income supplement, been very effective in decreasing poverty among seniors. Canadians over sixty-five years of age experience half of the prevalence of food insecurity of low-income Canadians under sixty-five (McIntyre et al. 2016). Similar attempts at alleviating poverty have been made with the national child tax benefit program: according to Statistics Canada the proportion of low-income persons who are children has been dropping since the mid-1990s, decreasing faster than the decrease in the number of children in the total population. Though this is good news, still nearly two in five children living in lone-parent families (38.9 percent) lived in a low-income household in 2015 (Statistics Canada 2017).

There was great promise for the benefits of the guaranteed basic income pilot project that was initiated in Ontario to cover a three-year period (2017 to 2020). Guaranteed basic income is also being tested elsewhere, such as Utrecht, Netherlands (Ostroff 2015). In Ontario, the basic income (BI) guaranteed individuals and couples was $16,989 or $24,027, less 50 percent of any earned income per year and up to an additional $6,000 per year for a person on disability (Ontario Government 2017). The BI was available to anyone who met the income eligibility criterion, even those who were working but earning below the basic income level. Unfortunately, the $150 million BI pilot was ended prematurely by the Progressive Conservative government that came into power in Ontario in 2018. Premier Ford cancelled the experiment before the first annual follow-up survey of four thousand research subjects could be conducted, so there was no formal evaluation of this project, calling into question Canadian policy for the ethical conduct of experiments with human participants (Monsebraaten 2018).

One of the outcomes that was going to be measured in the evaluation of the Ontario BI pilot project was food insecurity – and there were many who were hopeful that it would reduce it (Ghebreslassie 2017). Fortunately, the evaluation was salvaged by a group of researchers at McMaster University, who conducted an online survey (217 respondents) and qualitative interviews (forty individuals) with participants of the BI program. Outcomes related to diet and food security indicated that approximately two-thirds of study participants reported that the frequency of skipping a meal

(68.6 percent) or using a food bank (67.8 percent) was "somewhat or much less often" after receiving BI. Conversely, 85.2 percent of recipients reported that they were "somewhat or much more often" buying nutritious food after the receipt of BI and 86.2 percent of recipients reported that they had a "somewhat or much better" diet (Ferdosi et al. 2020). While these are only self-reported findings, they do indicate compelling reasons household food insecurity could be reduced with programs such as BI.

What is different about the approach to food insecurity in the US, as opposed to Canada, is that the US has federally funded programs that specifically address household food insecurity. These programs are administered by the US Department of Agriculture and include: the Women, Infant, and Children Program, which provides nutrition supplements to pregnant women and children up to age five (USDA n.d.b); what was known formerly as "food stamps" and is now called the Supplemental Nutrition Assistance Program for low-income households (USDA n.d.c); and the National School Lunch Program (see Chapter 4) as well as the School Breakfast Program, the Special Milk Program, and the Summer Food Service Program. These programs have a long-standing history with the USDA, born out of the Great Depression of the 1930s (Power, Little, and Collins 2014).

By comparison, Canada has never had any formal government programs at any level – federal, provincial, or municipal – that recognize or address food insecurity. All current programs in Canada geared to child hunger and household food insecurity – namely, food banks and breakfast programs – are run by charitable, non-government agencies, with in some cases a small amount of government funding, particularly in Quebec and New Brunswick (Martorell 2017). Studies of food bank users show that food banks are not sufficient to alleviate household food insecurity (Loopstra and Tarasuk 2012) and may also contribute to poor nutritional outcomes due to the low nutritional quality of donated foods that do not meet Canada's Food Guide recommendations for healthy eating (Irwin et al. 2007). It is also clear that many families who require food assistance do not use food banks for a variety of reasons, including shame and stigma, inability to gain access to food banks due to lack of transportation, or not even knowing that they are eligible to use them (Loopstra and Tarasuk 2012). Breakfast programs at schools or in community centres can be very helpful for many children who may not get breakfast at home due to financial or even time constraints of working parents. But there is also the problem of children not having access to school food programs on school holidays and summer vacation (Nord and Romig 2006).

Global Malnutrition and Children's Food (In)security   135

Clearly the government programs in the US are not sufficient to relieve food insecurity. Food banks and other types of charitable emergency food assistance programs are ubiquitous in the United States, just as they are in Canada, and the US has overall higher levels of food insecurity than Canada. What's concerning in Canada, however, is the lack of recognition at all levels of government that food insecurity is prevalent and growing. This is very problematic among pregnant women and children, the groups that one might argue most requires high-quality and nutritious food for growth, development, and future health and well-being. One exception to the lack of federal funding in food and nutrition support is the Canada Prenatal Nutrition Program, which funds centres across Canada to support breastfeeding, food preparation training, and education. Although it is mostly geared to education, it offers free prenatal vitamins and grocery gift cards for women who attend the weekly group meetings. While this is certainly much needed, it is still limited in the face of widespread food insecurity among women, particularly lone parents (Government of Canada n.d.).

Community Food Security and the Global Food System

Most of the discussion in this chapter focuses on household food (in)security; this is because it is at the household level that people feel the most acute effects of food insecurity on their individual health and well-being. In the past decade, however, there has been a growing discussion and focus on food security at the wider level of the community. One of the first to address this concept, Hamm and Bellows (2003, 37), proposed the following definition:

"Community food security (CFS) is defined as a situation in which all community residents obtain a safe, culturally acceptable, nutritionally adequate diet through a sustainable food system that maximizes community self-reliance and social justice." This definition encompasses a systems-level approach that addresses issues related to food security that involve more than just the individual and household, extending to food production and distribution by engaging and supporting, for example, local farmers and food markets. While the focus is on the low-income part of the population that experiences household food insecurity, the idea behind community food security is that it engages all citizens. This has also been conceptualized as the Community Food Security Continuum (Figure 5.2), whereby the food system in Stage 3 would be redesigned for sustainability for the whole

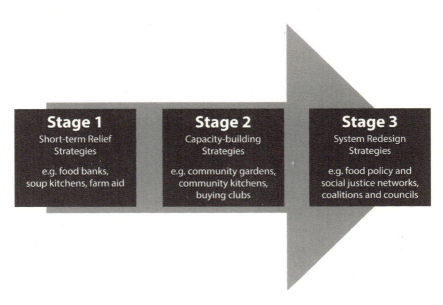

FIGURE 5.2 The food security continuum. | Adapted from Kalina (2001).

population to enable it to reach community food self-reliance, social justice, and population nutrition goals (McCullum et al. 2005). This approach would, of course, apply to the whole community, including children; however, as Hamm and Bellows (2003) suggest, points of entry could include public schools and community centres, where children could be involved in food and nutrition programs, community gardening, as well as other cooperative food and nutrition programs.

Larger food system approaches, such as sugar or soda pop taxes, taken up in Chapter 7, include food policy interventions at state/provincial and national government levels. These also must involve international-level systems changes to food tariffs and trade regulations that could limit the power of multinational corporations that market to children – such as Nestlé and Coca-Cola to name just two – and allow nations to be sustainable and self-reliant food producers in the face of globalizing food markets (Winson 2013). These global food system changes would not only have a positive impact on moving towards community food security but would also contribute to decreasing childhood overweight and obesity, the topic of the next chapter.

6

Childhood Obesity

A Twenty-First-Century Nutritional Dilemma

In 2005 I stood before an audience of concerned parents, at an end-of-year home and school council meeting, to which I was invited as a keynote speaker to report on the research I had done in three public elementary schools over the past two years examining children's diet, overweight and obesity, activity levels, and the schools' food and recreation environments. The study schools were selected through the school board to examine contrasting schools within Hamilton, Ontario: the first in an affluent and multi-ethnic neighbourhood; a second in a low-income, less ethnically diverse neighbourhood; and a third in a low-income, multi-ethnic neighbourhood (Moffat, Galloway, and Latham 2005; Moffat and Galloway 2007). I reported on the results of the study, focusing mostly on obesity findings. This was what I thought parents would want to hear about, since the early 2000s marked the beginning of heightened concern about childhood obesity and the so-called obesity epidemic. In my talk I reported on overweight and obesity prevalence for boys and girls found collectively at all three schools. I showed the dietary and activity level data that we had collected. After presenting these findings I talked about various issues related to the school environment. This was just prior to the establishment of the provincewide nutrition policy for school boards to remove vending machines selling sugar-sweetened drinks as well as the insertion into the elementary (kindergarten to Grade 8) curriculum of mandatory daily physical activity (DPA). Ontarians were on the cusp of making positive changes to the school environment, and I thought my presentation would inspire parents to demand more from the Ministry of Education and their school board.

At the end of my talk, I invited questions from the audience. The first question I received was from a concerned parent who asked me what I thought caused obesity. She said she had two children at home, one "normal" weight and the other "overweight." She was confused because she had raised them the same way and they were going to the same school, so why did she have an "overweight" child? As an anthropologist who examines cultural and societal "causes" of problems, I was completely taken aback by her more personal question. I can't remember how I answered it – I'm sure she wasn't satisfied with my response and neither was I – but her question stuck with me because the scientific community is no further along in deciphering what causes obesity today than it was in 2005. If, as this parent had stated, two people from the same family eat and live in the same environment, why is one individual's body more prone to store fat and another's is not?

In this chapter I attempt to answer that question within the context of perhaps the more pressing question: Why has the prevalence of overweight and obesity been increasing among children worldwide since the 1980s? Obesity is a complex phenomenon, not only biologically but culturally and socially. One chapter cannot begin to unravel its biocultural complexity, and in fact whole books have been devoted to the topic. The book that does this best in my opinion is Alexandra Brewis's (2011) *Obesity: Cultural and Biocultural Perspectives*, which I draw on for this chapter. As Brewis explains at the beginning of Chapter 1, "Defining Obesity," "Most generally, obesity refers to an excess of fat (adipose tissue) storage on the body ... Of course, what constitutes an excess of fat – how much fat is too much and when it negatively affects people – is open to considerable debate in both scientific and social terms" (11). In this chapter I review the many biocultural pieces of this complex puzzle to address and to reframe this problem through a consideration of child overweight and obesity as part of a larger problem of a flawed food system and the need for more governance to proactively effect positive change for future generations.

Defining the Problem

From a physiological perspective obesity can be defined as disruptions to the balance between food intake and energy expenditure that is regulated by multiple complex systems, mainly the gastrointestinal tract, adipose (fat) tissue, the stomach, and the pancreas. These are all coordinated centrally by the hypothalamus in the brain through signalling of hormones such as insulin, leptin, and ghrelin that give cues to our bodies, through short and long time frames, about appetite (hunger and satiety) and fat deposition. This regulatory system is designed to protect against weight loss, necessary for survival, but not against weight gain (Bell, Walley, and Froguel 2005). From an evolutionary perspective, humans, like most mammals, are very efficient at storing energy that is necessary not only for survival but also for reproduction (Brewis 2011; Ellison 2003). Humans in particular reserve fat (adipose tissue) during pregnancy, infancy, and early childhood, which is directly related to the need for high energy stores for our rapid brain growth during these developmental periods (Kuzawa 2010). So why is excess adiposity, however we define it, a problem for children?

Up until the last thirty years, obese children were rare, and there was not much focus on them in medical research or literature. Only recently has there been a more consolidated effort to understand and document the health and well-being of children living with overweight and obesity – in all realms, including physical, psychological, and social. Previously there were mostly concerns about obese children becoming obese adults, with the attendant chronic NCDs, but there was no evidence to determine whether that was actually the case. Two decades into the twenty-first century it can be empirically tested as to whether or not childhood obesity tracks into adulthood with longitudinal cohort studies. A systematic review and meta-analysis of fifteen of these cohort studies indicates that approximately 55 percent of obese children go on to be obese in adolescence, and around 70 percent of obese adolescents will be obese at age thirty, though we still don't know whether obesity tracks into older adulthood, after age thirty. From a public health perspective, moreover, targeting obese children to reduce the overall burden of adult obesity may not be an effective strategy since this same meta-analysis found that 70 percent of obese adults were not obese in childhood or adolescence (Simmonds et al. 2016).

Co-morbidities associated with obesity affect almost every system in the body, including endocrine, GI, pulmonary, cardiovascular, and musculoskeletal. What is new is the increase in co-morbidities associated with obesity in childhood, adolescence, and early adulthood – such as type 2 diabetes mellitus (T2DM), dyslipidemia, obstructive sleep apnea, and steatohepatitis (fatty liver disease) – that were previously seen only among adults. Those with T2DM during adolescence have more rapid progression of diabetes-related complications like dyslipidemia and hypertension (Kumar and

Kelly 2017). While psychological issues such as poor self-esteem, anxiety, and depression are often cited as being associated with obesity, as Assari (2014) points out, there has been very little research done to date on the link between child and adolescent mental health and obesity. One study out of the US, based on cross-sectional data from the 1996 National Longitudinal Study of Adolescent Health, found a link between obesity and poor physical quality of life, but no statistically significant relationship between body mass index (BMI) and psychosocial outcomes (Swallen et al. 2005). Mental health is complex and is mediated by gender, age, and ethnicity, among other variables (Assari 2014). The causal relationship between obesity and mental health is not necessarily understood either; obesity may in fact be a by-product of mental health problems, due to eating disorders brought on by anxiety and/ or depression rather than the inverse. More research – and not just large quantitative surveys but smaller qualitative and population-specific studies – are required to better understand the health consequences and associations between youth mental health, food, obesity stigma, and body image.

Measuring and Categorizing Childhood Obesity

Childhood obesity, like adult obesity, has been for the most part measured by the body mass index. The BMI is calculated as body mass over height squared (kg/m^2) and is a quick, convenient, and non-invasive measure employed in population studies. Adults are classified as overweight if their BMI is above twenty-five, and obese if it is above thirty. There are some problems with using BMI to classify overweight and obesity, including enhanced muscularity, large head size, and high torso-to-leg ratio, which may result in a falsely elevated BMI, especially for children under three years of age (Roberts and Dallal 2001). There are more precise measures of body composition, including waist measurements to estimate abdominal fat thickness, and fat thickness at various points of the body, as well as direct measures of fat using high-tech equipment such as dual energy x-ray absorptiometry (DXA). However, DXA lacks normal reference data for children and has some limitations for accuracy (Wells and Fewtrell 2006). BMI, though just an estimate, correlates well with direct measures of fat; it is fast, convenient, and non-invasive and thus, while limited for clinical use with individuals, it is ideal for population studies (Mei et al. 2002).

For children, the use of the BMI is more complicated, as the distribution and amount of body fat changes as children's bodies grow and develop (CDC n.d.). Moreover, unlike fixed adult BMI cutoffs that are related to health risks, there are no risk-based cutoffs for children. This is because the health risks for children are unknown since, apart from a small sample of youth who experience cardiovascular disease and type 2 diabetes, most problems occur later in adulthood (Flegal, Tabak, and Ogden 2006). The US Centers for Disease Control and Prevention (n.d.) recommends the use of the CDC/National Center for Health Statistics growth reference for children aged two to twenty years of age with statistical cutoffs of the 85th percentile and above for the classification of "overweight" and the 95th percentile and above as "obese," using US national reference data. The International Obesity Task Force created an alternative, internationally standardized classification of childhood overweight and obesity aligned with percentile cutoffs with the adult standards (BMI > 25 and 30) (Cole et al. 2000). And in 2007 the World Health Organization developed a new growth reference for children aged five to nineteen years using a multi-country WHO reference population (de Onis et al. 2007). To date, however, no universal standard has been adopted and all three are used in different studies.

Trends in Childhood and Adolescent Obesity

A recent review of worldwide trends in childhood and adolescent obesity (ages five to nineteen) found that the number of children with obesity increased from 5 and 6 million for girls and boys, respectively, in 1975 to 50 and 74 million for girls and boys, respectively, in 2016. Seventy-three percent of that increase was due to the increase in prevalence alone, as opposed to population growth. The good news is that in the year 2000 the prevalence of child obesity plateaued in high-income countries, though it continued to increase in many low- and middle-income countries (NCD Risk Factor Collaboration 2017). In the US in 2015–16, 18.5 percent of youth were classified as obese, with the highest prevalence among adolescents and the lowest among preschool children, two to five years of age (Hales et al. 2017). In Canada, in the US, obesity among children and youth doubled over the past forty years, though that proportion remained stable or slightly declined from 2004 to 2013 (Rao et al. 2016; Rodd and Sharma 2016). An estimated 13 percent of children were classified as obese as measured in Canadian Health Measures Surveys from 2009 to 2013 (Statistics Canada 2015).

It is noteworthy that there are still more children worldwide who are severely and moderately underweight than obese, mostly in South Asia and East Africa – though if increases in average BMI continue in the lower- and middle-income countries, this is expected to reverse (NCD Risk Factor Collaboration 2017). See Chapter 5 for more discussion of global child malnutrition and the double burden of under- and overnutrition in low- and middle-income nations.

What Causes Childhood Obesity?

The Role of Genetics

It is clear that the recent increase in obesity over the last four decades cannot be explained by any dramatic changes to the genome of the human species or any subgroups of our species – this would not be possible in such a short time frame. There are some rare genetic mutations that encode proteins that regulate appetite and that result in obese phenotypes, known as monogenic forms of obesity. As well, there are at least twenty rare syndromes caused by genetic defects or chromosomal anomalies that result in obesity. These are known as syndromic forms of obesity. The most common of these syndromic forms is Prader-Willi syndrome, characterized by an obese body form, excessive consumption of food, developmental disabilities, and short stature, among other phenotypic traits (Bell, Walley, and Froguel 2005).

While genetics does not play a role in the recent rise in obesity, it most certainly does in individual variation in body mass distribution. This speaks to the parent's question with which I open this chapter: Why is one of my kids overweight and the other not? Body mass, like, height is normally distributed in a population, so some individuals will be at the lower end of that bell curve and others at the higher end. BMI and obesity exhibit a high level of inheritance, as indicated by twin studies (Bell, Walley, and Froguel 2005; Albuquerque et al. 2015). The genetics of monogenic and syndromic forms of obesity (discussed above) are differentiated from "common obesity" – for which the underlying genetic basis is polygenic, meaning that effects are due to multiple altered genes that may vary from one individual to the next. This makes the study of the genetic risk for common obesity more complex, but future research is promising with new techniques to allow analysis of several gene loci at the same time (Albuquerque et al. 2015).

Individual variation in obesity risk may also be explained by epigenetic regulation of gene expression – that is, effects that do not involve changes in the DNA sequence but that do affect gene function. Unlike DNA genotypes, epigenetic markers, the most well known of which is DNA methylation, can affect the expression of genes, which can then change a person's phenotype

Childhood Obesity 143

within their lifetime. Preconceptual, in utero, and post-conceptual developmental environments can all affect the epigenome, which in turn will influence one's risk for obesity in childhood and adulthood. There is now growing evidence that parental peri-conceptual (just before, during, and after conception) environmental exposures, including those that affect parental nutrition and physical activity patterns, may influence both childhood and adult body composition. This means that epigenetic changes can be transferred from one generation to the next and that heritability in the form of epigenetics may indeed play a role in child obesity (Gluckman, Hanson, and Mitchell 2010; Godfrey, Gluckman, and Hanson 2010).

What is clear about the genetic, and especially epigenetic, underlying bases for obesity is that neither genes (nature) nor environment (nurture) alone can be implicated in obesity, even in terms of individual variation within a population. While some individuals may be at higher risk for obesity due to genetic or epigenetic factors, it is the interaction with the environment that allows for the obese phenotype to be expressed. In the case of epigenetics, environmental exposures to stress, toxins, and poor-quality food before conception, in utero, and postnatally may actually change the expression of the child's genotype even before they have reached the age of one year. Thus, even though it is necessary to understand the biological and physiological basis of obesity, it is equally imperative to fully map the environmental context of this multifactorial and complex phenomenon.

Diet and Physical Activity
While diet is obviously a factor related to the increase in childhood overweight and obesity, which aspect of dietary change is driving the increase in the average BMI, particularly in obesity, is not completely apparent. At a macro level there have been worldwide changes in diet since 1970, what Barry Popkin coins the "nutrition transition," consisting of a sweeter and more energy-dense diet. This has also been accompanied by higher consumption of animal and partially hydrogenated fats and lower intakes of fibre. Popkin argues that these changes are linked to the worldwide increase in urbanization, the decrease in food prices, particularly for meat and edible oils, and the increase in access to supermarkets (Popkin 2006). What has been fuelling these changes is the industrialization of our diets linked to the global growth of capitalism, which limits individuals' food choices and floods the market with energy-dense, low-nutrient foods (Wells 2012b).

The nutrition transition is illustrated empirically in the analysis of a twenty-one-year (1989–2010) dietary trends in food and beverage consumption data set for US children and adolescents (two to eighteen years) that shows clear and significant increases in mean overall energy intake. Specific intakes of foods that were found to decrease during this time were: high-fat milk, meats and processed meat products, ready-to-eat cereals, burgers, fried potatoes, fruit juice, and vegetables. Foods that were found to increase in intake over that time were: low-fat milk, poultry, sweet snacks and candies, and tortilla and corn-based dishes. Foods that were stable contributors to overall energy intake among children during the twenty-one-year period were: sugar-sweetened beverages (SSBs), pizza, grain-based desserts, breads, pasta dishes, and savoury snacks. A closer look by the authors at total energy intake in the first decade of the twenty-first century shows that, across the period 2003–8, total energy intake decreased to 1989–91 levels, and remained stable through 2009–10. Only preschool children (two to five years) and children in low-income families had higher total energy intakes in 2009–10 compared to those in 1989–91 (Slining, Mathias, and Popkin 2013). This general decline (with the above-mentioned groups excepting) in overall energy intakes correlates with the plateau of the mean BMI and child obesity that occurred in the first decades of the twenty-first century. Thus, these dietary trends among US youth documented by Slining and colleagues (2013) may account for the dramatic rise and then plateau of child and adolescent obesity.

There has been debate about the contribution of fat versus sugar in the rise in both childhood and adult obesity. As Robert Lustig (2012) details in his book *Fat Chance: Beating the Odds against Sugar, Processed Food, Obesity and Disease*, saturated fat was initially vilified as the cause of heart disease, the number one killer of adults in high-income countries; however, trans fats that were used as a substitute for saturated fats have now been implicated in contributing to higher risk for coronary heart disease (de Souza et al. 2015). Trans fats, also known as trans unsaturated fatty acids, or partially hydrogenated oils, are made from vegetable fats and are used in many processed foods such as margarines, crackers, and baked foods. They are what Lustig calls "disasters" because the mitochondria, the powerhouses in our cells, cannot break them down completely for energy, and fat remnants get into arterial walls causing hardening of the arteries (Lustig 2012, chap. 10). In the 1980s, major health and nutrition organizations in the US advised Americans to decrease dietary fat by 30 to 40 percent, and the food

Childhood Obesity 145

industry began marketing new low-fat products that replaced fats with refined carbohydrates, low in fibre and high in sugar. Many, like Lustig (2012), think that this increase in food products containing refined carbohydrates, specifically sugar, precipitated an increase in insulin production, leading to more fat storage. Lustig argues that this is the main driver of the rise in obesity after 1980: "And thus the obesity epidemic was born in the aftermath of this seemingly logical and well-meaning, yet tragically flawed, understanding of our biochemistry" (133).[1]

Sugar, its health effects, its association with children's foods, and its prominent place in the industrialization of children's foods is discussed in detail in Chapter 3. Here, however, I spend some time on sugar-sweetened beverages (SSBs) since they have been implicated by some as the cause of childhood obesity. As Ludwig, Peterson, and Gortmaker (2001) explain, numerous studies indicate that the consumption of SSBs does not displace calories in the diet but only adds to the number of calories consumed. Their prospective study over nineteen months of 548 school children (mean age 11.7 years) found that both baseline SSB consumption and change in consumption of SSBs independently predicted change in BMI. Retrospective studies also implicate SSBs in the rise of childhood obesity. A large study of national dietary data from the US National Health and Nutrition Examination Surveys collected between 1988 and 2004 found that per-capita daily caloric contribution from SSBs increased in that time period from 242 kilocalories to 270 kilcalories per day, with the largest increase, approximately 20 percent, occurring among children aged six to eleven years (Wang, Bleich, and Gortmaker 2008). While the average increase in kilocalories from SSBs is not huge, these are kilocalories that probably were consumed on top of, rather than in replacement of, energy from foods, thereby increasing total energy intake. There is also some evidence that refined carbohydrates in liquid form may not give the body the signal that it's feeling full (known as satiety) the way they might if eaten as a solid, so that more energy can be consumed with SSBs (Pan and Hu 2011).

Another obvious driver of child obesity over the past few decades, in addition to dietary change, is the increase in sedentary behaviour or the decrease in physical activity. Given that this is a book about children's food and nutrition, I will not go into much detail on this topic, except to say that it is an important factor that must be given consideration in balancing energy intake and output as part of maintaining a healthy body weight. There is a tendency, however, on the part of the food industry to overemphasize the role of physical activity in childhood obesity: witness the alacrity with which fast food franchises sponsor children's sports teams. Anyone who has tried to lose weight by exercising more and not changing their diet will find that weight loss doesn't necessarily occur. This is because it takes an extreme amount of physical activity to expend any significant number of calories; moreover, with increased physical activity muscle mass increases, so that on the weigh scale, even if the individual is becoming more toned, they are not necessarily losing weight. In the long run, however, physical activity maintains body weight balance by building muscle mass that enhances the body's metabolism, specifically resting metabolism, through which the majority of energy expenditure occurs throughout the day and night. Some experts argue that, in terms of prevention and even recovery from chronic diseases such as type 2 diabetes and heart disease, physical activity is as important to focus on as decreasing BMI (Sigal et al. 2006; Lustig 2012).

Studies of survey data that measure children's activity levels – measured as vigorous physical activity (VPA) and moderate-to-vigorous physical activity (MVPA) – demonstrate that both VPA and MVPA are independently and positively associated with decreased risk of obesity. This upholds the recommendation that all children engage in at least fifty-five minutes of MVPA per day (Katzmarzyk et al. 2015). An innovative approach to considering children's activity in relation to obesity, but, more important, in terms of overall holistic health, is the consideration of a variety of movement-related behaviours, including sleep and sedentary behaviour. This has been incorporated in the *Canadian 24-Hour Movement Guidelines for Children and Youth: An Integration of Physical Activity, Sedentary Behaviour, and Sleep*. These guidelines recommend nine to eleven uninterrupted hours of sleep per night for children aged 5 to 13 years and eight to ten hours per night for those aged 14 to 17 years; at least sixty minutes per day of MVPA with VPA and muscle- and bone-strengthening activities at least three days per week; several hours of structured and unstructured light physical activities; no more than two hours per day of recreational screen time; and limited sitting for extended periods (Tremblay et al. 2016). Any intervention program aimed at improving children's health and lowering levels of obesity must incorporate both eating and daily physical activity, including sleep, as an important part of enabling children to lead healthy lifestyles.

The Obesogenic Environment

While a consideration of diet and activity at the individual level is necessary in addressing child overweight and obesity, a focus on individuals and

Childhood Obesity 147

families leads to the construction of population changes in obesity as being caused by "poor lifestyle" choices. An investigation of the obesogenic environment, in contrast, helps to remove the responsibility of obesity away from the individual and put it on structural elements of the built environment that may compel people to eat more and to engage in less physical activity. The concept of the obesogenic environment has been formulated and theorized mostly by social geographers (Hill and Peters 1998; Swinburn, Egger, and Raza 1999) and has been embraced by many nutritionists as well as public health and urban planning policy-makers. Aspects of the physical environment that are considered to be obesogenic include: urban and suburban sprawl with residential areas that are devoid of opportunities for people to safely engage in walking and other forms of physical activity (Ewing et al. 2014); "food deserts" – neighbourhoods in which there is a lack of food outlets for purchasing healthy and affordable food (Walker, Keane, and Burke 2010); and "food swamps" – neighbourhoods in which there is an abundance of food outlets selling energy-dense and nutrient-poor fast food relative to healthier food options (Cooksey-Stowers, Schwartz, and Brownell 2017). For children, obesogenic environments can also include schools and daycare centres that promote unhealthy foods or that do not provide healthy foods and opportunities for physical activity (Carter and Swinburn 2004), and even supermarkets that, among other strategies, promote the spatial arrangement of junk foods at eye level and at the checkout counter (Winson 2004).

Using foraging theory from behavioural ecology, Leslie Sue Lieberman explains how and why the obesogenic environment may operate for humans. Optimal foraging theory posits that, since food is essential for survival, growth, and reproduction, all living species, including humans, will optimize their food foraging to gain as much energy as possible for the least amount of energy or time expended. Lieberman (2006, 483) argues that, in an obesogenic environment, since there is an endless supply of food, "there is no decreasing rate of return for time invested." This becomes obvious when one considers the modern, North American foodscape with fast-food convenience that includes pick-up, delivery, and drive-through modes of acquiring food, in addition to super-sizing, ready-to-eat, energy-dense, and low-fibre food that requires very little to no time or energy in terms of preparation or even digestion. Lieberman also points out that humans, like all primates, derive food cues visually since we have excellent depth perception, colour vision, and visual memory – something that serves monkeys and apes well when foraging for food, and early humans as well as modern-day hunter-gatherers. We continue to depend on visual cues as the food industry and its marketers have inundated the built environment and the media with visual representations of food as well as iconic images and logos such as McDonald's Golden Arches (485).

One aspect of child and adolescent food consumption that has changed significantly over the last thirty years and may have contributed to the rise in obesity is the increase in the consumption of food prepared away from home. Another US study using the data on children aged two to eighteen years from 1977 to 2006 showed that the percentage of kilocalories eaten per day away from home increased from 23.4 percent to 33.9 percent. From 1994 to 2006, the percentage of kilocalories from fast food increased to surpass intake of food from schools; for all age groups it was the largest contributor to foods prepared away from home (Poti and Popkin 2011). Food prepared away from home generally has higher amounts of sugar, fat (mostly saturated and trans fats), and sodium. The positive association between consumption of fried foods away from home and BMI among children aged nine to fourteen years has been demonstrated in a prospective cohort study (Taveras et al. 2005). Certainly "food swamps" could be implicated in some of this increase in the consumption of unhealthy foods prepared away from home, but I would argue that most people in North America – even in many parts of Mexico, where food swamps have also been identified (Bridle-Fitzpatrick 2015) – have easy access to fast/junk food. The obesogenic environment, then, is one factor among many, but others could include increasing time spent on work in dual-parent or single-parent families, leading to less time to prepare foods at home, as well as the trending downturn in food skills to enable families to cook and prepare foods at home (Anderson and Butcher 2006; Rosenkranz and Dzewaltowski 2008).

Julie Guthman, a critical medical geographer, argues that, while the obesogenic environment hypothesis is ethical in its focus on structural factors rather than on blaming people for their lack of self-discipline, the hypothesis does have some problematic aspects. Specifically, Guthman (2011, 75) critiques its focus on the built environment as overly deterministic. She argues that the approach "can easily give the impression that the environment simply acts on people in unmediated ways, as if once you find yourself living in the sprawling suburbs the fat will pile on." But, as Guthman reveals in her analysis of class, race, and political-economic structures in the United States, the problem with this framework is that the converse of the obesogenic environment, what she calls the "leptogenic environment" (*lepto* is Greek for thin), can be created only by addressing class and racial inequalities (87).

Childhood Obesity 149

Guthman's focus on the leptogenic neighbourhood raises the larger issue that the characteristics of these neighbourhoods – excellent access to public transportation and walking distances to amenities, including food outlets with healthy food; safe and convenient areas for children to play outdoors; lower density of fast-food restaurants – are usually neighbourhoods characterized by residents of middle to high socioeconomic status, with a lower proportion of racialized groups. These socioeconomic characteristics enable people living in these neighbourhoods to buy high-quality food, have gym memberships, enrol their children in sports and dance activities, and the list goes on. It is thus difficult to separate the qualities of the built environment from the socio-demographic characteristics of the neighbourhood (Guthman 2011).

Social and Cultural Determinants of Child Obesity

There have been a multitude of studies that have examined poverty and food insecurity as a determinant or risk factor for obesity, specifically child obesity. It appears that in the United States social and racial inequalities in health have risen over the past few decades, and that is starting to manifest in differential rates of child obesity. According to one study by Singh, Siahpush, and Kogan (2010), from 2003 to 2007 obesity prevalence increased by 10 percent for all US children but increased by 23 to 33 percent for children in low-education, low-income, and high-unemployment households. In 2007, children from low-income and low-education households had 3.3 to 4.3 times higher odds of being obese than children from higher socioeconomic households. They also report that, in 2007, Black and Hispanic children were about twice as likely to have overweight or obesity as did non-Hispanic, white children. In an effort to disentangle area effects from socioeconomic status (SES) variables, Janssen and colleagues (2006) conducted a multi-level analysis in a study of eleven to fifteen-year-old children who were part of the Canadian sample from the Health Behaviour in School-Aged Children Survey (2001 to 2002), part of a cross-national study of adolescents facilitated by the World Health Organization. Their outcome variables were obesity, unhealthy eating, and physical inactivity. The authors found that adolescents from what they characterize as "deprived families" were more likely to be obese, independent of neighbourhood SES, but they also found that adolescents living in poorer neighbourhoods comprised of mixed household incomes were more likely to be obese, regardless of household income, indicating that both individual and area variables have some effect on adolescent obesity. They did not find that individual characteristics of socioeconomic status were related to dietary habits, but both individual-level and area-level variables of SES were positively associated with physical activity, suggesting that this may be one important pathway linking SES with obesity among adolescents. The authors do caution that this is not a randomized controlled study, something that would be impossible to do when examining individual and area-related variables together (Janssen et al. 2006). The findings, however, are interesting and reveal just how complicated it is to uncover how factors such as household and area poverty, body weight, and dietary and physical activity variables are related to one another.

A more direct way to look at the relationship between diet, SES, and obesity is to directly measure the effects of food insecurity on child obesity. Food insecurity is discussed in more depth in Chapter 5, with a general discussion of the negative effects of household food insecurity on health, including obesity. Here I note that, although there is a strong and positive relationship between household food insecurity and obesity among women (but not men) in the US and Canada, that relationship is less apparent for children. Part of the difficulty in studying the relationship between food insecurity and obesity is that food insecurity is often reported for the household and not necessarily for the children living in the household (Eisenmann et al. 2011). The reason that the association between household food insecurity and obesity is stronger among adult women, however, may be due to the household management of food insecurity, with mothers working hard to prevent hunger among their children. Mothers may buffer their children from many of the mechanisms by which food insecurity leads to weight gain, including consuming energy-dense and low-nutrient, low-cost foods, eating irregular meals and skipping breakfast (Martin and Lippert 2012). This phenomenon is also found in a variety of settings around the world; for example, there is strong evidence of food buffering within low-income Amazonian households (Piperata et al. 2013).

If adults are buffering children to some extent from the very pernicious effects of household food insecurity in the short term, that is a good thing. That does not mean, of course, that there are not going to be repercussions for these children in the long term, and this is especially true in light of understandings of intergenerational transmission of obesity (discussed later in this chapter). In considering cultural variables in child obesity, all too often researchers conflate notions of "culture" with higher levels of deprivation in terms of income and education among racialized groups. As Brewis

(2011) points out, however, obesity can be viewed as an "index of injustice" that connects with a more politically aware vision of the obesogenic environment as an issue of "environmental injustice." In Canada, for example, there are environmental injustices related to child obesity within Indigenous communities. Willows, Hanley, and Delormier (2012) advocate that when addressing obesity among Indigenous children in Canada, researchers should go beyond just dietary and physical activity or the so-called lifestyle causes. Rather, researchers must build a larger socioecological model that includes historical trauma due to colonization, including assimilation policies and dispossession of traditional lands leading to, among other factors, lower formal educational attainment, poverty, and food insecurity, and impoverished foodscapes that limit traditional food and subsistence activities. Evidence arising from the Truth and Reconciliation Commission in Canada uncovers that hunger was a common experience of Indigenous children at residential schools (Mosby and Galloway 2017). Residential schools were first established in Canada in the 1880s and continued through the twentieth century, with the last one to close in 1995. They were part of the assimilationist program in Canada and were modelled on those in the US (MacDonald and Hudson 2012). Mosby and Galloway (2017) argue that, in large part due to the nutritional neglect and in some cases semi-starvation of children living in residential schools, there have been generations of Indigenous people who experienced malnutrition as children. These children grew up to experience a higher prevalence of obesity and metabolic disease relative to non-Indigenous Canadians – a prevalence that continues the intergenerational transmission of obesity and related metabolic diseases.

With the caveat that poverty and inequality are often at the basis of cultural or ethnic differences, culture must still be considered in relation to obesity. As Brewis (2011, 84) explains: "Ultimately, our bodies represent cultural facts, just as they do biological ones. Body size is imbued with cultural meaning in all human societies, perhaps because it is such an obvious physical trait." Cultural meanings around body size are mediated by gender and age – what constitutes a fit, healthy, or beautiful body will certainly vary from infancy through childhood and adolescence and will be judged differently for boys and girls. In her review of culture and body ideals Brewis (2011) demonstrates that, at least for adult women, preferred and acceptable body sizes have become much slimmer with modernization in most developing countries around the world. In a cross-national study of obesity stigmatization, Brewis and colleagues demonstrate that this obesity stigma is increasing in a diverse number of countries from low- to high-income and in different regions of the world (Brewis 2014; Brewis et al. 2011). Obesity stigma may in some cases be more harmful than the physical effects of being obese. An intriguing analysis of adults aged twenty to seventy-nine years who participated in the US National Health and Nutrition Examination Survey (1999–2006) showed that perceiving one's weight as "overweight," as opposed to "just about right," was associated with a significantly higher risk of cardiovascular disease over ten years, regardless of body composition (Cullin and White 2020). The tyranny of the "normal body" connected to what Wiley and Cullin (2020) call "biological normalcy" may have pernicious effects on long-term health outcomes. The implications for this are still unknown for youth, and more research is required into the changing normative acceptability and stigmatization of overweight and obese youth.

Finally, the prevalence of obesity and the way it is treated is gendered, even for young children and certainly for adolescents. In Canada in 2011 the prevalence of obesity differed between males and females aged five to nineteen (15.1 percent versus 8.0 percent, respectively), and between the ages of five and eleven there were three times as many boys categorized as obese (19.5 percent) compared to girls (6.3 percent) (Roberts et al. 2012). This gender difference in levels of child and adolescent obesity may be due to gendered approaches to children's bodies mediated through media, caregiver, and peer influences (Galloway 2007). In their book *Acquired Tastes: Why Families Eat the Way They Do*, Beagan and colleagues (2015) address gendered approaches to body weight among youth and in relation to their families. Based on their conversations with 105 families and their teenage children across Canada, they found that body weight issues were most commonly discussed among women and girls and that, while men and boys were also interested, boys were mostly focused on health discourse. In general, they found that teen girls were more likely to be concerned about maintaining body weight through diet and exercise as "disciplinary techniques through which women may create and articulate their identities, by engaging in practices that are perceived as feminine and by the resultant production of feminized bodies" (Beagan et al. 2015, 122). Parental pressure regarding body weight was more frequently targeted at teen girls in the study group, and boys were more relaxed about weight concerns; if boys did engage in weight loss it was more covert. Based on these findings health promotion efforts may need to take gender into account. A study by Simen-Kapeu and Veugelers (2010) of Grade 5 students in Alberta determined that, in general, boys were more physically active than girls and that girls were more concerned about healthy eating. Utmost sensitivity to the burden that girls and women bear in terms of body image and feminine ideals must be accounted for in any gendered health promotion approaches as there is potential for disordered eating patterns at a young age, as discussed in the last section of this chapter.

Beyond Diet and Physical Activity: Exploring the Road Less Travelled

When I lecture about obesity in my anthropology of food and nutrition course at McMaster University, I like to show a graph from Keith and colleagues' (2006) article from the *International Journal of Obesity* titled "Putative Contributors to the Secular Increase in Obesity: Exploring the Road Less Traveled." The graph illustrates that, along with the increase in the prevalence of adult obesity from 1960 to 2000, there have also been increases in some key environmental and behavioural variables – average home temperature, prevalence of air conditioning, hours awake, antidepressant prescriptions, mean age at mother's first birth, non-smoker prevalence, and the blood concentration of polybrominated diphenyl ethers (PBDEs) – that closely track the rise in adult obesity during the same time frame. While correlation does not equal causation, Keith and colleagues make the case that these variables have plausible physiological mechanisms for increasing body weight. It is difficult for students to see the fine details of this busy graph from the back of the large classroom in which I teach, but it's not the details I want to impress upon them. Rather, it's the sheer enormity of factors that have changed in our lives in the last quarter of the twentieth century and into the twenty-first that may be driving, or at least contributing to, the rise in overweight and obesity. Two leading and serious contenders for putative contributors to the rise in obesity, specifically related to children, are: (1) synthetic organic and inorganic chemicals called "obesogens" and (2) the increase in exposure to antibiotics.

Obesogens

The term "obesogens" was coined by Grün and Blumberg (2006, S50), who defined it as referring to "molecules that inappropriately regulate lipid metabolism and adipogenesis to promote obesity." More specifically they are called "endocrine disruptors" or "endocrine disrupting chemicals (EDCs)," a term that explains their physiological effects. The endocrine system is comprised of glands – the thyroid, pituitary, and hypothalamus

– and the pathways that emit hormones that signal information to other parts of the body. Changes in the endocrine system that occur prenatally or in early childhood can affect development and physiology through epigenetic changes – changes in the expression of inherited genes. Some studies have found that EDCs can disrupt body weight homeostasis by changing insulin response, brain-body signalling, and appetite; hormonal disturbances can also stimulate the production and growth of fat cells (Guthman 2011). Foetuses, infants, and young children may be more sensitive and have higher exposure to EDCs because they consume more water and greater quantities of certain foods, have higher ventilation (breathing) rates and higher intestinal absorption, and engage in more hand-to-mouth activity. Breastfed infants may have higher blood concentrations of EDCs than their mothers because of a concentration of EDCs in breast milk (Braun 2017).

A list of EDC candidates includes diethylstilbestrol (DES), bisphenol A (BPA), phthalates, organotins, polybrominated diphenyl ethers (PBDEs), per- and poly-fluoroalkyl substances (PFASs), organochlorine (OC) pesticides, and polychlorinated biphenyls (PCBs), and the list is growing (Hatch et al. 2010). There are potentially hundreds of these EDCs, both natural and synthetic, that humans are exposed to over their lifespans. Most epidemiological studies have examined the health effects of EDCs in isolation from one another, but it may be a mixture of EDCs that has synergistic or cumulative health effects (Braun 2017).

One class of synthetic EDCs that shows compelling evidence as obesogens is perfluoroalkyl substances. PFASs are used extensively in many industrial and consumer products, like food packaging (e.g., microwaveable popcorn packets), paper and textile coatings, and non-stick cookware. Even if a person does not use these products, PFASs have been found to exceed health advisory limits in some sources of drinking water, though there are still gaps in the existing science regarding acceptable levels, and there is no systematic testing of drinking water (Health Canada 2018). Evidence from animal studies indicates that PFASs perturb energy metabolism and thyroid hormone homeostasis, but evidence from human studies is still needed to prove this (Liu et al. 2017). A review of studies examining the effects of prenatal PFAS exposure on child obesity indicates that altered foetal growth patterns related to PFAS exposure may increase the risk of subsequent obesity, higher waist-to-height ratio, and cardiometabolic disorders among both children and adults (Braun 2017).

Childhood Obesity

Paediatric Antibiotic Overuse

In his book *Missing Microbes*, Martin Blaser (2014), a physician researcher at New York University, outlines his theory that exposure to antibiotics early in life during a critical window of organ and system development can perturb the balance of microbes in the body. The human microbiome – an invisible organ made up of the trillions of microbes, including bacteria and fungi, that live commensally with us – is only recently being appreciated as vital to many important functions in our bodies, such as our immune and nervous systems and our metabolism. Microbiomes can be found on the skin, mouth, nose, ears, esophagus, stomach, gut, and in the vagina. The microbiota in our digestive system are essential for our metabolism – by digesting food, extracting energy, and in some cases creating nutrients from our food for our body's use. Studies of both animal models and humans demonstrate that obesity is associated with changes in the relative abundance in two types of bacteria, the *Bacterioidetes* and the *Firmicutes*. The profile of this microbiome is called the "obese microbiome." The obese microbiome has been demonstrated to harvest more energy from the diet than a non-obese microbiome. Experiments with mice show that germ-free mice can be colonized with the obese microbiota, leading to an increase in total body fat after colonization compared to the mice that were colonized by the "lean microbiota" (Turnbaugh et al. 2006).

Blaser argues that the overuse of antibiotics may be causing weight gain in children, making this practice "the missing link in the obesity epidemic." Blaser compares this phenomenon to the practice of regular application of antibiotics in feed to rapidly increase growth in industrially farmed chickens and pigs. While children in North America are not given regular doses of antibiotics, they are treated therapeutically throughout their childhood, even before birth, as is common in many hospitals during labour and delivery. Blaser (2014) estimates that

> the average American child received nearly 3 courses of antibiotics in his or her first two years of life. They go on to receive, on average, another 8 courses in the next eight years. Extrapolating from the current Centers for Disease Control and Prevention statistics, the data suggest that on average our children receive about 17 courses of antibiotics before they are twenty years old. This is a big number, but it is in line with prior studies in the United States and other developed countries.

Essentially, Blaser argues that, by using antibiotics therapeutically – in addition to exposure to trace residues of antibiotics from other sources such as meats, farmed fish, and dairy – children's gut microbiomes can be rendered into a state of dysbiosis, the opposite of symbiosis, or balance and diversity of microbes (Cox and Blaser 2015).

More epidemiological studies are needed to test Blaser's theory. One large cohort study spanning from 2001 to 2013 in Philadelphia found that 69 percent of the children in the cohort were exposed to antibiotics before twenty-four months of age. Within that group of children, they found that repeated exposure to broad-spectrum antibiotics (the effect was much weaker for narrow-spectrum drugs) was positively associated with early childhood obesity. The authors admit, however, that a positive association does not prove causality. An alternative explanation may be that there are underlying health problems that cause the obesity that are associated with repeated use of antibiotics (Bailey et al. 2014). Given that antibiotic use is highly prevalent in early childhood and that there are other serious concerns regarding bacterial resistance associated with overuse of antibiotics, it behooves us to continue to research this association between antibiotic use and obesity.

The Early Life Environment and Child Obesity

"The First 1,000 Days" is a catchy phrase adopted by UNICEF and many other child-welfare organizations to drive home the point that the period from conception to two years of age is a time of very rapid growth and development for children. This period is both sensitive to perturbations and a window of opportunity for excellent nutrition during both pregnancy and early childhood (Lake 2017). Another important concept, though harder to translate to the public, is the importance of the peri-conceptual period – this includes the period before, during, and immediately after the conception and birth of the child (Stephenson et al. 2018). While there are a number of environmental toxins, such as EDCs, that appear to influence metabolism in utero or early life, as this book is about food and nutrition, I focus here on the effects of diet as an important early life determinant of obesity risk.

As discussed in Chapter 1, the developmental origins of health and disease is gaining traction in biomedical sciences, particularly when it comes to making links between maternal nutrition and child obesity. A mother's pregnancy weight is associated with higher risk for child obesity, and this

Childhood Obesity 157

applies to not only pre-pregnancy BMI of the mother but also gestational (pregnancy) weight gain. Most of the evidence for this comes from animal studies that experimentally feed or do not feed animal mothers high-fat diets. Findings from these experiments show that there is indeed a critical window of pregnancy that affects the weight outcomes of the offspring. Maternal overnutrition may influence the development of foetal cells and organs, resulting in an increase in foetal adipose tissue, or may act on the foetal epigenome, changing the expression of genes that are related to the offspring's metabolism (Oken 2009). It is important to note, however, that not only is high gestational weight gain (GWG) resulting in high birthweight a risk factor for child obesity, but low GWG and resulting low birthweight also predispose offspring to obesity, though it appears to occur later in the individual's life (Oken and Gillman 2003). Lest it is thought that mothers are all to blame for childhood obesity, there is also mounting evidence that the preconception nutritional status of men, including high-fat induced obesity and low vitamin status, influences sperm development and function, which can alter the metabolism of offspring in animal models (Soubry 2018; Hur, Cropley, and Suter 2017; Fleming et al. 2018). Thus, it is important to consider both parents peri-conceptually, as well as the in utero environment, in preventing child obesity.

Infant Feeding

There are multiple studies that have examined the effects of breast- versus formula-feeding on BMI outcomes of children. As Amanda Thompson (2012) explains, there are some plausible reasons breastfeeding may reduce the risk of obesity, including the fact that infant formula has a higher total energy density than breast milk, and formula-fed infants on average consume 20 to 30 percent higher volumes per feed, though by four months they feed less frequently than infants consuming breast milk. Infant formula also contains more protein and less fat than breast milk; variations in these nutrients, along with energy differences, may alter energy balance among formula-fed infants and promote hyperinsulinemia, with more rapid growth of fat relative to lean tissue. Indeed, a large epidemiological study found that formula-fed infants in affluent countries are 600 to 650 grams heavier than infants who were breast-fed for twelve months (Dewey 2001). Breast milk also contains bioactive substances such as leptin, ghrelin, and adiponectin that are associated with short-term regulation of infant weight and longer-term programming of neuroendocrine pathways that control appetite regulation. Nevertheless, as Thompson (2012) explains, how the presence of these identified hormones in breast milk might affect these short- and long-term pathways is still theoretical.

While there has been some debate over the past few decades as to whether breastfeeding is indeed protective against child obesity, a more recent meta-analysis of twenty-five studies in twelve countries showed that breastfeeding did significantly reduce the risk of obesity in children (Yan et al. 2014). Connected to the impact of breastfeeding on obesity is the role of the early diet in shaping the intestinal microbiome. An individual's gut microbiome is established in the first three years, after which point it stabilizes (Rodriguez et al. 2015). Breast milk provides a continuous source of bacteria and promotes growth of beneficial microbiota, in particular *Bifidobacteria*, which are associated with better glucose tolerance (Sela et al. 2008; Thompson 2012). But breastfeeding does not happen in a vacuum and is not uniform for all mothers and infants. Breastfeeding duration varies and is often mixed with formula-feeding. In addition, the early life consumption of antibiotics may mitigate the beneficial effects of breastfeeding (Paolella and Vajro 2016). In a study of 226 healthy Finnish children aged two to six years, breastfeeding had a protective effect in reducing the BMIs only for infants who were not early antibiotic users and who also had reduced lifetime antibiotic use (Korpela et al. 2016). There may even be individual variation in the quality of breast milk, possibly mediated through diet, that may influence the establishment of the infant's microbiome, though this is still speculative within an emerging area of research.

~

A final note to this discussion of alternative and early life origins of childhood obesity is that a consideration of environmental factors, such as the role of obesogens and antibiotics, must also consider their interplay with children's diet and physical activity. Obesogens and changes to the human gut microbiota are not necessarily sufficient to increase the prevalence of childhood obesity and the mean BMI of children; rather, infant and childhood environmental and dietary factors probably work synergistically with prenatal obesogens to produce this rapid and massive change in children's bodies. It is very difficult, moreover, to disentangle sociodemographic variables (income, ethnicity, education) as well as environmental variables related to place of residence that may influence behavioural practices like breastfeeding and antibiotic use that are implicated in reducing or increasing the risk of childhood obesity. This is why for all studies researchers need to always consider factors such as social and environmental inequities.

Moreover, a consideration of the preconceptual period to the first thousand days necessitates a consideration of the transgenerational transmission of obesity – what future grandparents and parents eat influences the health of future generations. With this comes the ethical responsibility to address gender inequalities and access to healthy food for all people, including and especially youth, expecting parents, and postpartum people (Barker 2015; Barker et al. 2018; McKerracher et al. 2019).

A Need to Reframe the Issue

I have written elsewhere (Moffat 2010) about the problematic framing of obesity as an epidemic and the moral panic that has ensued since the beginning of the late 1990s and early 2000s when childhood overweight and obesity became a hot topic. I continue to contend that we need to be concerned about this issue. In my 2010 article "The 'Childhood Obesity Epidemic': Health Crisis or Social Construction?" I argue that the framing of obesity as an epidemic is problematic because it brings on a panic mentality and a tendency to jump to quick fixes, like short-term behavioural modifications. While these programs are well-intentioned, the meta-analytic reviews have indicated that behaviourally based interventions that focus on getting children to eat healthier food and exercise with the goal of losing weight do not result in long-term weight loss for children. In fact, some researchers have argued that anti-obesity campaigns may do more harm than good by stigmatizing overweight youth, lowering their self-esteem, and ultimately leading to eating disorders that may increase the likelihood of them becoming very obese in adulthood (Greenhalgh 2016).

The fallout from the blame-and-shame approach, and what I think is an overreaction to the so-called obesity epidemic, is the effects it has on all children, even the so-called normal weight children. In her California Body Politics Project anthropologist Susan Greenhalgh (2016) asked students in her "Woman in the Body" undergraduate class at the University of California, Irvine, to write an essay about how issues of diet, weight, and the BMI played out in their life or that of someone they knew well. Of the essays featuring experiences of 234 individuals from diverse ethnic backgrounds, 25 percent of these students wrote about individuals with anorexia and eating disorders, but mostly she found that troubled or disordered eating was normalized for all youth no matter their body size. Many of them revealed the intense pressure they felt to conform to certain body standards, and that meant they heavily patrolled and controlled their own eating. Most of the stories focus on close or extended family members who criticized the way their body looked or made comments about their eating; sometimes it was a family physician or another health care provider. While rushing to "fix" childhood obesity, a corollary is the current rise in eating disorders that often results in binge-eating, bulimia, or the extreme other end of the spectrum – anorexia nervosa. Anorexia nervosa continues to be a problem in North America and Europe, and it is growing in many Asian countries. It is the mental illness with the highest incidence of mortality, and survivors may experience long-term health issues such as heart disease and osteoporosis (Arcelus et al. 2011). It is important to remember that many children fear becoming obese, to the point at which it becomes a mental illness – a large part of this fear is connected to obesity stigma and antipathy towards larger body size and fat. "Thin at all cost" is the mantra.

The focus on overweight and obesity means that health messages become connected solely to physical appearance. There has always been and will continue to be normal variation in both height and weight – as evidenced by the Gaussian, or "normal," distribution of both measurements. Admittedly, as described by an analysis of national survey data of BMI for children in the US between 1976–80 and 1988–94, there was an increase in skewness, with large shifts in the upper part of the distribution curve for body mass index with little change at the lower end (Flegal and Troiano 2000). Nevertheless, there will always be those at the lower and higher ends of that distribution. It's important to remember that what a person eats is not always reflected in their body weight, and body weight is just one indicator of a person's nutritional and health status. A person may have a low to normal body weight for their age and height and eat a nutritionally poor diet; conversely, a person who is overweight may have a perfectly healthy diet – the two don't always correlate. A lifetime of eating a low-quality diet will probably result in some serious, long-term health problems; yet an unhealthy person with a lower BMI may pass under the radar of their family doctor because they are not overweight. Clearly, we need to reflect as a society on what may be considered an "unhealthy" obsession with body fat and obesity.

What is considered an ideal body size and shape varies across nations and among ethnic groups within nations. The ideal thin body type is a relatively recent phenomenon and is not universal (Brewis 2011). In the United States and Canada many of the programs that have declared "war" on child obesity are implicitly focused on and often imposed upon the

Childhood Obesity 161

minority body, bodies of colour, and lower socioeconomic class groups. As Laura Azzarito (2009) explains in her chapter titled "The Rise of the Corporate Curriculum: Fatness, Fitness and Whiteness," schools have become a place to normalize and regulate the body: read "white and fit body." Azzarito describes projects that claim to include cultural sensitivity (such as Dance for Health and Hip-Hop for Health) and that are focused on low-income Latino and African American youth as being devoid of relevant historical and cultural education, with the only focus being on weight control. Azzarito advocates "the need to decolonize young people's bodies by opening up conversations about the body, fatness, health, race, class, and gender" (194).

Understanding Child Obesity from a Systems Perspective

In considering how to approach child obesity I concur with Julie Guthman (2011, 9) that obesity is "an ecological condition" that requires an understanding of the wider political, economic, and cultural contexts that influence individual bodies. When focusing on individuals, we risk missing the larger problems inherent in our systems. For example, the industrial food system prioritizes cheap, fast, and processed food, leaving a significant proportion of the world's population to live with food insecurity and/or time constraints that necessitate the consumption of nutrient-poor and energy-dense food. It's a system that produces food through factories, with large inputs of chemical preservatives and other additives, pesticides and fertilizers, growth hormones, and antibiotics, as is the case in the production of meat in North America. Rather than looking to critique and improve the food system, however, we often blame children and their caregivers for consuming too much junk food or screen time. In the end, children who are overweight or obese may grow up feeling very bad about themselves, assuming that they are doing something wrong, when in fact they may just be the ones who are more sensitive to the environment – the proverbial canaries in the coalmine. This circles back to the mother at my school meeting discussed at the beginning of this chapter: Why this child and not that one? The parent was looking for an explanation that pinpointed what they or their child did wrong, as opposed to considering that some children's bodies are more sensitive to the environment than are others.

Many may see the systems approach as a cop-out, as a way to avoid tackling a thorny and sensitive problem. I argue, however, that, in the face of all the known and unknown risk factors for obesity that are not under the control of individuals and families, it is the only way to effectively move forward. In the next and concluding chapter, I present some of the ways we can address children's food and nutrition, including child obesity, from this systems approach.

7

New Directions in Children's Food and Nutrition

Where We've Come From

From the moment children are conceived until their second birthday (the first thousand days), they are completely and utterly dependent on adults for their food and feeding. Particularly during pregnancy and usually through the first four to six months postpartum, the mother is pivotal, though not exclusively. Even pregnancy diet is highly influenced by surrounding family and friends as well as by the environmental foodscape, the community, and governmental social supports (McKerracher et al. 2020). As a species we have evolved to be cooperative breeders, which entails cooperative care and feeding of our children (Blaffer Hrdy 2009). In the late twentieth and early twenty-first centuries, however, the burden of responsibility for child feeding has been laid on mothers, with little effort to support women who wish to embrace the responsibility of child feeding in the form of breastfeeding, for example, but who also engage in other forms of labour. At the same time that the value of women's roles in child feeding is acknowledged, the important work of feeding children should be distributed among other members of the family as well as social institutions such as daycares and schools. Though schools have historically played a role in feeding children in many countries, they have not always provided children with the most nutritious food, and sometimes they do not provide any food at all, as is mostly the case in Canada. In many countries, schools — where children spend the better part of their days – have become key players in feeding children nutritious and reliable food. Thus, rather than view schools as a fallback source of food, the opportunity for schools to nourish children and play a key public health role in preventing diet-related diseases should be supported to make them a central pillar of child feeding alongside families.

One food that has been highlighted in this book is sugar. Sugar is a strange, almost non-food, or "drug-food," as it has been called by Sidney Mintz (1985), because it contains only energy with no nutrients. It is added to most of the food items that are produced and marketed to children, with the result that it has been implicated as the number-one offender in the rise of obesity and diet-related diseases. Although as humans, particularly as infants and young children, we have an innate predisposition for sweet tastes, I argue that the almost insatiable recent desire to consume sugar-sweetened products has been culturally and socially manufactured by the food industry with the rising use of sugar, increasingly in the form of high-fructose corn syrup added to processed foods. Indeed, so-called children's foods – apart from breast milk, breast milk substitutes, and weaning foods – are not documented in anthropological accounts of preindustrial populations prior to the emergence of industrialized food and global food markets for processed and fast foods. The way and what children eat is shaped by cultural views of children and the institution of childhood. In the case of the industrial food system that emerged in many late-twentieth-century societies, a special category of children's food products was created. Breakfast cereals are an excellent example of this; unlike the original breakfast cereals that were designed to be health foods (and some that continue in that tradition), breakfast cereals specifically marketed to children are laden with sugar. Except for their fortification with vitamins and minerals, they are no more nutritious for children than candy or sweetened baked goods.

While there is great concern about child obesity, particularly in high-income countries, we still live in a world in which many children are chronically undernourished, something that is physically manifested by stunting and more acute undernourishment, measured by underweight for age and wasting. In addition to energy and protein deficits, children also experience a multitude of vitamin and mineral deficiencies, iron and vitamin A being two of the most serious micronutrient deficiencies experienced among children living in low-income nations. There has been some progress in addressing chronic malnutrition. I detail the experience of the nation of Nepal, where child growth indicators have improved over the last fifteen years,

New Directions in Children's Food and Nutrition 165

mainly as a result of household economic development and the improvement of health care services and other infrastructure, such as sewerage and water supply. Nepal still has a long way to go though, particularly in improving environmental hygiene and water quality and access to services in remote rural areas; but it is heartening to see the nation's improvement in child health indicators. Sadly, with these successes, there is now growing evidence in many low- and middle-income countries of the double burden of malnutrition (both undernutrition and obesity). This is an enormous strain on health care systems in regions of the world that continue to deal with infectious disease, often a result of undernutrition, and now in addition more chronic, NCDs such as type 2 diabetes mellitus.

Though frank child undernutrition is not an issue in high-income regions, there are many children who live in food-insecure households – a shocking fact given the enormous wealth available in high-income countries. Child malnutrition, both undernutrition and obesity, arise fundamentally from poverty, resulting in household food insecurity and larger food system flaws. Until there is a collective will to reduce poverty, improve infrastructure and social welfare systems, and improve our food systems with better governance, these problems will continue in the future.

I address child obesity head-on, albeit reluctantly, because I believe many people are too focused on obesity as a disease or outcome rather than as just one of multiple symptoms of child malnutrition and nutritionally poor diets. I review, moreover, other causal variables in addition to poor diets related to child obesity, such as the role of environmental toxins and the ubiquity of therapeutic antibiotic use. While these non-diet/activity-related phenomena may not be exclusively causal in the global rise of child obesity, they have arisen at the same time as dramatic changes in the global food system that have allowed us, and, in many cases, forced us, to eat increasingly lower-quality foods less expensively. All these variables may be interacting synergistically to produce the relatively recent uptick in child overweight and obesity.

By viewing the effects of nutrition transition and environmental change through a developmental origins of health and disease lens, it becomes reframed as an intergenerational phenomenon that started with our grandparents and may continue with future generations. Focusing on children's obesity at the individual level may do more harm than good, due to the psychological effects of obesity stigma that may actually exacerbate a child's problems by precipitating a marginally overweight child to go on a calorie-restricted diet as an adolescent, only to develop disordered eating patterns and become morbidly obese as an adult. This problem cannot be tackled entirely with an individual focus on managing children's diets and physical activity levels; we must create policies that will govern the way the food industry produces and sells foods, and the way that children are fed in family units and in larger institutions such as daycares and schools. Uppermost in consideration must be vulnerable groups who may be less resilient and may suffer more nutrition and health inequities. Therefore, we must address child obesity from environmental and food justice perspectives.

Throughout this book I touch on a variety of nutritional issues for children, including the most severe forms of malnutrition, such as undernutrition and obesity, but I also address concerns and debates about supplementation of solids or non-milk foods, allergies, and longer-term health outcomes related to diet-related diseases. Despite the focus on these debates and conditions, I try to make the point that children's food and feeding should be topics valued in their own right, apart from their health and nutrition-related outcomes. As Hannah Landecker (2011, 179) warns, we need to be wary of a "biologically determinist backlash" emerging from frameworks like developmental origins of health and disease and nutrition science: "an obsession with 'manipulating long-term health through diet,' with food envisaged as a kind of molecular delivery system to be incorporated into social engineering." Food is and should be conceived of as more than a collection of nutrients: it is also a fundamental part of our economies; it is tied to our sociocultural, ethnic, and national identities; and it creates and maintains social bonds that produce and maintain our mental and physical health and well-being. Food is and should be pleasurable to eat. This is true for all people, but perhaps more so for children who are trying new foods for the first time, often with delight – and sometimes with disgust – experiencing new smells, tastes, and textures. I argue that cultural perspectives on children and food can affect the way we feed our children, fuelling anxieties about children's nutritional health and the way they eat, sometimes leading us to construct children as "picky eaters" or requiring different kinds of food from adults. Though there may be some developmental stages during which children are more discerning eaters, if we reflect on the way children eat and are fed in other societies, we gain more insight into our own cultural approaches to child feeding and why they may not be the only or the best ones.

New Directions in Children's Food and Nutrition

Where We're Going

Up until this point, this book has looked to our evolutionary history for cues and parameters about how we feed children, allowing that both biology and culture shape those fundamental patterns. I have argued for being attuned to our biocultural evolution, but not necessarily being limited by it. I have also reviewed the rise of the capitalist, industrial food system, which has become increasingly global, to understand the underpinnings of more contemporary historical roots of child malnutrition, including the more recent rise of child obesity. Armed with this perspective and the knowledge of where things have gone right and gone wrong, we must begin to consider ways to move forward to support what we fundamentally value and to change what is not working. Though not reviewed in previous chapters, what has been going well in human history – and more recently, with the overall decrease in famines since the rise of agriculture some ten thousand years ago – is the trend, since the medieval period, towards increasing food supply, with concomitant improvements in human nutritional well-being. Despite the persistence of social inequalities in many nations, in the past century there have been overall improvements in human nutrition, along with a decrease in infectious disease epidemics. This is manifest in the rise in average human height/stature from the end of the nineteenth century onwards in many high-income countries (Fogel 1991) and, more recently, in the latter part of the twentieth century, in countries (like China) with rapidly emerging global economies (Ji and Chen 2008). Though food supply may again become an issue in coming decades, we are currently at a point at which the quality of food and issues of access are more of a problem than the food supply quantity.

Food Insecurity Is an Income Issue

We live in an increasingly urbanizing world. Today 55 percent of the world's population lives in urban areas, and by 2050 the urban population is expected to grow to 68 percent (United Nations 2018). Even in rural regions, where most food is produced, the majority of the world's food production (about 70 percent) is grown on farms that are greater than two hectares – the definition of a small producer farm is less than two hectares (Ricciardi et al. 2018). This isn't to diminish the importance of household food production or practices of foraging and hunting that continue in many parts of the world, including the

Canadian North, where "country food" is an invaluable and healthy means of ensuring food security (Power 2008). Rather, this is an acknowledgment of the reality that most people procure their food through industrial agriculture and market transactions that require sufficient income. The case study of Nepal encapsulates what can be done to improve child nutrition through a relatively stable government, after the end of the Maoist insurgency in 2006, and concerted efforts by NGOs, international government organizations like UNICEF, and the people of Nepal themselves to increase household incomes and to improve their nation's infrastructure. More national and international efforts are required to quell global conflicts and displacement of peoples, leading to growing numbers of refugees and concomitant food insecurity. Low-income countries must not only have food sovereignty – that is, the ability to produce their own food and govern how they do so – but they must also have stable and responsible governments that allow people to develop their economies, including food economies, to produce sufficient household incomes to afford food. Realistically, in an interconnected and globalized world no nation can be completely self-sufficient, and all food systems, especially those in low-income countries, may be profoundly shaken by global events such as, for example, the global economic recession of 2008 (Himmelgreen and Romero-Daza 2009). The COVID-19 pandemic had a severe impact on maternal-child nutrition through major increases in unemployment, the disruption of food supply chains, especially in low-income countries, and the closure of schools and school meal programs. Instead of lapsing into despair and remaining passive in the face of global pandemics, we need to bolster intersectoral programming and policies to improve food security and to make our food systems more resilient for the most vulnerable members of the population (Pérez-Escamilla, Cunningham, and Hall Moran 2020).

In the case of high-income nations, there are increasing numbers of children who are living in food-insecure households due to rising wealth disparities and the retrenchment of social services and social assistance, which do not keep pace with inflation and the rise in the cost of living (Lambie-Mumford and Green 2017; Mendly-Zambo and Raphael 2018). Researchers and governments are getting better at counting and classifying food-insecure families but are not so good at figuring out how to address the problem and to come up with solutions. In a review of interventions to address household food insecurity in high-income countries, Rachel Loopstra (2018) argues that, to date, the most effective ones for families with children are income and cash transfers (like the Canada Child Benefit) to families living in

New Directions in Children's Food and Nutrition 169

poverty. In a report outlining the potential impact of a basic income guarantee (BIG) program on food insecurity, Valerie Tarasuk (2017) argues that, in Canada, it is the households at the lowest end of the income spectrum that experience the most and the most severe food insecurity. Since BIG would have the biggest effect on these households, it makes sense that it would also have the highest impact with regard to reducing food insecurity. While I just stated that governments are good at counting but not necessarily at acting on food insecurity, it's worth noting that current tools to count or measure household food insecurity, such as the Canadian Community Health Survey in Canada, are blunt as they don't specifically measure food insecurity among vulnerable groups such as racialized minorities, homeless people, LGBTQ+, students attending postsecondary institutions, Indigenous peoples living in reserve communities, and refugees. Because the Canadian Community Health Survey is only conducted in English, newcomers to Canada who do self-identify on it probably experience a prevalence of household food insecurity that is higher than reported. As Tarasuk (2017) points out, the advantage of an all-encompassing program like BIG is that it applies to all people in a nation (with the exception, perhaps, of homeless people). This would of course include all children and potential parents.

Loopstra (2018) and Tarasuk (2017) argue that food assistance benefits that are directed towards families with insufficient government income transfers, such as the United States Department of Agriculture's SNAP (Supplemental Nutrition Assistance Program, formerly called Food Stamps), do not significantly improve food insecurity among families who receive them. These types of programs, however, have yet to be tested and evaluated in countries like Canada, where government assistance for people living with low income is higher, though obviously not high enough to prevent food insecurity. A review of SNAP by Power, Little, and Collins (2014) finds that there are some benefits to this program in that it does somewhat alleviate food insecurity in the US and ensures that recipients spend the money specifically on food, which, in turn, stimulates the food economy. These authors argue, however, that the disadvantages of recipients incurring stigma, the disempowering paternalism of the program (the government will decide how people spend their money), and the fact that poverty persists even with SNAP in place outweigh the benefits of adequate cash transfers to families. In addition to criticizing food subsidy benefits, Rachel Loopstra and Valerie Tarasuk (2012) demonstrate that food banks, which first appeared in the 1980s, are not an effective solution to improving household food insecurity. This is due to the limited availability and quality of food bank food and the associated social stigma. Nevertheless, food banks persist and are flourishing in the US and Canada, and, more recently, in the UK (Loopstra 2018). And while, ultimately, it would be best to reach a point at which food banks are no longer needed, right now they are needed and therefore must be improved to provide higher-quality, more nutritious food. Food banks must move beyond the model that relies on donations, which often consist of processed foods rather than, for example, rice, dried legumes, and beans – all items that are sought by many newcomers from countries where these are staples (Moffat, Mohammed, and Newbold 2017). One of the ways that food banks have been transformed is by turning them into community food centres that are more welcoming and encompassing hubs for families, including children, to gain access to healthier food options through community gardening, meals, and subsidized food markets. Community food centres also provide food programming, such as cooking in community kitchens, that enables people to connect and combat social isolation (a problem in many urban communities) (Levkoe and Wakefield 2011; Saul and Curtis 2013).

Kirkpatrick and Tarasuk (2008) and Collins, Power, and Little (2008) make excellent arguments as to why community food programs – usually funded at the municipal level and really the only response to household food insecurity in Canada beyond charity programs – do not alleviate household food insecurity. I take issue, however, with the argument that community food programs impede addressing food insecurity as an income rather than as a food issue. Those who run and advocate for community food programs are well aware of the social inequities that lead to household food insecurity: community food programs do not and should not take the place of poverty reduction. They do, however, serve a role in addressing larger issues of *community* food security and food justice as well as social inclusion and the role that food can play in that process. These programs have many more benefits that must also be considered (more on this below).

Food and Nutrition Policy

In keeping with one of the central arguments of this book – that contemporary nutrition problems of children must not be individualized and must be addressed by larger institutions (such as governments) – I present here some recently evolving food legislation relevant to children. Historically, government oversight of the food supply, particularly in the areas of food safety and food fortification, has had profound effects on children's health.

New Directions in Children's Food and Nutrition

Some examples that stand out are the mandatory pasteurization of milk, instituted in the early 1900s in the US and Canada, that prevented millions of child deaths from bacterial contamination (Carstairs, Schell, and Quaile 2016; Wiley 2016). The other is the fortification of commonly consumed items in the food supply. Fortification began in the US in 1924 with the iodization of salt to prevent goitres, followed by the addition of vitamin D to milk to prevent childhood rickets, and, more recently, the fortification of flour with folic acid to prevent the development in utero of neural tube defects. These are a few of the important instances of food legislation, but there are many other examples of vitamin and mineral fortification to prevent nutritional deficiencies in children and in the general population (Backstrand 2002). Today we must also be concerned about overnutrition as well as undernutrition and food safety; therefore, much of future food legislation will focus on preventing children from consuming unhealthy foods.

Taxes and Bans

The industrialized food system that is regulated by capitalist market forces is not going away anytime soon. Any efforts to stem the nefarious effects of this food system must therefore be implemented through government oversight using regulation and legislation (Nestle 2002). I present a detailed discussion of limits and bans placed on children's food advertising in Chapter 3, so I will not review this here, except to point out that there is considerable opposition to this type of legislation from the food industry. In Canada, Bill S-228, which would restrict the marketing of unhealthy food to children, was delayed and eventually quashed by the Senate, purportedly due to food industry fears that unhealthy foods would include items such as bread, which would be deleterious to Canada's agricultural sector (Johnson 2018). In addition to industry attempts to thwart advertising bans, there are also limits to the effectiveness of these bans, in part due to the complexity of globalized forms of new media. Several types of food legislation that focus on reducing the consumption of unhealthy foods have recently been advanced and are outlined in the following sections.

Sugary Drink Taxes

Sugar, in particular sugar-sweetened beverages (SSBs), has been implicated as a major contributor to the rise in child obesity and diet-related diseases such as type 2 diabetes and heart disease. Within the past decade there have been many governments that have proposed or have recently instituted a tax on

SSBs. These include governments in the UK, France, Finland, Hungary, Fiji, Samoa, Nauru, French Polynesia, South Africa, and Mexico, as well as in American cities such as Berkeley and Philadelphia (Hagenaars et al. 2017). As noted by Hagenaars and colleagues (2017) in their review of the policy motivations and operationalization of the taxation of unhealthy energy-dense foods and/or SSBs in thirteen different localities, though most of these taxes were promoted through public health policy, the impetus for some was simply that they would be revenue generators. They further state that the governments that instituted these taxes were not all left-leaning on the political spectrum; the rationale behind such taxation can be conceived of as either to keep the soft drink/snack food industry in line (left wing) or to place the onus of curtailing consumption of unhealthy foods/beverages on the individual (centre to right wing) (Hagenaars et al. 2017). One of the longest-standing (since 2014) and most studied SSB taxes is in Mexico, which implemented a tax of one peso per litre (roughly a 10 percent increase) on all non-alcoholic beverages containing added sugar. Mexico is among the countries with the highest prevalence of diabetes and overweight and obesity (Colchero et al. 2016). The focus on reducing the consumption of SSBs in Mexico is warranted since, according to an analysis of the Mexican National Health Nutrition Survey (2012), 69 percent of added dietary sugar comes from SSBs (Sánchez-Pimienta et al. 2016). A number of studies on the effects of this tax have shown positive results, including an average decrease of 6 percent (12 mL/capita/day) in SSB consumption in the first year (Colchero et al. 2016), with even higher average reductions among households that had higher purchases of SSBs at baseline before the tax was implemented (Ng et al. 2019). It appears that this type of taxation is promising and is growing in popularity across the world, with many countries increasing the SSB tax amount, and the United Arab Emirates, Portugal, and Sri Lanka most recently instituting SSB taxes (Wan, Watson, and Arthur 2017).

Trans Fatty Acid Bans

Trans fats were discovered in the mid-2000s to be a major contributor to cardiovascular disease due to their deleterious effect on low-density lipoprotein and high-density lipoprotein cholesterol levels. As discussed in Chapter 3, trans fats, found in small quantities naturally in meat and milk, have been manufactured artificially by the food industry in the form of partially hydrogenated oils, first introduced by Procter and Gamble in 1911 with the vegetable shortening product called Crisco. Because hydrogenated

New Directions in Children's Food and Nutrition 173

oil has a long shelf life, is tasty, and works well for deep-frying, it has been used in large quantities in many processed foods, including many foods that children commonly eat, such as baked goods, crackers, and deep-fried foods (Dietz and Scanlon 2012; Brownell and Pomeranz 2014).

Despite the toxic nature of trans fats, there has been a long struggle by nutritionists and healthy food advocates to try to eliminate them completely from the food supply. In 2005, the Food and Drug Administration (FDA) in the US required that trans fat content appear on the nutrient labels of all food products (Brownell and Pomeranz 2014). In 2005, Canada also instituted mandatory labelling, and in 2007 Health Canada required that, in two years' time, the food industry voluntarily reduce trans fats (Dietz and Scanlon 2012). Though most of the food industry complied, there were still enough trans fats in some sectors of the processed food industry that Canada decided to follow the United States's lead, and, as of 2018, there has been a total ban on the use of trans fats in manufactured foods in both the US and Canada (Beck 2018). Denmark was the first country to ban trans fats in 2004, and many other European nations followed, but trans fats are still ubiquitous in low- and middle-income nations. The WHO has included the elimination of industrially produced trans fatty acids from the global food supply as one of the priority targets of its strategic plan from 2019 to 2023. It estimates that 500,000 deaths from cardiovascular disease will be prevented at the global level if it achieves this goal (WHO 2019).

Education, Youth Food Programs, and Food Justice

Educating children and youth about food and nutrition is something we have done as humans throughout our history as a species, though in the past it was done experientially through children's participation in hunting and gathering as observed in foraging societies and through children's participation and labour in household food production, processing, and culinary activities. Though this continues today for many children in the world, an increasing number, especially those living in high-income, urban settings, are not practising these skills in their daily lives and thus are not learning them "naturally," so to speak, as they would have previously.

As I argue, an excellent way to incorporate experiential learning about food and nutrition into children's everyday lives is through school meal programs. In the case of school meal programs in France and Japan, children are fed well-balanced and healthy school meals that incorporate not only nutrition lessons but also lessons on how to serve and eat food – in Japan, for example, children take turns serving and cleaning up after the lunches. In these countries, children all partake in the same meal, which they eat in a social manner, unlike in Canada, where school children usually eat their packed lunches at their desks, are discouraged from talking and sharing food, and are hurried from their lunch period to go to outdoor recess (Galloway and Moffat 2013). France and Japan also promote farm-to-table organic foods in their meal programs, which teach children about sustainable food production systems as well as national food heritage. Linking school meals with the wider food system has been developed even more fully in Rome, Italy; Bogota, Colombia; and Brazil, where a substantial proportion of school food is procured from local farms to promote sustainable economic development in the food and agricultural sectors (Ashe and Sonnino 2013; Sonnino 2009; Wittman and Blesh 2017). The federal government of Canada recently announced details about the nation's first national food policy, with a promise to create a national student food program. Hernandez and colleagues (2018) outline the case for a national school food program in Canada based on a review of international school food programs as well as specific research examples from Canadian case studies. From this review they distill six key characteristics that should be incorporated into the development of a national school food program. Such a program must be: (1) universal – offered at no cost or a subsidized cost; (2) health promoting – serving nutritious food; (3) respectful – culturally appropriate and locally adapted with stakeholder input; (4) connected – drawing on local communities and food sources; (5) multi-component – integrating education with an emphasis on sustainable by drawing on "farm to fork to food waste"; and (6) sustainability – with solid funding, training of staff, and monitoring of the program (Hernandez et al. 2018, 219). It remains to be seen whether the Canadian government will follow through on the national school food program by following these well-researched and thoughtful recommendations.

To date one of the main tools for educating children and youth about nutrition and eating in Canada and many nations is national food guides. The Canada Food Guide (CFG) was first created in 1949 and has been updated periodically every five to ten years (Mosby 2012). The CFG is used as the main resource for teaching nutrition as part of the elementary school health curriculum. In 2019, Canada updated its food guide from the previous 2007 version. The most recent CFG is visually similar to the United States Department of Agriculture's *Choose My Plate*, with some differences, as seen in Figures 7.1 and 7.2. The CFG features photos of real food, mostly

New Directions in Children's Food and Nutrition

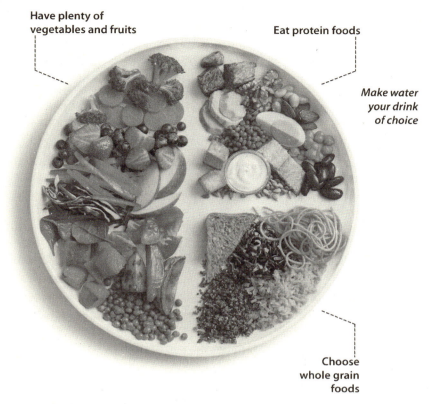

FIGURE 7.1 The *Canada Food Guide*. | (Government of Canada 2019a).

plant-based, and does not list dairy as a specific food group, with a suggestion on the side of the plate, where one would normally find a cup or glass, that water should be the beverage of choice. The development of the new version, unlike previous ones, was undertaken without consultation or input from food industry representatives, which is why dairy did not get categorized as a separate food group, as in past CFGs. This is also why the half cup of fruit juice as a substitute for one serving of fruit was removed from the 2019 CFG (Hui 2018). Note that dairy, specifically milk, in what looks like a cup at the side of the plate labelled dairy, is featured in the USDA's *Choose My Plate* graphic (Wiley 2016) (Figure 7.2). Milk and fruit juice are both part of so-called children's food products; the removal of these items from the new CFG as well as the very adult-like appearance of the new guide (featuring photos of real food rather than graphic pictures) is something of a revolution in food

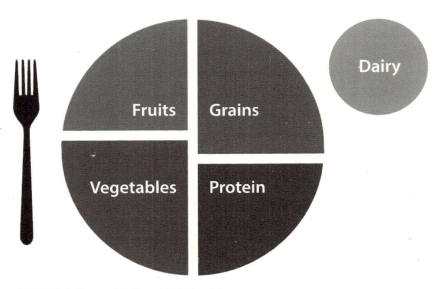

FIGURE 7.2 Choose My Plate | (USDA n.d.a).

guide history. The CFG also follows the lead of the Brazilian Food-Based Dietary Guidelines revised in 2014, recommending, among other things, limiting the consumption of processed foods and avoiding "ultra-processed" foods; whenever possible eating in company; and, as much as possible, cooking at home (FAO 2019).

The recommendation in the Brazilian Dietary Guidelines to cook as much food as possible in its unprocessed state has been lauded by many food advocates, such as Michael Pollan (Belluz 2016), and makes good nutrition sense from the standpoint of the documented increase in the amount of food that children eat outside of the home resulting in a higher consumption of processed fast-foods, one of the contributing factors to the rise in child obesity. It is also a way of returning to the model of teaching children about food (rather than just nutrients) and food skills through modelling and having them engage in food preparation. Along with this push for more cooking from scratch, however, there needs to be more awareness about the challenges of balancing domestic work with other forms of productive labour and the squeeze on time, which seems to be a decreasing commodity in today's fast-paced world. Women, moreover, continue to support the lion's share of food production, processing, and preparation work around the world, despite the fact that they have been steadily increasing their role in the formal economy for over a century. As Michelle Szabo (2011, 549) argues, re-engagement with food "cannot take place unless employment conditions, the shifting make-up of the household, and the gendered (as well as racialized and classed) division of labor are also considered." Szabo makes a number of suggestions for moving forward with these challenges, including state-wide initiatives such as those found in France, where people can work fewer hours and maintain the benefits and stability that come with full-time employment. While Canada does not offer such programs, it does offer parental-leave benefits for up to eighteen months, which not only supports breastfeeding but also allows more time for both parents to cook for their young families. Another of Szabo's recommendations is to promote cooking among men and boys, both formally through school curriculum and programs, and informally in the household. This also requires, as she points out, that women share the kitchen with men, something younger generations of women are probably more open to, as more opportunities for other spheres of influence and power, beyond the domestic one, open up to them.

Current reality is that many families do not have the time, financial resources, or skills to teach children how to cook and eat healthy, unprocessed foods, and they need support from community organizations to do so. Unfortunately, due to budget cuts and admonishments to return to the three Rs (reading, writing, and 'rithmetic), many non-academic subjects (like music, art, and what used to be called "home economics") have been removed from public school curricula. Many food and nutrition advocates, however, call for a return to mandatory food skills classes for students (Sadegholvad et al. 2017). As well, there are a number of community organizations that offer food literacy programs to youth, often those targeted as "at-risk," to help them engage more with cooking and budgeting skills (Thomas and Irwin 2011; Brooks and Begley 2014; Vaitkeviciute et al. 2015). Food literacy, broadly defined, encompasses food knowledge, skills, and behaviours (Vaitkeviciute et al. 2015), and, in the case of youth, the impact of these programs is usually evaluated by measuring dietary behaviour change (e.g., increase in fruit and vegetable consumption) in the individuals after they've completed the programs. A review of multiple studies of these programs shows mixed results in changing dietary behaviours; some show improvements in healthy food consumption and others do not, and adolescents are deemed to be generally harder to connect with to change their dietary habits than other children (Brooks and Begley 2014; Vaitkeviciute et al. 2015; Racey et al. 2016). As I argue in the discussion of childhood obesity, however, short-term behaviour modification interventions, whether to reduce body weight or to change dietary behaviours, miss the longer-term and intergenerational opportunities for systemic change. These kinds of programs may not have an immediate impact on children and adolescents, but they can carry the knowledge and experience through their lives, maybe using it at another point along the way. The focus should be not on changing children's food behaviour or body size but, rather, on changing their engagement with food and food systems.

To that end, I argue that the kinds of food programming developed for children and adolescents should engage at a deeper level than teaching them how to budget, shop, and cook a nutritious meal. The type of programming that is being developed by Community Food Centres Canada, for example, brings people together, often those living in marginalized or vulnerable circumstances, to garden, cook, and eat together in social settings that cultivate empowering awareness and activism about social and food system inequities. The Hamilton Community Food Centre (HCFC), part of Neighbour to Neighbour (N2N) in Hamilton, has created a program specifically targeted to teens (twelve to eighteen years) called Cookin' Up Food Justice. Not only do teens cook together to develop their food literacy and food skills, they also discuss food justice issues related to the food they are preparing so as to engage in a more comprehensive understanding of food systems and community food security (HCFC n.d.). This type of program shifts the attention away from the individual as a consumer and a body that must be maintained in good nutritional health and towards a more systems and outward-facing approach, with the goal being to change the food system and move towards more community food security. This is called *critical food literacy*, which is described by Lina Yamashita and Diane Robinson (2015, 270) as "the ability to examine one's assumptions, grapple with multiple perspectives and values that underlie the food system, understand the larger sociopolitical contexts that shape the food system, and take action towards creating just, sustainable food systems." While these types of programs may not be a quick fix for solving current paediatric nutrition issues or improving health outcomes, they address larger structures that are the underlying drivers of and solutions to these nutrition problems.

The Future of Children's Food

We are now living in what is referred to by many scientists – including those in social sciences, the arts, and humanities – as the Anthropocene. The

New Directions in Children's Food and Nutrition

term Anthropocene points to humans and their agency, due to unprecedented population growth and use of resources, as a major force in changing the planet through climate change and biodiversity loss (Moore 2015). Though the Anthropocene has not yet been formally designated as an epoch (following the Holocene epoch that began about eleven thousand years ago), the Anthropocene Working Group agreed, after long debate, to mark its inception at the mid-twentieth century, a time of accelerated industrial production, use of agricultural chemicals, and the first atomic bomb (Subramanian 2019). Archaeologists and anthropologists argue that the Anthropocene began long before the mid-twentieth century, potentially as far back as the advent of agriculture, some ten thousand years ago in the Middle East and in other parts of the globe thereafter (Moore 2015). For the purposes of considering children's food and nutrition and larger food system change, however, the mid-twentieth century, due to the uptick in the industrialization of food, marks a turning point in the way we feed our children.

Of course, when considering children's food and nutrition in the Anthropocene, we are really talking about everyone's food and nutrition. Biophysical changes associated with climate change – like increasing temperatures and more extreme rainfall and drought – will affect crop production, livestock, and fisheries, and will ultimately threaten human food security. Gains that have been made in increasing food production and distribution to decrease the prevalence of famine and undernutrition may be reversed in the future (Myers et al. 2017). Agriculture is also a major contributor to the rapid environmental change on our planet due to greenhouse-gas emissions (methane and nitrous oxide from animals and land tillage and carbon dioxide from fossil fuel use), land and water use, nitrogen and phosphorous applications of fertilizers, biodiversity loss, and herbicide and pesticide chemical pollution (IPCC 2019). Eating an unhealthy and highly processed diet – high in red meat, refined carbohydrates, and saturated fats – not only contributes to a decline in population health but also to the environmental unsustainability of food production (Willett et al. 2019). The EAT-*Lancet* Commission on healthy diets from sustainable food systems argues that our food system as it is currently configured is not only contributing to premature death and morbidity but is also a major force behind the decline of the Earth's system. The commission sets out five strategies to guide what it calls the "Great Food Transformation" towards eating a healthy diet consisting of "a diversity of plant-based foods, low in animal sourced foods, unsaturated rather than saturated fats, and small amounts of refined grains, highly processed foods, and added sugars (Willett et al. 2019, 448).

The strategies are as follows: (1) seek international and national commitment to shift towards healthy diets; (2) reorient agricultural priorities from producing large quantities of food to producing healthy food; (3) sustainably intensify agricultural production, generating high-quality output; (4) implement strong and coordinated governance of land and oceans; (5) at least halve food loss and waste, in line with the United Nations sustainable development goals.

While this sounds like a formidable task, we should remind ourselves that, as humans, we have developed many sustainable agricultural methods and food production methods that we can look back to in order to transform our food system in the future. This is already something that is happening among those who are part of the growing local food movement, which prioritizes people-centred food production and distribution, and which is also more environmentally sustainable (Connelly, Markey, and Roseland 2011). As Amanda Little (2019) points out in *The Fate of Food: What We'll Eat in a Bigger, Hotter, and Smarter World*, as well as looking to ancient food knowledge, we must not be afraid of new food technology. Little reviews a number of these technologies, such as post-organic indoor and vertical farming and lab-based meat production. These are only the food production technologies that are in the pipe now: there are many more to come. Human ingenuity is boundless, and while technology shouldn't be relied upon as a panacea – it clearly hasn't always been so in our history – it has been a part of human food systems for a very long time, ever since hunter-gatherers first developed tools to extract food from the environment. In the future our children will, through innovation or necessity, be living with a very different food system from that which exists today.

While we look to technology for solutions, however, we must remember that many of the world's food problems can be improved by focusing on alleviating poverty and distributing food more equitably. A valid criticism of the EAT-*Lancet* Commission's report is that it does not examine the affordability of such a recommended diet for those living in low- and middle-income countries (Zagmutt, Pouzou, and Costard 2019) – not to mention those living in food-insecure households in high-income countries. Furthermore, they point out that the commission's analysis did not take into account children under two years of age, effectively ignoring pregnant and lactating women, infants, and young children, one of the sectors most vulnerable to malnutrition. In order to guide and have a positive influence on our planet's diet and food production, we must start with our children. Like children, who take "small bites," we, too, must take "small bites," or incremental steps,

New Directions in Children's Food and Nutrition

to change our food system to make it more sustainable, equitable, and nourishing for everyone. We took hundreds of years to develop this industrial food system and our current way of feeding children, which has clearly gone awry. Now it's time to pivot, using policy and community action, to set it on the right course for the future.

Notes

Introduction

1 This difference in terminology reflects the varying traditions of anthropology, where North America followed Boasian "cultural anthropology" and the UK and Europe followed "social anthropology" (Layton and Kaul 2006). Here I follow Canadian and some American scholars, using the term "sociocultural anthropology" with equal recognition of both social and cultural processes.

Chapter 1: Baby Steps

1 There is another good reason to do this. Since the cord blood is full of iron stores, it has been demonstrated that, even if the cord cutting is delayed for only two to three minutes, the neonate's blood hemoglobin level is much higher (Chaparro 2011).

2 For an exception to this, see Baksh and colleagues (1994), who evaluate the influence of women's reproductive status on rural Kenyan women's time use.

3 It should be pointed out that, even if the researcher is from the low- or middle-income country in question, they may still hold a postindustrial perspective, since many middle-class and university-educated academics do not share the worldviews of their research subjects.

Chapter 4: It Takes a Village

1 Parts of the remainder of this chapter were originally published by Routledge, Taylor and Francis in *Critical Public Health* and, on behalf of the Association for the Study

Notes 183

of Food and Society, as an article in *Food, Culture and Society* in 2018. doi: http://www.tandfonline.com/.

2 Assman (2015, 173) points out that this emphasis on local foods occurred after the 2011 accident at the Fukushima nuclear reactor; yet, they are still portrayed as safe in the food education campaign.

3 Ironically, every school meal is accompanied by a carton of milk, a practice begun after the Second World War, with American food aid to Japan (Assman 2015, 178). This has perhaps been maintained in the meal program because of the rising trend in the promotion of milk in East Asia as a health- and growth-promoting beverage for children, despite the fact that milk has never been part of Japanese cuisine and that many people of East Asian descent are lactase impersistent, lacking the genetic variant that enables digestion of lactose in milk after early childhood (Wiley 2007, 2011). Given the recent impetus to move away from Western food items and towards more traditionally defined Japanese meals (Assman 2015), it will be interesting to see if milk maintains its place in Japanese school meals in the future.

Chaper 5: Global Malnutrition and Children's Food (In)security

1 Despite using the same questions, Canada uses a broader system for classifying households as food insecure; if the US classification system were used, the prevalence of food insecurity in Canada would be lower (Power 2014; Power, Little, and Collins 2014).

Chaper 6: Childhood Obesity

1 The jury still isn't out, however, on saturated fats and its links to coronary heart disease. A recent study by a group of Harvard nutritionists summarized as follows: "Higher dietary intakes of major saturated fatty acids (SFAs) are associated with an increased risk of coronary heart disease. Owing to similar associations and high correlations among individual SFAs, dietary recommendations for the prevention of coronary heart disease should continue to focus on replacing total saturated fat with more healthy sources of energy" (Zong et al. 2016, 1).

References

Abrams, Elissa M., Kyla Hildebrand, Becky Blair, and Edmond S. Chan. 2019. "Timing of Introduction of Allergenic Solids for Infants at High Risk." *Paediatrics and Child Health* 24, no. 1: 56. doi: 10.1093/pch/pxy195.

Adams, Jean, Rachel Tyrrell, Ashley J. Adamson, and Martin White. 2012. "Effect of Restrictions on Television Food Advertising to Children on Exposure to Advertisements for 'Less Healthy' Foods: Repeat Cross-Sectional Study." *PLoS ONE* 7, no. 2: e31578. doi: 10.1371/journal.pone.0031578.

Agliano Sanborn, Alexis. 2013. "Flavoring the Nation: School Lunch in Japan." MA thesis, Harvard University.

Alberta Government. 2017. *Alberta Education School Nutrition 2016/17 Pilot Summary*. Edmonton: Alberta Education School Nutrition Program.

Albuquerque, David, Eric Stice, Raquel Rodríguez-López, Licíno Manco, and Clévio Nóbrega. 2015. "Current Review of Genetics of Human Obesity: From Molecular Mechanisms to an Evolutionary Perspective." *Molecular Genetics and Genomics* 290: 1191–221. doi: 10.1007/s00438-015-1015-9.

Allison, Anne. 1991. "Japanese Mothers and Obentōs: The Lunch-Box as Ideological State Apparatus." *Anthropological Quarterly* 64, no. 4: 194–208.

Anderson, Patricia M., and Kristin F. Butcher. 2006. "Childhood Obesity: Trends and Potential Causes." *Future of Children* 16, no. 1: 19–45. 10.1353/foc.2006.0001.

Andreas, Nicholas J., Beate Kampmann, and Kirsty Mehring Le-Doare. 2015. "Human Breast Milk: A Review on Its Composition and Bioactivity." *Early Human Development* 91, no. 11: 629–35. https://doi.org/10.1016/j.earlhumdev.2015.08.013.

Arcelus, Jon, Alex J. Mitchell, Jackie Wales, and Søren Nielsen. 2011. "Mortality Rates in Patients with Anorexia Nervosa and Other Eating Disorders." *Archives of General Psychiatry* 68, no. 7: 724–31. doi: 10.1001/archgenpsychiatry.2011.74.

Ashe, Leah M., and Roberta Sonnino. 2013. "At the Crossroads: New Paradigms of Food Security, Public Health Nutrition and School Food." *Public Health Nutrition* 16, no. 6: 1020–27. doi: 10.1017/S1368980012004326.

Assari, Shervin. 2014. "The Link between Mental Health and Obesity: Role of Individual and Contextual Factors." *International Journal of Preventative Medicine* 5, no. 3: 247–49.

Assman, Stephanie. 2015. "The Remaking of a National Cuisine: The Food Education Campaign in Japan." In *The Globalization of Asian Cuisines: Transnational Networks and Culinary Contact Zones*, ed. James Farrer, 165–85. New York: Palgrave Macmillan.

Backstrand, Jeffrey R. 2002. "The History and Future of Food Fortification in the United States: A Public Health Perspective." *Nutrition Reviews* 60, no. 1: 15–26.

Bailey, L. Charles, Christopher B. Forrest, Peixin Zhang, Thomas M. Richards, Alice Livshits, and Patricia A. DeRusso. 2014. "Association of Antibiotics in Infancy with Early Childhood Obesity." *Journal of the American Medical Association Pediatrics* 168, no. 11: 1063–69. doi: 10.1001/jamapediatrics.2014.1539.

Baksh, Michael, Charlotte G. Neumann, Michael Paolisso, Richard M. Trostle, and A.A.J. Jansen. 1994. "The Influence of Reproductive Status on Rural Kenyan Women's Time Use." *Social Science and Medicine* 39, no. 3: 345–54. http://dx.doi.org/10.1016/0277-9536(94)90130-9.

Ball, Helen. H., and Alan C. Swedlund. 1996. "Poor Women and Bad Mothers: Placing the Blame for Turn-of-the-Century Infant Mortality." *Northeast Anthropology* 52: 31–52.

Ballantyne, Sarah. 2012. "Paleo Baby Foods – What to Introduce When." *Dr. Sarah Ballantyne's* The Paleo Mom. https://www.thepaleomom.com/paleo-baby-foods -what-to-introduce-when/.

Barker, David, J.P. 1995. "Fetal Origins of Coronary Heart Disease." *British Medical Journal* 311: 171–74.

Barker, David J.P., Johan G. Eriksson, Tom Forsén, and Clive Osmond. 2002. "Fetal Origins of Adult Disease: Strength of Effects and Biological Basis." *International Journal of Epidemiology* 31: 1235–39.

Barker, David J.P., and Clive Osmond. 1986. "Infant Mortality, Childhood Nutrition, and Ischaemic Heart Disease in England and Wales." *Lancet* 10, no. 1: 1077–81.

Barker, Mary. 2015. "Developmental Origins, Behaviour Change, and the New Public Health." *Journal of the Developmental Origins of Health and Disease* 6, no. 5: 428–33.

Barker, Mary, Stephan U. Dombrowski, Tim Colbourn, Caroline H.D. Fall, Natasha M. Kriznik, Wendy T. Lawrence, Shane A. Norris, Gloria Ngaiza, Dilisha Patel, Jolene Skordis-Worrall, Falko F. Sniehotta, Régine Steegers-Theunissen, Christina Vogel, Kathryn Woods-Townsend, and Judith Stephenson. 2018. "Intervention Strategies to Improve Nutrition and Health Behaviours before Conception." *Lancet* 391, no. 10132: 1853–64. https://doi.org/10.1016/S0140-6736(18)30313-1.

Barrett, Christopher B. 2010. "Measuring Food Insecurity." *Science* 327: 825–28.

BBC. n.d. *Fast Food Factory. Attracting Customers.* BBC World Service. http://www.bbc.co.uk/worldservice/specials/1616_fastfood/page6.shtml.

BBC News. 2015. "French MP Yves Jego Calls for Vegetarian School Meals." 21 August. http://www.bbc.com/news/world-europe-34019374.

Beagan, Brenda L., Gwen E. Chapman, Josée Johnston, Deborah McPhail, Elaine M. Power, and Helen Vallianatos. 2015. *Acquired Tastes: Why Families Eat the Way They Do*. Vancouver: UBC Press.

Beauchesne, P. and S. Agarwal, eds. 2018. *Children and Childhood in Bioarcheology*. University of Florida Press.

Beck, Leslie. 2018. "What You Need to Know about Trans Fats and Why They Are Being Banned." *Globe and Mail*, 17 September. https://www.theglobeandmail.com/life/health-and-fitness/health/what-you-need-to-know-about-trans-fats-and-why-they-are-being-banned/article36317373/.

Becker, Stan, Robert E. Black, Kenneth H. Brown. 1991. "Relative Effects of Diarrhoea, Fever and Dietary Intake on Weight Gain in Rural Bangladesh Children." *American Journal of Clinical Nutrition* 53: 1499–503.

Bell, Christopher G., Andrew J. Walley, and Philipp Froguel. 2005. "The Genetics of Human Obesity." *Nature Reviews Genetics* 6: 221–34. doi: 10.1038/nrg1556.

Bellis, Mary. 2019. "The History of Who Invented Breakfast Cereal." ThoughtCo, 25 May. http://thoughtco.com/who-invented-breakfast-cereal-1991781.

Belluz, Julia. 2016. "Michael Pollan on How America Got So Screwed Up about Food." *Vox.com*. https://www.vox.com/2015/12/16/10227456/michael-pollan-interview.

Belsky, Daniel W., Terrie E. Moffitt, Louise Arseneault, Maria Melchior, and Avshalom Caspi. 2010. "Context and Sequelae of Food Insecurity in Children's Development." *American Journal of Epidemiology* 172, no. 7: 809–18. doi: 10.1093/aje/kwq201.

Bentley, Amy. 2014. *Inventing Baby Food: Taste, Health, and the Industrialization of the American Diet*. Oakland: University of California Press.

Bentley, Margaret E., Heather M. Wasser, and Hilary M. Creed-Kanashiro. 2011. "Responsive Feeding and Child Undernutrition in Low- and Middle-Income Countries." *Journal of Nutrition* 141, no. 3: 502–7.

Bertin, Mélanie, Lionel Lafay, Gloria Calamassi-Tran, Jean-Luc Volatier, and Carine Dubuisson. 2012. "School Meals in French Secondary State Schools: Do National Recommendations Lead to Healthier Nutrition on Offer?" *British Journal of Nutrition* 107: 416–27.

Birch, Leann L. 1999. "Development of Food Preferences." *Annual Review of Nutrition* 19: 41–62.

Bird, Douglas W., and Rebecca Bliege Bird. 2005. "Martu Children's Hunting Strategies in the Western Desert, Australia." In *Hunter-Gatherer Childhoods: Evolutionary, Developmental and Cultural Perspectives*, ed. Barry S. Hewlett and Michael E. Lamb, 129–46. New Brunswick, NJ: Transaction Publishers.

Black, Robert E., Kenneth H. Brown, and Stan Becker. 1984. "Effects of Diarrhea Associated with Specific Enteropathogens on the Growth of Children on Rural Bangladesh." *Pediatrics* 73, no. 6: 799–805.

References

Blaffer Hrdy, Sarah. 2009. *Mothers and Others: The Evolutionary Origins of Mutual Understanding*. Cambridge, MA: Harvard University Press.

Blaser, Martin J. 2014. *Missing Microbes: How the Overuse of Antibiotics Is Fueling Our Modern Plagues*. New York: Henry Holt.

Bluebond-Langner, M., and J.E. Korbin. 2007. "Challenges and Opportunities in the Anthropology of Childhoods: An introduction to 'Children, Childhoods, and Childhood Studies.'" *American Anthropologist* 109, no. 2: 241–46.

Bock, John, and Daniel Sellen. 2002. "Childhood and the Evolution of the Human Life Course: An Introduction." *Human Nature* 13, no. 2: 153–59.

Bogin, Barry. 1999. *Patterns of Human Growth*. 2nd ed. Cambridge: Cambridge University Press.

–. 2010. "Evolution of Human Growth." In *Human Evolutionary Biology*, ed. Michael P. Muehlenbein, 379–95. Cambridge: Cambridge University Press.

Boseley, Sarah. 2018. "Schools Are Not the Answer to Childhood Obesity Epidemic, Study Shows." *Guardian*, 8 February. https://www.theguardian.com/society/2018/feb/08/schools-are-not-the-answer-to-childhood-obesity-epidemic-study-shows.

Bourdieu, Pierre. 1984. *Distinction: A Social Critique of the Judgement of Taste*. London: Routledge and Kegan Paul.

Bowman, Shanthy A., Steven L. Gortmaker, Cara B. Ebbel, Mark A. Pereira, and David S. Ludwig. 2004. "Effects of Fast-Food Consumption on Energy Intake and Diet Quality among Children in a National Household Survey." *Pediatrics* 113, no. 1: 112–18.

Boyland, Emma, and Jennifer L. Harris. 2017. Regulation of Food Marketing to Children: Are Statutory or Industry Self-Governed Systems Effective? *Public Health Nutrition* 20, no. 5: 761–64.

Braun, Joseph M. 2017. "Early Life Exposure to Endocrine Disrupting Chemicals and Childhood Obesity and Neurodevelopment." *Nature Reviews Endocrinology* 13, no. 3: 161–73. doi: 10.1038/nrendo.2016.186.

Bray, George A., Samara Joy Nielsen, and Barry M. Popkin. 2004. "Consumption of High-Fructose Corn Syrup in Beverages May Play a Role in the Epidemic of Obesity." *American Journal of Clinical Nutrition* 79: 537–43.

Breastfeeding Committee for Canada. 2017. The Baby-Friendly Initiative in Canada Status Report 2017. The National Authoriy for the Baby-Friendly Initiative. https://breastfeedingcanada.ca/wp-content/uploads/2020/03/Status_report_Sept2017-English.pdf.

Brewis, Alexandra. 2011. *Obesity. Cultural and Biocultural Perspectives*. New Brunswick, NJ: Rutgers University Press.

–. 2014. "Stigma and the Perpetuation of Obesity." *Social Science and Medicine* 118:152–58. https://doi.org/10.1016/j.socscimed.2014.08.003.

Brewis, Alexandra A., Amber Wutich, Ashlan Falletta-Cowden, and Isa Rodriguez-Soto. 2011. "Body Norms and Fat Stigma in Global Perspective." *Current Anthropology* 52, no. 2: 269–76.

Brewis, Alexandra A., B. Piperata, and Amanda L. Thompson. 2020. "Localizing Resource Insecurities: A Biocultural Perspective on Water and Wellbeing." *WIREs Water* e1400. doi: 10.1002/wat2.1440.

Bridle-Fitzpatrick, Susan. 2015. "Food Deserts or Food Swamps? A Mixed-Methods Study of Local Food Environments in a Mexican City." *Social Science and Medicine* 142: 202–13. https://doi.org/10.1016/j.socscimed.2015.08.010.

Brooks, Natalie, and Andrea Begley. 2014. "Adolescent Food Literacy Programmes: A Review of the Literature." *Nutrition and Dietetics* 71: 158–71. doi: 10.1111/1747-0080.12096.

Brownell, Kelly D., and Jennifer L. Pomeranz. 2014. "The Trans-Fat Ban – Food Regulation and Long-Term Health." *New England Journal of Medicine* 370, no. 19: 1773–75.

Buijzena, Moniek, Joris Schuurman, and Elise Bomhof. 2008. "Associations between Children's Television Advertising Exposure and Their Food Consumption Patterns: A Household Diary – Survey Study." *Appetite* 50: 231–39.

Cairns, Kate, and Joseé Johnston. 2015. *Food and Femininity*. London: Bloomsbury Academic.

Canadian Food Inspection Agency (CFIA). 2019. "Notice of Modification: Prohibiting the Use of Partially Hydrogenated Oils (PHOS) in Foods." Ottawa: Government of Canada. https://www.inspection.gc.ca/food/requirements-and-guidance/food-safety-standards-guidelines/notice-of-modification-phos/eng/15 36939719584/1536939792275.

Carbone, Sarah, Elaine Power, and Mary Rita Holland. 2020. "Canada's Missed Opportunity to Implement Publicly Funded School Meal Programs in the 1940s." *Critical Public Health* 30, no. 2: 191–03. doi: 10.1080/09581596.2018.1524849.

Cardoso, Hugo F.V., and Susanna Garcia. 2009. "The Not-So-Dark Ages: Ecology for Human Growth in Medieval and Early Twentieth Century Portugal as Inferred from Skeletal Growth Profiles." *American Journal of Physical Anthropology* 138: 136–47.

Carstairs, Catherine, Paige Schell, and Sheilagh Quale. 2016. "Making the 'Perfect Food' Safe: The Milk Pasteurization Debate." In *How Canadians Communicate VI: Food Promotion, Consumption and Controversy*, ed. Charlene Elliott, 163–84. Athabasca, AB: Athabasca University Press.

Carter, Mary-Ann, and Boyd Swinburn. 2004. "Measuring the 'Obesogenic' Food Environment in New Zealand Primary Schools." *Health Promotion International* 19, no. 1: 15–20. doi: 10.1093/heapro/dah103.

Caviness, Jr., V.S., D.N. Kennedy, C. Richelme, J. Rademacher, and P.A. Filipek. 1996. "The Human Brain Age 7–11 Years: A Volumetric Analysis Based on Magnetic Resonance Images." *Cerebral Cortex* 6: 726–36.

CBC News. 2017a. "Food Insecurity in Nunavut 'Should Be Considered a National Crisis,' Expert Says." 19 May. https://www.cbc.ca/news/health/food-insecurity-1.4122103.

–. 2017b. "Why Canada Could Benefit from a National School Food Program." 5 September. https://www.cbc.ca/news/health/school-food-1.4275520.

CDC. n.d., *About Child and Teen BMI*. https://www.cdc.gov/healthyweight/assessing/bmi/childrens_bmi/about_childrens_bmi.html.

Chaparro, Camila M. 2011. "Timing of Umbilical Cord Clamping: Effect on Iron Endowment of the Newborn and Later Iron Status." *Nutrition Reviews* 69 (suppl. 1): S30–36.

References 189

Chee, Bernadine W.L. 2000. "Eating Snacks and Biting Pressure: Only Children in Beijing." In *Feeding China's Little Emperors: Food, Children, and Social Change*, ed. Jun Jing, 48–70. Stanford, CA: Stanford University Press.

Chen, Lincoln C. 1983. "Interactions of Diarrhea and Malnutrition." In *Diarrhea and Malnutrition*, ed. Lincoln C. Chen and Neville S. Scrimshaw. Boston: Springer.

Chisholm, James S. 1993. "Death, Hope, and Sex: Life-History Theory and the Development of Reproductive Strategies." *Current Anthropology* 34, no. 1: 1–24.

Choi, Yoon Y., Alexis Ludwig, and Jennifer L. Harris. 2020. "US Toddler Milk Sales and Associations with Marketing Practices." *Public Health Nutrition* 23, no. 6: 1127–35. doi: 10.1017/S1368980019003756.

Chrisafis, Angelique. 2015. "Pork or Nothing: How School Dinners Are Dividing France." *Guardian*, 13 October. https://www.theguardian.com/world/2015/oct/13/pork-school-dinners-france-secularism-children-religious-intolerance.

Chung, Mei, Jiantao Ma, Kamal Patel, Samantha Berger, Joseph Lau, and Alice H. Lichtenstein. 2014. "Fructose, High-Fructose Corn Syrup, Sucrose, and Nonalcoholic Fatty Liver Disease or Indexes of Liver Health: A Systematic Review and Meta-Analysis." *American Journal of Clinical Nutrition* 11: 833–49.

City of Toronto. 2019. "Food Insecurity in Toronto." https://www.toronto.ca/community-people/health-wellness-care/health-programs-advice/nutrition-food-basket/.

Clark, Melissa, and Mary Kay Fox. 2009. "Nutritional Quality of the Diets of US Public School Children and the Role of the School Meal Programs." *Journal of the American Dietetic Association* 109: S44-S56.

Coalition for Healthy School Food. n.d. "For a Universal Healthy School Food Program." https://foodsecurecanada.org/sites/foodsecurecanada.org/files/coalition_document_en.compressed.pdf.

Colchero, M. Arantxa, Barry M. Popkin, Juan A. Rivera, and Shu Wen Ng. 2016. "Beverage Purchases from Stores in Mexico under the Excise Tax on Sugar Sweetened Beverages: Observational Study." *British Medical Journal* 352: h6704. doi: 10.1136/bmj.h6704.

Cole, Tim J. 1989. "Relating Growth Rate to Environmental Factors – Methodological Problems in the Study of Growth-Infection Interaction." *Acta Paediatrica* 78, no. s350: 14–20. https://doi.org/10.1111/j.1651–2227.1989.tb11194.x.

Cole, Tim J., Mary C. Bellizzi, Katherine M. Flegal, and William H. Dietz. 2000. "Establishing a Standard Definition for Child Overweight and Obesity Worldwide: International Survey." *British Medical Journal* 320: 1240

Coleman-Jensen, Alisha, Matthew P. Rabbitt, Christian A. Gregory, and Anita Singh. 2018. *Household Food Security in the United States in 2017, ERR-256.* US Department of Agriculture, Economic Research Service.

Collier, Roger. 2015. "Free Lunch Is a Good Thing for Children." *Canadian Medical Association Journal* 187, no. 1: E11. doi: https://doi.org/10.1503/cmaj.109–4952.

Collins, Patricia A., Elaine M. Power, and Margaret H. Little. 2014. "Municipal-Level Responses to Household Food Insecurity in Canada: A Call for Critical, Evaluative Research." *Canadian Journal of Public Health* 105, no. 2: e138–41.

Connell, Carol L., Kristi L. Lofton, Kathy Yadrick, and Timothy A. Rehner. 2005. "Children's Experiences of Food Insecurity Can Assist in Understanding Its Effect on Their Well-Being." *Journal of Nutrition* 135, no. 7: 1683–90.

Connelly, Sean, Sean Markey, and Mark Roseland. 2011. "Bridging Sustainability and the Social Economy: Achieving Community Transformation through Local Food Initiatives." *Critical Social Policy* 31, no. 2: 308–24.

Cook, John T., Deborah A. Frank, Carol Berkowitz, Maureen M. Black, Patrick H. Casey, Ciana B. Cutts, Alan F. Meyers, Nieves Zaldivar, Anne Skalicky, Suzette Levenson, Tim Heeren, and Mark Nord. 2004. "Food Insecurity Is Associated with Adverse Health Outcomes among Human Infants and Toddlers." *Journal of Nutrition* 134, no. 6: 1432–38.

Cooksey-Stowers, Kristen, Marlene B. Schwartz, and Kelly D. Brownell. 2017. "Food Swamps Predict Obesity Rates Better Than Food Deserts in the United States." *International Journal of Environmental Research and Public Health* 14, no. 11: 1366. https://doi.org/10.3390/ijerph14111366.

Couillard, Lucie. 2019. "Global Fast Food Restaurants." IBISWorld Industry Report G4621-GL. https://clients1.ibisworld.com/reports/gl/industry/industryoutlook. aspx?entid=1480.

Cox, Laura M., and Martin J. Blaser. 2015. "Antibiotics and Early Life Obesity." *Nature Reviews Endocrinology* 11, no. 3: 182–90. doi: 10.1038/nrendo. 2014.210.

Crider, Krista S., Lynn B. Bailey, and Robert J. Berry. 2011. "Folic Acid Food Fortification – Its History, Effect, Concerns, and Future Directions." *Nutrients* 3, no. 3: 370–84.

Crooks, Deborah. 2003. "Trading Nutrition for Education: Nutritional Status and the Sale of Snack Foods in an Eastern Kentucky School." *Medical Anthropology Quarterly* 17, no. 2: 182–99. doi: 10.1525/maq.2003.17.2.182.

Cross, Brian. 2013. "Outlawed Junk Food Means Dramatic Sales Drop at High-school Cafeterias." *Windsor Star.* https://windsorstar.com/news/local-news/ outlawed-junk-food-means-dramatic-sales-drop-at-high-school-cafeterias.

CTV News. 2011. "Caterer Says No Profit in Serving Healthy School Meals." https://www.ctvnews.ca/caterer-says-no-profit-in-serving-healthy-school-meals-1.696524.

Cullin, Jennifer M., and Kurt E. White. 2020. "Weight Perception among US Adults Predicts Cardiovascular Risk When Controlling for Body Fat Percentage." *American Journal of Human Biology* 32, no. 4: e23384. https://doi.org/10.1002/ ajhb.23384.

Cummins, Steven, and Sally Macintyre. 2002. "'Food Deserts' – Evidence and Assumption in Health Policy Making." *British Medical Journal* 325: 436–38.

Cunningham, Kenda, Derek Headey, Akriti Singh, Chandni Karmacharyad, and Rana Pooja Pandey. 2017. "Maternal and Child Nutrition in Nepal: Examining Drivers of Progress from the Mid-1990s to 2010s." *Global Food Security* 13: 30–37.

Dahl, Roald. 1964. *Charlie and the Chocolate Factory.* New York: Alfred A. Knopf.

References

Daily Mail Reporter. 2014. "'Eat Pork or Go Hungry': France's National Front Leader Tells School Canteens to Stop Offering Religious Alternatives to Muslim Children." *Daily Mail Online,* 14 April. http://www.dailymail.co.uk/news/article-2597082/Eat-pork-hungry-Frances-far-right-National-Front-leader-tells-schools-stop-offering-religious-alternatives-canteen.html.

de Benedictis, Sara. 2012. "'Feral' Parents: Austerity Parenting under Neoliberalism. *Studies in the Maternal* 4, no. 2: 1–21. doi: 10.16995/sim.40.

De Coopman, J. 1993. "Breastfeeding after Pituitary Resection: Support for a Theory of Autocrine Control of Milk Supply?" *Journal of Human Lactation* 9, no. 1: 35–40.

de Onis, Mercedes, Adelheid W. Onyango, Elaine Borghi, Amani Siyam, Chizuru Nishida, and Jonathan Siekman. 2007. "Development of a WHO Growth Reference for School-Aged Children and Adolescents." *Bulletin of the World Health Organization* 85, no. 9: 660–67.

de Souza, Russell J., Andrew Mente, Adriana Maroleanu, Adrian I. Cozma, Vanessa Ha, Teruko Kishibe, Elizabeth Uleryk, Patrick Budylowski, Holger Schünemann, Joseph Beyene, and Sonia S. Anand. 2015. "Intake of Saturated and Trans Unsaturated Fatty Acids and Risk of All Cause Mortality, Cardiovascular Disease, and Type 2 Diabetes: Systematic Review and Meta-Analysis of Observational Studies." *British Medical Journal* 351: h3978. doi: 10.1136/bmj.h3978.

Decaro, Jason A., Mange Manyama, and Warren Wilson. 2016. "Household-Level Predictors of Maternal Mental Health and Systemic Inflammation among Infants in Mwanza, Tanzania." *American Journal of Human Biology* 28, no. 4: 461–70. doi: 10.1002/ajhb.22807.

Dettwyler, Katherine A. 1986. "Infant Feeding in Mali, West Africa: Variations in Belief and Practice." *Social Science and Medicine* 23, no. 7: 651–64.

–. 1989. "Styles of Infant Feeding: Parental/Caretaker Control of Food Consumption in Young Children." *American Anthropologist* 91, no. 3: 696–703.

Development Initiatives. 2018. *2018 Global Nutrition Report: Shining a Light to Spur Action on Nutrition.* Bristol, UK: Development Initiatives.

Dewey, Kathryn G. 2001. "Nutrition, Growth, and Complementary Feeding of the Brestfed Infant." *Pediatric Clinics of North America* 48, no. 1: 87–104. https://doi.org/10.1016/S0031-3955(05)70287-X.

Dewey, Kathryn G., and Seth Adu-Afarwuah. 2008. "Systematic Review of the Efficacy and Effectiveness of Complementary Feeding Interventions in Developing Countries." *Maternal and Child Nutrition* 4: 24–85.

Dhar, Tirtha, and Kathy Baylis. 2011. "Fast-Food Consumption and the Ban on Advertising Targeting Children: The Quebec Experience." *Journal of Marketing Research* 48, no. 5: 799–813.

Dietz, William H., and Kelley S. Scanlon. 2012. "Eliminating the Use of Partially Hydrogenated Oil in Food Production and Preparation." *Journal of the American Medical Association* 308, no. 2: 143–44.

DiFelice, Josie. 2015. "A Model for Healthy Food in Ontario Schools: FoodShare's Good Food Café." Sustain Ontario. 19 January. https://sustainontario.com/2015/01/19/a-model-for-healthy-food-in-ontario-schools-foodshares-good-food-cafe/.

Dixon, Helen G., Maree L. Scully, Melanie A. Wakefield, Victoria M. White, and David A. Crawford. 2007. "The Effects of Television Advertisements for Junk Food versus Nutritious Food on Children's Food Attitudes and Preferences." *Social Science and Medicine* 65: 1311–23.

Dovey, Terence M., Paul A. Staples, E. Leigh Gibson, and Jason C.G. Halford. 2008. "Food Neophobia and 'Picky/Fussy' Eating in Children: A Review." *Appetite* 50: 181–93.

Drewnowski, Adam, and S.E. Specter. 2004. "Poverty and Obesity: The Role of Energy Density and Energy Costs." *American Journal of Clinical Nutrition* 79, no. 1: 6–16. https://doi.org/10.1093/ajcn/79.1.6.

Drèze, Jean, and Amartya Sen. 1989. *Hunger and Public Action*. Delhi: Oxford University Press.

Druckerman, Pamela. 2012. *Bringing Up Bébé: One American Mother Discovers the Wisdom of French Parenting*. New York: Penguin Press.

Dubuisson, Carine, Sandrine Lioret, Ariane Dufour, Jean-Luc Volatier, Lionel Lafay, and Dominique Turck. 2012. "Associations between Usual School Lunch Attendance and Eating Habits and Sedentary Behaviour in French Children and Adolescents." *European Journal of Clinical Nutrition* 66: 1335–41. doi: 10.1038/ejcn.2012.137.

Dunne, J., K. Rebay-Salisbury, R.B. Salisbury, A. Frisch, C. Walton-Doyle, and R.P. Evershed. 2019. "Milk of Ruminants in Ceramic Baby Bottles from Prehistoric Child Grave." *Nature* 574, no. 7777: 246–48

Dupras, Tosha L., Henry P. Schwarcz, Scott I. Fairgrieve. 2001. "Infant Feeding and Weaning Practices in Roman Egypt." *American Journal of Physical Anthropology* 115: 204–12.

DuToit, George, Peter H. Sayre, Graham Roberts, Michelle L. Sever, Katie Lawson, Henry T. Bahnson, Helen A. Brough, Alexandra F. Santos, Kristina M. Harris, Suzana Radulovic, Monica Basting, Victor Turcanu, et al., for the Immune Tolerance Network LEAP-On Study Team. 2016. "Effect of Avoidance on Peanut Allergy after Early Peanut Consumption." *New England Journal of Medicine* 374: 1435–43.

Eicher-Miller, Heather, April C. Mason, Connie M. Weaver, George P. McCabe, and Carol J. Boushey. 2011. "Food Security Is Associated with Diet and Bone Mass Disparities in Early Adolescent Males but Not Females in the United States." *Journal of Nutrition* 141: 1738–45.

Eisenmann, Joey C., Craig Gundersen, Brenda J. Lohman, S. Garasky, and S.D. Stewart. 2011. "Is Food Insecurity Related to Overweight and Obesity in Children and Adolescents? A Summary of Studies, 1995–2009." *Obesity Reviews* 12, no. 5: e73–83. doi: 10.1111/j.1467-789X.2010.00820.x.

Elliott, Charlene. 2008. "Assessing 'Fun Foods': Nutritional Content and Analysis of Supermarket Foods Targeted at Children." *Obesity Reviews* 9: 368–77. doi: 10.1111/j.1467-789X.2007.00418.x.

–. 2010. "Eatertainment and the (Re)classification of Children's Foods." *Food, Culture and Society* 13, no. 4: 539–53. doi: 10.2752/175174410X12777254289385.

Elliott Cooper, Elizabeth. 2013. "Does Child Food Exist for Rural Malays? A Mixed Methods Approach to Food and Identity." *Food and Foodways* 21: 211–35. https://doi.org/10.1080/07409710.2013.821298.

References

Ellison, Peter T. 2003. "Energetics and Reproductive Effort." *American Journal of Human Biology* 15: 342–51. doi: 10.1002/ajhb.10152.

–. 2005. "Evolutionary Perspectives on the Fetal Origins Hypothesis." *American Journal of Human Biology* 17: 113–18. doi: 10.1002/ajhb.20097.

Ellison, Peter T., Meredith W. Reiches, Heather Shattuck-Faegre, Alicia Breakey, Martina Konecna, Samuel Urlacher, and Victoria Wobber. 2012. "Puberty as a Life History Transition." *Annals of Human Biology* 39, no. 5: 352–60. doi: 10.3109/03014460.2012.693199.

Estima, Camilla C.P., Meg Bruening, Peter J. Hannan, Marle S. Alvarenga, Greisse V.S. Leal, Sonia T. Philippi, and Dianne Neumark-Sztainer. "A Cross-Cultural Comparison of Eating Behaviors and Home Food Environmental Factors in Adolescents From São Paulo (Brazil) and Saint Paul–Minneapolis (US)." *Journal of Nutrition Education and Behavior* 46, no. 5: 370–75.

Evans, Charlotte E.L., Darren C. Greenwood, Janice D. Thomas, and Janet E. Cade. 2010. "A Cross-Sectional Survey of Children's Packed Lunches in the UK: Food- and Nutrient-Based Results." *Journal of Epidemiology and Community Health* 64, no. 11: 977–83. doi: 10.1136/jech.2008.085977.

Ewing, Reid, Gail Meakins, Shima Hamidi, and Arthur C. Nelson. 2014. "Relationship between Urban Sprawl and Physical Activity, Obesity, and Morbidity – Update and Refinement." *Health and Place* 26: 118–26. http://dx.doi.org/10.1016/j.healthplace.2013.12.008.

Fallon, Anne, Deidre Van der Putten, Cindy Dring, Edina H. Moylett, Gerarad Fealy, and Declan Devane. 2016. "Baby-Led Compared with Scheduled (or Mixed) Breastfeeding for Successful Breastfeeding." *Cochrane Database of Systematic Reviews* 31, no. 7: CD009067. doi: 10.1002/14651858.CD009067.

Ferdosi, Mohammad, Tom McDowell, Wayne Lewchuk, and Stephanie Ross. 2020. *Southern Ontario's Basic Income Experience.* https://labourstudies.mcmaster.ca/documents/southern-ontarios-basic-income-experience.pdf.

Fildes, Valerie A. 1986. *Breasts, Bottles and Babies.* Edinburgh: Edinburgh University Press.

Fitchen, Janet M. 1988. "Hunger, Malnutrition, and Poverty in the Contemporary United States: Some Observations on Their Social and Cultural Context." *Food and Foodways* 2: 309–33.

Flegal, Katherine M., Carolyn J. Tabak, and Cynthia L. Ogden. 2006. "Overweight in Children: Definitions and Interpretation." *Health Education Research* 21, no. 6: 755–60.

Flegal, Katherine M., and R.P. Troiano. 2000. "Changes in the Distribution of Body Mass Index of Adults and Children in the US Population." *International Journal of Obesity* 24: 807–18.

Fleming, Tom P., Adam J. Watkins, Miguel A. Velazquez, John C. Mathers, Andrew M. Prentice, Judith Stephenson, Mary Barker, Richard Saffery, Chittaranjan S. Yajnik, Judith J. Eckert, Mark A. Hanson, Terrence Forrester, Peter D. Gluckman, and Keith M. Godfrey. 2018. "Origins of Lifetime Health around the Time of Conception: Causes and Consequences." *Lancet* 391: 1842–52. https://doi.org/10.1016/S0140-6736(18)30312-X.

Fogel, Robert W. 1991. "The Conquest of High Mortality and Hunger in Europe and America: Timing and Mechanisms." In *Favorites of Fortune: Technology, Growth, and Economic Development since the Industrial Revolution*, ed. Patrice Higgonet, David S. Landes, and Henry Rosovsky, 33–71. Cambridge, MA: Harvard University Press.

Food and Agriculture Organization (FAO). n.d. *Food-Based Dietary Guidelines – Brazil.* http://www.fao.org/nutrition/education/food-dietary-guidelines/regions/asia-pacific/en/.

–. 2003. *Trade Reforms and Food Security. Conceptualizing the Linkages.* Rome: Food and Agriculture Organization of the United Nations.

–. 2008. *An Introduction to the Basic Concepts of Food Security.* Food Security Information Action. Practical Guides. Rome: EC-FAO Food Security Programme. www.foodsec.org/docs/concepts_guide.pdf.

–. 2019. *The State of Food Security and Nutrition in the World.* Rome: FAO. http://www.fao.org/3/y4671e/y4671e00.htm#Contents.

Food Secure Canada. n.d. "Health School Food." https://foodsecurecanada.org/community-networks/healthyschoolfood.

Frizzell, Sara. 2018. "Iqaluit High School Fights Food Insecurity with Free Hot Lunch Program." CBC News, 10 January. https://www.cbc.ca/news/canada/north/inuksuk-high-school-lunch-program-1.4480160.

Fujita, Masako, Eric Roth, Yun-Jia Lo, Carolyn Hurst, Jennifer Vollner, and Ashley Kendell. 2012. "In Poor Families, Mothers' Milk Is Richer for Daughters Than Sons: A Test of Trivers–Willard Hypothesis in Agropastoral Settlements in Northern Kenya." *American Journal of Human Biology* 149: 52–29.

Fulkerson, Jayne A., Mary Story, Dianne Neumark-Sztainer, and Sarah Rydell. 2008. "Family Meals: Perceptions of Benefits and Challenges among Parents of 8- to 10-Year-Old Children." *Journal of the American Dietetic Association* 108: 706–9.

Galloway, Tracey. 2007. "Gender Differences in Growth and Nutrition in a Sample of Rural Ontario Schoolchildren." *American Journal of Human Biology* 19: 774–88. doi: 10.1002/ajhb.20637.

–. 2014. "Is the Nutrition North Canada Retail Subsidy Program Meeting the Goal of Making Nutritious and Perishable Food More Accessible and Affordable in the North?" *Canadian Journal of Public Health* 105, no. 5: e395–97.

–. 2017. "Canada's Northern Food Subsidy *Nutrition North Canada:* A Comprehensive Program Evaluation." *International Journal of Circumpolar Health* 76, no. 1: 1–19. doi: 10.1080/22423982.2017.1279451.

Galloway, Tracey, and Tina Moffat. 2013. "'Not Neutral Ground': Exploring School as a Site for Childhood Obesity Intervention and Prevention Programs." In *Anthropology of Food and Nutrition Series: Interdisciplinary Approaches to Obesity Research*, ed. Meghan McCullough and Jessica Harding, 161–96. New York: Berghahn Press.

Garner, Richard. 2009. "Jamie's School Dinners for All." *Independent*, 30 August. https://www.independent.co.uk/news/education/education-news/jamies-school-dinners-for-all-1779635.html.

References

Ghebreslassie, Makda. 2017. "Food Banks Are 'Short-Term Band-Aid' on 'Huge Gaping Wound,' Says Mary Ellen Prange." *CBC News.* 29 November. https://www.cbc.ca/news/canada/toronto/programs/metromorning/food-banks-security-1.4424443.

Gibson, Rosalind S. 1990. *Principles of Nutritional Assessment.* New York: Oxford University Press.

Giedd, Jay N. 2015. "The Amazing Teen Brain." *Scientific American* 312, no. 6: 32–37.

Gionet, Linda. 2013. "Breastfeeding Trends in Canada." *Health at a Glance.* November. Statistics Canada Catalogue no. 82–624-X. https://www150.statcan.gc.ca/n1/pub/82-624-x/2013001/article/11879/cite-eng.htm.

Gitlin, Martin, and Topher Ellis. 2012. *The Great American Cereal Book: How Breakfast Got Its Crunch.* New York: Harry N. Abrams.

Gluckman, Peter D., Mark A. Hanson, and Murray D. Mitchell. 2010. "Developmental Origins of Health and Disease: Reducing the Burden of Chronic Disease in the Next Generation." *Genome Medicine* 2, no. 14.

Godfrey, Keith M., Peter D. Gluckman, and Mark A. Hanson. 2010. "Developmental Origins of Metabolic Disease: Life Course and Intergenerational Perspectives." *Trends in Endocrinology and Metabolism* 21, no. 4: 199–205.

Godin, Katelyn M., Sharon I. Kirkpatrick, Rhona M. Hanning, Jackie Stapleton, and Scott T. Leatherdale. 2017. "Examining Guidelines for School-Based Breakfast Programs in Canada: A Systematic Review of the Grey Literature." *Canadian Journal Dietetic Practice and Research* 78: 92–100. doi: 10.3148/cjdpr-2016-037.

Goldberg, Joel. 2016. "It Takes a Village to Determine the Origins of an African Proverb." National Public Radio (NPR). "Goats and Soda." https://www.npr.org/sections/goatsandsoda/2016/07/30/487925796/it-takes-a-village-to-determine-the-origins-of-an-african-proverb.

Goldman, Jane A., and Lara Descartes. 2016. "Food Depictions in Picture Books for Preschool Children: Frequency, Centrality, and Affect." *Appetite* 96: 203–8. http://dx.doi.org/10.1016/j.appet.2015.09.018.

Goodall, Jane. 1964. "Tool-Using and Aimed Throwing in a Community of Free-Living Chimpanzees." *Nature* 201: 1264–66.

Goodman, Alan H., and Thomas L. Leatherman. 1998. "Traversing the Chasm between Biology and Culture: An Introduction." In *Building a New Biocultural Synthesis: Political-Economic Perspectives on Human Biology,* ed. Alan H. Goodman and Thomas L. Leatherman, 3–41. Ann Arbor: University of Michigan Press.

Gortmaker, Steven L., Aviva Must, Arthur M. Sobol, Karen Peterson, Graham A. Colditz, and William H. Dietz. 1996. "Television Viewing as a Cause of Increasing Obesity among Children in the United States, 1986–1990." *Archives of Pediatric Adolescent Medicine* 150, no. 4: 356–62. doi: 10.1001/archpedi.1996.02170290022003.

Government of Canada. n.d. *About CPNP.* https://www.canada.ca/en/public-health/services/health-promotion/childhood-adolescence/programs-initiatives/canada-prenatal-nutrition-program-cpnp/about-cpnp.html.

–. 2012. *The Household Food Security Survey Module.* https://www.canada.ca/en/health-canada/services/food-nutrition/food-nutrition-surveillance/health-nutrition-surveys/canadian-community-health-survey-cchs/household-food

-insecurity-canada-overview/household-food-security-survey-module-hfssm
-health-nutrition-surveys-health-canada.html

–. 2019a. *The Canada Food Guide*. https://food-guide.canada.ca/en/.

–. 2019b. *EI maternity and Parental Benefits: What These Benefits Offer*. Employment and Social Development Canada. https://www.canada.ca/en/services/benefits/ei/ei-maternity-parental.html.

Gravlee, Clarence C. 2009. "How Race Becomes Biology: Embodiment of Social Inequality." *American Journal of Physical Anthropology* 139, no. 1: 47–57.

Greenberg, Julia. 2015. "Exposing the Murky World of Online Ads Aimed at Kids." *Wired.com*. https://www.wired.com/2015/04/exposing-murky-world-online-ads-aimed-kids/.

Greenhalgh, Susan. 2016. "Disordered Eating/Eating Disorder: Hidden Perils of the Nation's Fight against Fat." *Medical Anthropology* 30, no. 40: 545–62. https://doi.org/10.1111/maq.12257.

Gregory, Laurel. 2017. "Baby-Led Weaning 101: Why Some Experts Advocate Solid Food at 6 Months." Global News, 12 September. https://globalnews.ca/news/3735249/baby-led-weaning-101-why-some-experts-advocate-solid-food-at-6-months/.

Grün, Felix, and Bruce Blumberg. 2006. "Environmental Obesogens: Organotins and Endocrine Disruption via Nuclear Receptor Signaling." *Endocrinology* 147, no. 6 (supplement): S50–55. doi: 10.1210/en.2005-1129.

Guthman, Julie 2011. *Weighing In: Obesity, Food Justice, and the Limits of Capitalism*. Berkeley: University of California Press.

Guthrie, Joanne F., Biing-Hwan Lin, and E. Frazao. 2002. "Role of Food Prepared Away from Home in the American Diet, 1977–78 versus 1994–96: Changes and Consequences." *Journal of Nutrition Education and Behavior* 34, no. 3: 140–50.

Hadley, Craig, and Deborah Crooks. 2012. "Coping and the Biosocial Consequences of Food Insecurity in the 21st Century." *Yearbook of Physical Anthropology* 55: 72–94. doi: 10.1002/ajpa.22161.

Hadley, Craig, and Crystal L. Patil. 2006. "Food Insecurity in Rural Tanzania Is Associated with Maternal Anxiety and Depression." *American Journal of Human Biology* 18: 359–68.

Hagenaars, Luc Louis, Patrick Paulus, Theodoor Jeurissen, and Niek Sieds Klazinga. 2017. "The Taxation of Unhealthy Energy-Dense Foods (EDFs) and Sugar-Sweetened Beverages (SSBs): An Overview of Patterns Observed in the Policy Content and Policy Context of 13 Case Studies." *Health Policy* 121: 887–94. http://dx.doi.org/10.1016/j.healthpol.2017.06.011.

Hales, C. Nicholas, and David, J.P. Barker. 1992. "Type 2 (Non-Insulin-Dependent) Diabetes Mellitus: The Thrifty Phenotype Hypothesis. *Diabetologia* 35, no. 7: 595–601.

Hales, Craig M., Margaret D. Carroll, Cheryl D. Fryar, and Cynthia L. Ogden. 2017. "Prevalence of Obesity among Adults and Youth: United States, 2015–2016." NCHS Data Brief No. 288. 17 October. US Department of Health and Human Services, Centers for Disease Control and Prevention, National Center for Health Statistics.

Hamilton Community Food Centre (HCFC). n.d. http://www.n2ncentre.com/hamilton-community-food-centre/.

Hamm, Michael W., and Anne C. Bellows. 2003. "Community Food Security and Nutrition Education." *Journal of Nutrition Education and Behavior* 35, no. 1: 37–43.

Hammons, Amber J., and Barbara H. Fiese. 2011. "Is Frequency of Shared Family Meals Related to the Nutritional Health of Children and Adolescents?" *Pediatrics* 127, no. 6: e1565–74. doi: 10.1542/peds.2010-1440.

Harrington, Daniel W., Jennifer Dean, Kathi Wilson, and Zafar Qamar. 2015. "'We Don't Have Such a Thing, That You May Be Allergic': Newcomers' Understandings of Food Allergies in Canada." *Chronic Illness* 11, no. 2: 126–39. doi: 10.1177/1742395314546136.

Harris, Jennifer L., K.S. Haraghey, M. Lodolce, and N.L. Semenza1. 2017. "Teaching Children about Good Health? Halo Effects in Child-Directed Advertisements for Unhealthy Food." *Pediatric Obesity* 13, no. 4: 256–64. doi: 10.1111/ijpo.12257.

Hatch, Elizabeth E., J.W. Nelson, R.W. Stahlhut, and T.F. Webster. 2010. "Association of Endocrine Disruptors and Obesity: Perspectives from Epidemiological Studies." *International Journal of Andrology* 33: 324–32. doi: 10.1111/j.1365-2605.2009.01035.x.

Hawkes, Kristen. 2003. "Grandmothers and the Evolution of Human Longevity." *American Journal of Human Biology* 15: 380–400.

–. 2004. "Human Longevity: The Grandmother Effect." *Nature* 428, no. 6979:128–29.

Hawkes, Kristen, James F. O'Connell, and Nicholas G. Blurton Jones. 1995. "Hadza Children's Foraging: Juvenile Dependency, Social Arrangements, and Mobility among Hunter-Gatherers." *Current Anthropology* 36, no. 4: 688–700.

Headey, Derek D., and John Hoddinott. 2015. "Understanding the Rapid Reduction of Undernutrition in Nepal, 2001–2011." *PLoS One* 10, no. 12: e0145738. https://doi.org/10.1371/journal.pone.0145738.

Health Canada. 2018. *Guidelines for Canadian Drinking Water Quality: Guideline Technical Document – Perfluorooctane Sulfonate (PFOS)* https://www.canada.ca/en/health-canada/services/publications/healthy-living/guidelines-canadian-drinking-water-quality-guideline-technical-document-perfluorooctane-sulfonate/document.html.

Heart and Stroke Foundation of Canada. 2014. *Sugar, Heart Disease and Stroke.* Position Statement. https://www.heartandstroke.ca/-/media/pdf-files/canada/2017-position-statements/sugar-ps-eng.ashx?rev=4d57a3adb1f24765aced70cc290ed27e&hash=321D8D356CACA369E6D5F26A20BFD965.

Heller, Chaia. 2007. "Techne Versus Technosciences: Divergent (and Ambiguous) Notions of Food 'Quality' in the French Debate over GM Crops." *American Anthropologist* 109, no. 4: 603.

Hendrick, Harry. 2015. "Constructions and Reconstructions of British Childhood: An Interpretative Survey, 1800 to the Present." In *Constructing and Reconstructing Childhood: Contemporary Issues in the Sociological Study of Childhood,* classic ed., ed. Allison James and Alan Prout, 29–53. Abingdon, UK: Routledge.

Henrich, Joseph, Steven J. Heine, and Ara Norenzayan. 2010. "The Weirdest People in the World?" *Behavioral and Brain Sciences* 33, nos. 2–3: 61–83; discussion 83–135. doi: 10.1017/S0140525X0999152X.

Hercberg, Serge, Stacie Chat-Yung, and Michel Chauliac. 2008. "The French National Nutrition and Health Program: 2001–2006–2010." *International Journal of Public Health* 53, no. 2: 68–77.

Hernandez, Kimberley, Rachel Engler-Stringer, Sara Kirk, Hannah Wittman, and Sasha McNicholl. 2018. "The Case for a Canadian National School Food Program." *Canadian Food Studies* 5, no. 3: 208–29.

Hertzman, C., and T. Boyce. 2010. "How Experience Gets under the Skin to Create Gradients in Developmental Health." *Annual Review of Public Health* 31: 329–47.

Hewlett, Barry S., and Michael E. Lamb. 2005. "Emerging Issues in the Study of Hunter-Gatherer Children." In *Hunter-Gatherer Childhoods: Evolutionary, Developmental and Cultural Perspectives*, ed. Barry S. Hewlett and Michael E. Lamb, 3–18. London: Routledge.

Hicks, Kathryn, and William R. Leonard. 2014. "Developmental Systems and Inequality: Linking Evolutionary and Political-Economic Theory in Biological Anthropology." *Current Anthropology* 55, no. 5: 523–50.

Hill, Andrew J. 2002. "Developmental Issues in Attitudes to Food and Diet." *Proceedings of the Nutrition Society* 61, no. 2: 259–66.

Hill, James O., and John C. Peters. 1998. "Environmental Contributions to the Obesity Epidemic." *Science* 280: 1371–74.

Hill Kim, and Hillard Kaplan. 1999. "Life History Traits in Humans: Theory and Empirical Studies." *Annual Review of Anthropology* 28: 397–430. doi: 10.1146/annurev.anthro.28.1.397.

Himmelgreen, David A., and Nancy Romero-Daza. 2009. "Anthropological Approaches to the Global Food Crisis: Understanding and Addressing the 'Silent Tsunami.'" *NAPA Bulletin* 32: 1–11.

Hinde, Katie, and Lauren A. Milligan. 2011. "Primate Milk: Proximate Mechanisms and Ultimate Perspectives." *Evolutionary Anthropology* 20: 9–23.

Hiroko, Takeda. 2008. "Delicious Food in a Beautiful Country: Nationhood and Nationalism in Discourses on Food in Contemporary Japan." *Studies in Ethnicity and Nationalism* 8, no. 1: 5–30.

Hoelscher, Deanna M., Andrew E. Springer, Nalini Ranjit, Cheryl L. Perry, Alexandra E. Evans, Melissa Stigler, and Steven H. Kelder. 2013. "Reductions in Child Obesity among Disadvantaged School Children with Community Involvement: The Travis County CATCH Trial." *Obesity* 18, no. S1: S36–S44. doi: 10.1038/oby.2009.430.

Holland, Allyson, and Tina Moffat. 2017. "Comparing Measured Calcium and Vitamin D Intakes with Perceptions of Intake in Canadian Young Adults: Insights for Designing Osteoporosis Prevention Education." *Public Health Nutrition* 20, no. 10: 1760–67.

–. 2020. "Gendered Perceptions of Osteoporosis: Implications for Youth Prevention Programs." *Global Health Promotion* 27, no. 2: 91–99.

Huang, R.-C., Susan L. Prescott, Keith M. Godfrey, and Elizabeth A. Davis. 2015. "Assessment of Cardiometabolic Risk in Children in Population Studies: Underpinning Developmental Origins of Health and Disease Mother-Offspring Cohort Studies." *Journal of Nutrition Science* 4, no. e12: 1–8. doi: 10.1017/jns.2014.69.

Hubbard, Kristie L., Aviva Must, Misha Elizsziw, Sara C. Folta, and Jeanne Goldberg. 2014. "What's in Children's Backpacks: Foods Brought from Home." *Journal of the Academy of Nutrition and Dietetics* 114, no. 9: 1424–31. doi: 10.1016/j.jand.2014.05.010.

Hughlett, Mike. 2013. "General Mills Settles Claim over Fruit Roll-Ups Label." *Star Tribune*. https://www.startribune.com/general-mills-settles-claim-over-fruit-roll-ups-label/184878301/.

Hui, Ann. 2018. "The Big Squeeze: Inside the Fight over Juice in Canada's Food Guide." *Globe and Mail*, 22 November. https://www.theglobeandmail.com/canada/article-the-big-squeeze-inside-the-fight-over-juice-in-canadas-food-guide/.

–. 2019. "Federal Budget 2019: Details Released on Long-Awaited National Food Policy." *Globe and Mail*, 20 March. https://www.theglobeandmail.com/canada/article-federal-budget-2019-details-released-on-long-awaited-national-food/.

Hur, Suzy, Jennifer Cropley, and Cath Suter. 2017. "Paternal Epigenetic Programming: Evolving Metabolic Disease Risk." *Journal of Molecular Endocrinology* 58, no. 3: 1–29.

Institute of Medicine (US). Committee to Review Dietary Reference Intakes for Vitamin D and Calcium. 2011. *Dietary Reference Intakes for Calcium and Vitamin D*. Washington, DC: National Academies Press. https://www.ncbi.nlm.nih.gov/books/NBK56060/.

Intergovernmental Panel on Climate Change (IPCC). 2019. *Climate Change and Land. Summary for Policy Makers*. Geneva: United Nations.

Irwin, Jennifer D., Victor, K. Ng, Timothy J. Rush, Cuong Nguyen, and Meizi He. 2007. "Can Food Banks Sustain Nutrient Requirements? A Case Study in Southwestern Ontario." *Canadian Journal of Public Health* 98, no. 1: 17–20. https://doi.org/10.1007/BF03405378.

James, Allison, and Alan Prout. 1997. *Constructing and Reconstructing Childhood: Contemporary Issues in the Sociological Study of Childhood*. 2nd ed. London: Routledge.

Janssen, Ian, William F. Boyce, Kelly Simpson, and William Pickett. 2006. "Influence of Individual- and Area-Level Measures of Socioeconomic Status on Obesity, Unhealthy Eating, and Physical Inactivity in Canadian Adolescents." *American Journal of Clinical Nutrition* 83: 139–45.

Ji, Cheng-Ye, and Tian-Jiao Chen. 2008. "Secular Changes in Stature and Body Mass Index for Chinese Youth in Sixteen Major Cities, 1950s–2005." *American Journal of Human Biology* 20: 530–37.

Jing, Jun, ed. 2000. *Feeding China's Little Emperors: Food, Children, and Social Change*. Stanford: Stanford University Press.

Joekes, S. 1989. "Women's Work and Social Support for Child Care in the Third World." In *Women, Work, and Child Welfare in the Third World* (AAAS Selected Symposium 110), ed. Joanne Leslie and Michael Paolisso, 59–84. Boulder, CO: Westview Press.

Johnson, Kelsey. 2018. "Health Canada Changes How Rules for Marketing Food to Kids Will Be Applied." *iPolitics*, 6 December. https://ipolitics.ca/2018/12/06/health-canada-changes-how-rules-for-marketing-food-to-kids-will-be-applied/.

Johnson, Rachel K., Lawrence J. Appel, Michael Brands, Barbara V. Howard, Michael Lefevere, Robert R. Lustig, Frank Sacks, Lyn M. Steffen, and Judith Wylie-Rosett, on behalf of the American Heart Association Nutrition Committee of the Council on Nutrition, Physical Activity, and Metabolism and the Council on Epidemiology and Prevention. 2009. "Dietary Sugars Intake and Cardiovascular Health: A Scientific Statement From the American Heart Association." *Circulation* 120: 1011–20.

Johnson, Richard. 2013. "Michael Pollan: Why the Family Meal Is Crucial to Civilization." *Guardian*, 25 May. https://www.theguardian.com/lifeandstyle/2013/may/25/michael-pollan-family-meal-civilisation.

Jones, Nicholas, and Frank Marlowe. 2002. "Selection for Delayed Maturity: Does It Take 20 Years to Learn to Hunt and Gather?" *Human Nature* 13, no. 2: 199–238.

Kalina, Laura. 2001. *Building Food Security in Canada: From Hunger to Sustainable Food Systems – A Community Guide*. Kamloops, BC: Kamloops FoodShare.

Katz, David L. 2010. "It Does, Indeed, Take a Village: Schools, Families, and beyond for Weight Control in Children." *Childhood Obesity* 6: 184–92. doi: 10.1089/chi.2010.0416.

Katzmarzyk, Peter T., Tiago V. Barreira, Stephanie T. Broyles, Catherine M. Champagne, Jean-Philippe Chaput, Mikael Fogelholm, Gang Hu, William D. Johnson, Rebecca Kuriyan, Anura Kurpad, Estelle V. Lambert, Carol Maher, Jose Maia, Victor Matsudo, Timothy Olds, Vincent Onywera, Olga L. Sarmiento, Martyn Standage, Mark S. Tremblay, Catrine Tudor-Locke, Pei Zhao, and Timothy S. Church. 2015. "Physical Activity, Sedentary Time, and Obesity in an International Sample of Children." *Medicine and Science in Sports and Exercise* 47, no. 10: 2062–69. https://doi.org/10.1249/MSS.0000000000000649.

Kauer, Jane, Marcia Pelchat, Paul Rozin, and Hana F. Zickgraf. 2015. "Adult Picky Eating: Phenomenology, Taste Sensitivity, and Psychological Correlates." *Appetite* 90: 219–28.

Kearney, John. 2010. "Food Consumption Trends and Drivers." *Philosophical Transactions of the Royal Society* B 365: 2793–2807. doi: 10.1098/rstb.2010.0149.

Keenleyside A., H. Schwarcz, L. Stirling, and N.B. Lazreg. 2009. "Stable Isotopic Evidence for Diet in a Roman and Late Roman Population from Leptiminus, Tunisia." *Journal of Archeological Science* 36: 1–63.

Keith, Scott W., D.T. Redden, Peter T. Katzmarzyk, M.M. Boggiano, E.C. Hanlon, R.M. Benca, D. Ruden, A. Pietrobelli, J.L. Barger, K.R. Fontaine, C. Wang, L.J. Aronne, S.M. Wright, M. Baskin, N.V. Dhurandhar, M.C. Lijoi, C.M. Grilo, M. DeLuca, A.O. Westfall, and D.B. Allison. 2006. "Putative Contributors to the Secular Increase in Obesity: Exploring the Road Less Traveled." *International Journal of Obesity* 30: 1585–94.

Kelly, Bridget, Jason C.G. Halford, Emma J. Boyland, Kathy Chapman, Inmaculada Bautista-Castaño, Christina Berg, Margherita Caroli, Brian Cook, Janine G. Coutinho, Tobias Effertz, Evangelia Grammatikaki, Kathleen Keller, Raymond Leung, Yannis Manios, Renata Monteiro, Claire Pedley, Hillevi Prell, Kim Raine, Elisabetta Recine, Lluis Serra-Majem, Sonia Singh, and Carolyn Summerbell. 2010. "Television Food Advertising to Children: A Global Perspective." *American Journal of Public Health* 100, no. 9: 1730–36.

Kennedy, Gail E. 2005. "From the Ape's Dilemma to the Weanling's Dilemma: Early Weaning and Its Evolutionary Context." *Journal of Human Evolution* 48: 123–45.

Keskitalo, Kaisu, Antti Knaapila, Mikko Kallela, Aarno Palotie, Maija Wessman, Sampo Sammalisto, Leena Peltonen, Hely Tuorila, and Markus Perola. 2007. "Sweet Taste Preferences Are Partly Genetically Determined: Identification of a Trait Locus on Chromosome 16." *American Journal of Clinical Nutrition* 86, no. 1: 55–63.

Kestens, Yan, and Mark Daniel. 2010. "Social Inequalities in Food Exposure around Schools in an Urban Area." *American Journal of Preventive Medicine* 39, no. 1: 33–40.

Khazan, Olga. 2020. "Baby-Formula Sales Are Slumping, So the Companies That Make It Have Turned to Supplements for 3-Year-Olds." *Atlantic*, 4 February. https://www.theatlantic.com/health/archive/2020/02/should-you-buy-toddler-milk/606028/.

Kirkpatrick, Sharon I., L. McIntyre, and Melissa L. Potestio. 2010. "Child Hunger and Long-term Adverse Consequences for Health." *Archives of Pediatric Adolescent Medicine* 164, no. 8: 754–62.

Kirkpatrick, Sharon I., and Valerie Tarasuk. 2008. "Food Insecurity Is Associated with Nutrient Inadequacies among Canadian Adults and Adolescents." *Journal of Nutrition* 138: 604–12.

–. 2009. "Food Insecurity and Participation in Community Food Programs among Low-Income Toronto Families." *Canadian Journal of Public Health* 100: 135–39.

Kline, Stephen. 2016. "Canaries in the Supermarket: Moral Panic, Food Marketing and Children's Eating." In *How Canadians Communicate VI. Food Promotion, Consumption and Controversy*, ed. Charlene Elliott, 273–96. Athabasca, AB: Athabasca University Press.

Knodel, John, and van de Walle, Etienne. 1967. "Breast Feeding, Fertility and Infant Mortality: An Analysis of Some Early German Data." *Population Studies* 21: 109–31.

Koç, Mustafa, Jennifer Sumner, and Anthony Winson. 2012. *Critical Perspectives in Food Studies*. Don Mills, ON: Oxford University Press.

Koirala, Madan, Resham B. Khatri, Vishnu Khanal, and Archana Amatya. 2015. "Prevalence and Factors Associated with Childhood Overweight/Obesity of Private School Children in Nepal." *Obesity Research and Clinical Practice* 9: 220–27.

Konner, Melvin. 2005. "Hunter-Gatherer Infancy and Childhood: The !Kung and Others." In *Hunter-Gatherer Childhoods: Evolutionary, Developmental and Cultural Perspectives*, ed. Barry S. Hewlett and Michael E. Lamb, 19–64. London: Routledge.

Korpela, Katri, Anne Salonen, Lauri J. Virta, Riina A. Kekkonen, Kristoffer Forslund, Peer Bork, and Willem M. de Vos. 2016. "Intestinal Microbiome Is Related to Lifetime Antibiotic Use in Finnish Pre-School Children." *Nature Communications* 7, no. 10410: 1–8. doi: 10.1038/ncomms10410.

Krieger, Nancy. 2005. "Embodiment: A Conceptual Glossary for Epidemiology." *Journal of Epidemiology and Community Health* 59, no. 5: 350–55.

–. 2016. "Living and Dying at the Crossroads: Racism, Embodiment, and Why Theory Is Essential for a Public Health of Consequence." *American Journal of Public Health* 106, no. 5: 832–33.

Kumar, Seema, and Aaron S. Kelly. 2017. "Review of Childhood Obesity: From Epidemiology, Etiology, and Comorbidities to Clinical Assessment and Treatment." *Mayo Clinic Proceedings* 92, no. 2: 251–65.

Kuzawa, Chistopher W. 2010. "Beyond Feast–Famine: Brain Evolution, Human Life History, and the Metabolic Syndrome." In *Human Evolutionary Biology*, ed. Michael P. Muehlenbein, 518–27. Cambridge: Cambridge University Press.

Kuzawa, Christopher W., Harry T. Chugani, Lawrence I. Grossman, Leonard Lipovich, Otto Muzik, Patrick R. Hof, Derek E. Wildman, Chet C. Sherwood, William R. Leonard, and Nicholas Lange. 2014. "Metabolic Costs and Evolutionary Implications of Human Brain Development." *Proceedings of the National Academy of Science* 111, no. 36: 13010–15.

Kuzawa, C.W., and E. Sweet. 2009. "Epigenetics and the Embodiment of Race: Developmental Origins of US Racial Disparities in Cardiovascular Health." *American Journal of Human Biology* 21, no. 1: 2–15.

Kuzawa, Christopher W., and Elizabeth A. Quinn. 2009. "Developmental Origins of Adult Function and Health: Evolutionary Hypotheses." *Annual Review of Anthropology* 38: 131–47.

Kuzma, Jessica N., Gail Cromer, Derek K. Hagman, Kara L. Breymeyer, Christian L. Roth, Karen E. Foster-Schubert, Sara E. Holte, David S. Weigle, and Mario Kratz. 2016. "No Differential Effect of Beverages Sweetened with Fructose, High-Fructose Corn Syrup, or Glucose on Systemic or Adipose Tissue Inflammation in Normal-Weight to Obese Adults: A Randomized Controlled Trial." *American Journal of Clinical Nutrition* 104: 306–14.

Labbok, Miriam, H. 2001. "Effects of Breastfeeding on the Mother." *Pediatric Clinics of North America* 48, no. 1: 143–58.

Lafraire, Jeremie, Camille Rioux, Agnès Giboreau, and Delphine Picard. 2016. "Food Rejections in Children: Cognitive and Social/Environmental Factors Involved in Food Neophobia and Picky/Fussy Eating Behavior." *Appetite* 96: 347–57.

Laitala, Marja-Liisa, Miira M. Vehkalahti, and Jorman I. Virtanen. 2018. "Frequent Consumption of Sugar-Sweetened Beverages and Sweets Starts at Early Age." *Acta Odontologica Scandinavica* 76, no. 2: 105–10. doi: 10.1080/00016357.2017.1387929.

Lake, Jonathan. 2017. "The First 1,000 Days: A Singular Window of Opportunity." *Unicef Connect*, https://blogs.unicef.org/blog/first-1000-days-singular-opportunity/.

Lambie-Mumford, Hannah, and Mark A. Green. 2017. "Austerity Welfare Reform and the Rising Use of Food Banks by Children in England and Wales." *Area* 49, no. 3: 273–79. doi: 10.1111/area.12233.

Landecker, Hannah. 2011. "Food as Exposure: Nutritional Epigenetics and the New Metabolism." *BioSocieties* 6: 167–94. doi: 10.1057/biosoc.2011.1.

Lang, Andrew, ed. 1965. *The Blue Fairy Book*. New York: Dover.

Laraia, Barbara A. 2013. "Food Insecurity and Chronic Disease." *Advances in Nutrition* 4, no. 2: 203–12.

Larsen, Kristian, and Jason Gilliland. 2008. "Mapping the Evolution of 'Food Deserts' in a Canadian City: Supermarket Accessibility in London, Ontario, 1961–2005." *International Journal of Health Geographics* 7: 1–16. doi: 10.1186/1476-072X-7-16.

Latham, James, and Tina Moffat. 2007. "Determinants of Variation in Food Cost and Availability in Two Socioeconomically Contrasting Neighbourhoods of Hamilton, Ontario, Canada." *Health and Place* 13: 273–87.

Layton, Robert, and Adam R. Kaul. 2006. "American Cultural Anthropology and British Social Anthropology." *Anthropology News*, January. https://www.augustana.edu/files/2017–10/American_Cultural_Anthropology_Connections_Differences_Layton_2008_Anthropology_News%20_Wiley_Online.pdf.

Le Billon, Karen. 2012. *French Kids Eat Everything (And Yours Can Too): How Our Family Moved to France, Cured Picky Eating, Banned Snacking and Discovered 10 Simple Rules for Raising Happy, Healthy Eaters*. Toronto: HarperCollins.

Leatherman, Thomas L., and Alan H. Goodman. 2019. "Building on the Biocultural Syntheses: 20 Years and Still Expanding." *American Journal of Human Biology* e23360. doi: 10.1002/ajhb.23360.

Leatherman, Thomas, Mogan K. Hoke, and Alan H. Goodman. 2016. "Local Nutrition in Global Contexts: Critical Biocultural Perspectives in the Nutrition Transition in Mexico." In *New Directions in Biocultural Anthropology*, ed. Molly K. Zuckerman and Debra L. Martin, 49–68. Hoboken, NJ: John Wiley and Sons.

Leonard, William R. 2002. "Food for Thought." *Scientific American* 287, no. 6: 106–15.

Leslie, Joanne. 1988. "Women's Work and Child Nutrition in the Third World. *World Development* 16, no. 11: 1341–62.

Levenstein, Harvey. 2013. *Fear of Food. A History of Why We Worry about What We Eat*. Chicago: University of Chicago Press.

Levine, Nancy. 1988. "Women's Work and Infant Feeding: A Case from Rural Nepal." *Ethnology* 27: 231–51

Levine, Susan. 2008. *School Lunch Politics: The Surprising History of America's Favorite Welfare Program*. Princeton, NJ: Princeton University Press.

Levkoe, Charles Z., and Sarah Wakefield. 2011. "The Community Food Centre: Creating Space for a Just, Sustainable, and Healthy Food System." *Journal of Agriculture, Food Systems, and Community Development*. http://dx.doi.org/10.5304/jafscd.2011.021.012.

Lewis, Mary E. 2002. "Impact of Industrialization: Comparative Study of Child Health in Four Sites from Medieval and Postmedieval England (A.D. 850–1859). *American Journal of Physical Anthropology* 119: 211–23.

–. 2006. *The Bioarchaeology of Children*. Cambridge: Cambridge University Press.

Leynse, Wendy L.H. 2006. "Journeys through 'Ingestible Topography': Socializing the 'Situated Eater' in France." In *Food, Drink and Identity in Europe: An Interdisciplinary Series in European Culture, History and Politics*, ed. Thomas M. Wilson, 129–58. Amsterdam: Rodopi.

Li, Codie. n.d. "Top 20 Childhood Snacks Every Kid Raised in Hong Kong Will Understand: Asian Kids Everywhere Rejoice." https://spoonuniversity.com/lifestyle/hong-kong-childhood-snacks.

Li, Minglan, Deborah Sloboda, Mark H. Vickers. 2011. "Maternal Obesity and Developmental Programming of Metabolic Disorders in Offspring: Evidence from Animal Models." *Experimental Diabetes Research* 1687–5214. doi: 10.1155/2011/592408.

Li, Yan, Anping Shi, Ying Wan, Masanaka Hotta, and Hiroshi Ushijima. 2001. "Child Behavior Problems: Prevalence and Correlates in Rural Minority Areas of China." *Pediatrics International* 43: 651–66.

Li, Ziyi, Klazine van der Horst, Lisa Edelson-Fries, Kai Yu, Lili You, Yumei Zhang, Gerard Vinyes-Pares, Peiyu Wang, Defu Ma, Xiaoguang Yang, Liqiang Qin, and Jiaji Wang. 2017. "Perceptions of Food Intake and Weight Status among Parents of Picky Eating Infants and Toddlers in China: A Cross-Sectional Study." *Appetite* 108: 456–63.

Lieberman, Leslie Sue. 2006. "Evolutionary and Anthropological Perspectives on Optimal Foraging in Obesogenic Environments." *Appetite* 47: 3–9.

Liem, Djin, and Gie Cees de Graaf. 2004. "Sweet and Sour Preferences in Young Children and Adults: Role of Repeated Exposure." *Physiology and Behavior* 83, no. 3: 421–29. https://doi.org/10.1016/j.physbeh.2004.08.028.

Little, Amanda. 2019. *The Fate of Food: What We'll Eat in a Bigger, Hotter, and Smarter World.* New York: Crown Publishing Group.

Liu, Gang, Klodian Dhana, Jeremy D. Furtado, Jennifer Rood, Geng Zong, Liming Liang, Lu Qi, George A. Bray, Lilian DeJonge, Brent Coull, Philippe Grandjean, and Qi Sun. 2017. "Perfluoroalkyl Substances and Changes in Body Weight and Resting Metabolic Rate in Response to Weight-Loss Diets: A Prospective Study." *PLoS Med* 15, no. 2: e1002502.

Lobstein, Tim, and Rachel Jackson-Leach. 2016. "Planning for the Worst: Estimates of Obesity and Comorbidities in School-Age Children in 2025." *Pediatric Obesity* 11: 321–25.

Lobstein, Tim, and S. Dibb. 2005. "Evidence of a Possible Link between Obesogenic Food Advertising and Child Overweight." *Obesity Reviews* 6: 203–8.

Lock, Margaret. 2017. "Recovering the Body." *Annual Review of Anthropology* 46: 1–14.

Lodge, Caroline J., D.J. Tan, M.X.Z. Lau, X. Dai, R. Tham, A.J. Lowe, G. Bowatte, K.J. Allen, and S.C. Dharmage. 2015. "Breastfeeding and Asthma and Allergies: A Systematic Review and Meta-Analysis." *Acta Paediatrica* 104: 38–53. doi: 10.1111/apa. 13132.

Loopstra, Rachel. 2018. "Interventions to Address Household Food Insecurity in High-Income Countries." *Proceedings of the Nutrition Society* 77: 270–81. doi: 10.1017/S002966511800006X.

Loopstra, Rachel, and Valerie Tarasuk. 2012. "The Relationship between Food Banks and Household Food Insecurity among Low-Income Toronto Families." *Canadian Public Policy* 38, no. 4: 497–514. doi: 10.1080/10796120600879582.

Lowndes, Joshua, Stephanie Sinnett, Sabrina Pardo, Von T. Nguyen, Kathleen J. Melanson, Zhiping Yu, Britte E. Lowther, and James M. Rippe. 2014. "The Effect of Normally Consumed Amounts of Sucrose or High Fructose Corn Syrup on Lipid Profiles, Body Composition and Related Parameters in Overweight/Obese Subjects." *Nutrients* 6: 1128–44. doi: 10.3390/nu6031128.

Lozada, Jr., and P. Eriberto. 2000. "Globalized Childhood: Kentucky Fried Chicken in Beijing." In *Feeding China's Little Emperors: Food, Children, and Social Change,* ed. Jun Jing, 114–34. Stanford: Stanford University Press.

References

Ludwig, David S., Karen E. Peterson, and Steven L. Gortmaker. 2001. "Relation between Consumption of Sugar-Sweetened Drinks and Childhood Obesity: A Prospective, Observational Analysis." *Lancet* 35, no. 9255: 505–8. https://doi.org/10.1016/S0140-6736(00)04041-1.

Lund-Blix, Nicolai A., Lars C. Stene, Trond Rasmussen, Peter A. Torjesen, Lene F. Andersen, and Kjersti S. Rønningen. 2015. "Infant Feeding in Relation to Islet Autoimmunity and Type 1 Diabetes in Genetically Susceptible Children: The MIDIA Study." *Diabetes Care* 38: 257–63. doi: 10.2337/dc14–113.

Lustig, Robert H. 2012. *Fat Chance: Beating the Odds against Sugar, Processed Food, Obesity, and Disease.* New York: Hudson Street Press.

MacDonald, David B., and Graham Hudson. 2012. "The Genocide Question and Indian Residential Schools in Canada." *Canadian Journal of Political Science/Revue canadienne de science politique* 45, no. 2: 427–49. doi: https://doi.org/10.1017/S000842391200039X.

Mah, Catherine L. 2010. "Shokuiku: Governing Food and Public Health in Contemporary Japan." *Journal of Sociology* 46: 393–412.

Maher, Vanessa. 1992. "Breast-Feeding and Maternal Depletion: Natural Law or Cultural Arrangements?" In *The Anthropology of Breast-feeding: Natural Law or Social Construct*, ed. Vanessa Maher, 151–80. Oxford: Berg.

Mann, Michael D., Iain D. Hill, and M.D. Bowie. 1990. "Absorption and Retention in Acute Diarrhea." *European Journal of Clinical Nutrition* 44: 629–35.

Martinez, Gilbert A., and John P. Nalezienski. 1979. "The Recent Trend in Breast-Feeding." *Pediatrics* 64, no. 5: 686–92.

Marlowe, Frank W. 2010. *The Hadza: Hunter-Gatherers of Tanzania.* Berkeley, CA: University of California Press.

Martin, Molly A., and Adam M. Lippert. 2012. "Feeding Her Children, but Risking Her Health: The Intersection of Gender, Household Food Insecurity and Obesity." *Social Science and Medicine* 74, no. 11: 1754–64. https://doi.org/10.1016/j.socscimed.2011.11.013.

Martorell, Reynaldo. 1999. "The Nature of Child Malnutrition and Its Long-Term Implications." *Food and Nutrition Bulletin* 20, no. 3: 288–92. https://doi.org/10.1177/156482659902000304.

Martorell, Reynaldo, C. Yarbrough, S. Yarbrough, and R.E. Klein. 1980. "The Impact of Ordinary Illnesses on the Dietary Intake of Malnourished Children." *American Journal of Clinical Nutrition* 33: 345–50.

McCann, Margaret F., and Deborah E. Bender. 2006. "Perceived Insufficient Milk as a Barrier to Optimal Infant Feeding: Examples from Bolivia." *Journal of Biosocial Science* 38, no. 3: 341–64. doi: 10.1017/S0021932005007170

McCullum, Christine, Ellen Desjardins, Vivica I. Kraak, Patricia, Ladipo, and Helen Costello. 2005. "Evidence-Based Strategies to Build Community Food Security." *Journal of the American Dietetic Association* 105, no. 2: 278–83. doi: 10.1016/j.jada.2004.12.015.

McDade, Thomas. 2001. Parent-Offspring Conflict and the Cultural Ecology of Breast-Feeding. *Human Nature* 12: 9–25. https://doi.org/10.1007/s12110-001-1011-0.

McDade, Thomas W., and Carol M. Worthman. 1998. "The Weanling's Dilemma Reconsidered: A Biocultural Analysis of Breastfeeding Ecology." *Journal of Developmental and Behavioral Pediatrics* 19: 286–99.

McIntyre, Lynn, Daniel J. Dutton, Cynthia Kwok, and J.C. Herbert Emery. 2016. "Reduction of Food Insecurity among Low-Income Canadian Seniors as a Likely Impact of a Guaranteed Annual Income." *Canadian Public Policy* 42, no. 3: 274–86. doi: 10.3138/cpp.2015-069.

McIntyre, Lynn, Suzanne Officer, and Lynne Robinson. 2003. "Feeling Poor: The Felt Experience Low-Income Lone Mothers." *Affilia* 18, no. 3: 316–31. doi: 10.1177/0886109903254581.

McKenna, James J., Helen Ball, and Lee T. Gettler. 2007. "Mother-Infant Cosleeping, Breastfeeding, and Sudden Infant Death Syndrome: What Biological Anthropology Has Discovered about Normal Infant Sleep and Pediatric Sleep Medicine." *Yearbook of Physical Anthropology* 50: 133–61.

McKenna, James J., and Lee Gettler. 2016. "There Is No Such Thing as Infant Sleep, There Is No Such Thing as Breastfeeding, There Is Only Breastsleeping." *Acta Paediatrica* 105: 12–17

McKenna, James J., and Thomas McDade. 2005. "Why Babies Should Never Sleep Alone: A Review of the Co-Sleeping Controversy in Relation to SIDS, Bed Sharing and Breastfeeding." *Paediatric Respiratory Reviews* 6, 134–52.

McKerracher, Luseadra J., Mark Collard, Rachel M. Altman, Daniel Sellen, and Pablo A. Nepomnaschy. 2017. "Energy-Related Influences on Variation in Breastfeeding Duration among Indigenous Maya Women from Guatemala." *American Journal of Physical Anthropology* 162, no. 4: 616–26.

McKerracher, Luseadra, Mary Barker, Tina Moffat, Sarah Oresnik, Dianna Williams, and Deborah Sloboda. 2020. "Addressing Embodied Inequities in Health: How Do We Enable Improvement in Women's Diet in Pregnancy? *Public Health Nutrition* 23, no. 16: 2994–3004. doi: 10.1017/S1368980020001093.

McKerracher, Luseadra, Tina Moffat, Mary Barker, D. Williams, and Deborah M. Sloboda. 2019. "Translating the Developmental Origins of Health and Disease Concept to Improve the Nutritional Environment for Our Next Generations: A Call for a Reflexive, Positive, Multi-Level Approach." *Journal of Developmental Origins of Health and Disease* 10: 420–28. doi: 10.1017/S2040174418001034.

McNew, Aimee. 2016. "Is the Paleo Diet Safe for Babies?" *PaleoPlan*. http://www.paleoplan.com/2016/11–30/is-the-paleo-diet-safe-for-babies/.

Mei, Zuguo, Laurence M. Grummer-Strawn, Angelo Pietrobelli, Ailsa Goulding, Michael I. Goran, and William H. Dietz. 2002. "Validity of Body Mass Index Compared with Other Body-Composition Screening Indexes for the Assessment of Body Fatness in Children and Adolescents." *American Journal of Clinical Nutrition* 75, no. 6: 978–85.

Melchior, Maria, Jean-François Chastang, Bruno Falissard, Cédric Galéra, Richard E. Tremblay, Sylvana M. Côté, and Michel Boivin. 2012. "Food Insecurity and Children's Mental Health: A Prospective Birth Cohort Study." *PLoSOne* 7, no. 12: 52615. http://dx.doi.org/10.1016/j.prrv.2005.03.006.

References

Mendly-Zambo, Zsofia, and Dennis Raphael. 2018. "Competing Discourses of Household Food Insecurity in Canada." *Social Policy and Society*, 1–20. doi: 10.1017/S1474746418000428.

Mennella, Julie A., Nuala K. Bobowski, and Danielle R. Reed. 2016. "The Biology of Sweet Taste: From Biology to Hedonics." *Review of Endocrinological Metabolic Disorders* 17: 171–78. doi 10.1007/s11154-016-9360-5.

Milward, Joe D. 2017. "Nutrition, Infection and Stunting: The Roles of Deficiencies of Individual Nutrients and Foods, and of Inflammation, as Determinants of Reduced Linear Growth of Children." *Nutrition Research Reviews* 30: 50–72. doi: 10.1017/S0954422416000238.

Mintz, Sidney W. 1979. "Time, Sugar and Sweetness." *Marxist Perspectives* 2, no. 4: 56–73.

–. 1985. *Sweetness and Power: The Place of Sugar in Modern History*. New York: Penguin Books.

Moffat, Tina. 1998. "Growing up among the Looms: The Growth and Nutrition of Children Living in a Peri-Urban Environment in Kathmandu, Nepal." PhD diss., McMaster University.

–. 2000. "Parents' Estimation of Their Children's Body Size Compared to Classification of Children's Nutritional Status Using the International Growth Reference." *Ecology of Food and Nutrition* 39, no. 4: 311–29. https://doi.org/10.1080/036702 44.2000.9991621.

–. 2001. "The Weaning Process as a Biocultural Practice: A Case Study of Peri-Urban Mothers and Infants in Nepal." *Journal of Biosocial Science* 33: 321–38.

–. 2002. "Breastfeeding, Wage Labor and Insufficient Milk in Peri-Urban Kathmandu, Nepal." *Medical Anthropology* 21: 207–30.

–. 2003. "Diarrhea, Respiratory Infections, Protozoan Gastrointestinal Parasites, and Child Growth in Kathmandu, Nepal." *American Journal of Physical Anthropology* 122, no. 1: 85–97. https://doi.org/10.1002/ajpa.10258.

–. 2010. "The 'Childhood Obesity Epidemic': Health Crisis or Social Construction?" *Medical Anthropology Quarterly* 24, no. 1: 1–21.

Moffat, Tina, and Elizabeth Finnis. 2010. "Dietary Diversity, Dietary Transitions, and Childhood Nutrition in Nepal." In *Human Diet and Nutrition in Biocultural Perspective: Past Meets Present*, ed. Tina Moffat and Tracy Prowse, 133–51. New York: Berghahn Press.

Moffat, Tina, and Tracey Galloway. 2007. "Adverse Environments: Investigating Local Variation in Child Growth." *American Journal of Human Biology* 19, no. 5: 676–83.

Moffat, Tina, Tracey Galloway, and James Latham. 2005. "Stature and Adiposity among Children in Contrasting Neighbourhoods in the City of Hamilton, Ontario, Canada." *American Journal of Human Biology* 17, no. 3: 355–67.

Moffat, Tina, and Danielle Gendron. 2019. "Cooking up the "Gastro-Citizen" through School Meal Programs in France and Japan." *Food, Culture and Society* 22, no. 1: 63–77. doi: 10.1080/15528014.2018.1547587.

Moffat, Tina, and Ann D. Herring. 1999. "The Historical Roots of High Rates of Infant Death in Aboriginal Communities in Canada in the Early Twentieth Century: The Case of Fisher River, Manitoba." *Social Science and Medicine* 48: 1821–32.

Moffat, Tina, Charlene Mohammed, and Bruce Newbold. 2017. "Cultural Food Security among Immigrants and Refugees." *Human Organization* 76, no. 1: 15–27.

Moffat, Tina, and Tracy L. Prowse. 2018. "Biocultural and Bioarchaeological Approaches to Infant and Young Child Feeding in the Past." In *Children and Childhood in Bioarchaeology*, ed. Patrick Beauchesne and Sabrina C. Agarwal, 98–126. Gainesville: University of Florida Press.

Moffat, Tina, and Danielle Thrasher. 2016. "School Meal Programs and Their Potential to Operate as School-Based Obesity Prevention and Nutrition Interventions: Case Studies from France and Japan." *Critical Public Health* 26, no. 2: 133–46.

Mohanty, Chandra T. 1991. "Under Western Eyes: Feminist Scholarship and Colonialist Discourse." In *Third World Women and the Politics Of Feminism*, ed. Chandra T. Mohanty, Ann Russo, and Lourdes Torres, 51–80. Bloomington: Indiana University Press.

Monsebraaten, Laurie. 2018. "Cancellation of Ontario's Basic Income Project Sparks Global Outrage." *Toronto Star*, 18 September. https://www.thestar.com/news/queenspark/2018/09/14/cancellation-of-ontarios-basic-income-project-sparks-global-outrage.html.

Moore, Amelia. 2015. "Anthropocene Anthropology: Reconceptualizing Contemporary Global Change." *Journal of the Royal Anthropological Institute* 22: 27–46.

Moore, Henrietta L. 2006. "The Future of Gender or the End of a Brilliant Career?" In *Feminist Anthropology. Past, Present, and Future*, ed. P.L. Geller and M.K. Stockett, 23–42. Philadelphia: University of Pennsylvania Press.

Morgan, Kevin, and Roberto Sonnino. 2008. *The School Food Revolution: Public Food and the Challenge of Sustainable Development*. London: Earthscan.

Mosby, Ian. 2012. "Making and Breaking Canada's Food Rules: Science, the State, and the Government of Nutrition, 1942–1949." In *Edible Histories, Cultural Politics: Towards a Canadian Food History*, ed. Franca Iacovetta, Valerie J. Korinek, and Marlene Epp, 409–2. Toronto: University of Toronto Press.

Mosby, Ian, and Tracey Galloway. 2017. "Hunger Was Never Absent": How Residential School Diets Shaped Current Patterns of Diabetes among Indigenous Peoples in Canada." 14, no. 189: E1043–45. doi: 10.1503/cmaj.170448.

Moss, Michael. 2013. *Salt Sugar, Fat: How the Food Giants Hooked Us*. New York: Random House.

Myers, Samuel S., Matthew R. Smith, Sarah Guth, Cristopher D. Golden, Bapu Vaitla, Nathaniel D. Mueller, Alan D. Dangour, and Peter Huybers. 2017. "Climate Change and Global Food Systems: Potential Impacts on Food Security and Undernutrition." *Annual Review of Public Health* 38, no. 1: 259–77. https://doi.org/10.1146/annurev-publhealth-031816-044356.

NCD Risk Factor Collaboration (NCD-RisC). 2017. "Worldwide Trends in Body-Mass Index, Underweight, Overweight, and Obesity from 1975 to 2016: A Pooled Analysis of 2416 Population-Based Measurement Studies in 128.9 Million Children, Adolescents, and Adults." *Lancet* 390: 2627–42. http://dx.doi.org/10.1016.

Nelson, Michael, K. Lowes, V. Hwang, and members of the Nutrition Group, School Meals Review Panel, Department for Education and Skills. 2007. "The

Contribution of School Meals to Food Consumption and Nutrient Intakes of Young People Aged 4–18 Years in England." *Public Health Nutrition* 10, no. 7: 652–62.

Nestle, Marion. 2002. *Food Politics*. Berkeley: University of California Press.

Ng, Shu Wen, Juan A. Rivera, Barry M. Popkin, and M. Arantxa Colchero. 2019. "Did High Sugar-Sweetened Beverage Purchasers Respond Differently to the Excise Tax on Sugar-Sweetened Beverages in Mexico?" *Public Health Nutrition* 22, no. 4: 750–56. doi: 10.1017/S136898001800321X.

Nguyen, P.K., S. Lin, and P. Heidenreich. 2016. "A Systematic Comparison of Sugar Content in Low-Fat vs Regular Versions of Food." *Nutrition and Diabetes* 6: 1–3. doi: 10.1038/nutd.2015.43.

NIH (National Institutes of Health). n.d. *Calcium: Fact Sheet for Health Professionals*. https://ods.od.nih.gov/factsheets/Calcium-HealthProfessional/.

Nisbett, Nicholas. 2019. "Understanding the Nourishment of Bodies at the Centre of Food and Health Systems – Systemic, Bodily and New Materialist Perspectives on Nutritional Inequity." *Social Science and Medicine* 228 (2019): 9–16.

Nord, Mark, and Kathleen Romig. 2007. "Hunger in the Summer: Seasonal Food Insecurity and the National School Lunch and Summer Food Service Programs." *Journal of Children and Poverty* 12, no. 2: 141–58. doi: 10.1080/10796120600879582.

O'Gara, Chloe. 1989. "Breastfeeding and Maternal Employment in Urban Honduras." In *Women, Work, and Child Welfare in the Third World* (AAAS Selected Symposium 110), ed. Joanne Leslie and Michael Paolisso, 113–30. Boulder, CO: Westview Press.

O'Gara, Chloe, Judy Canahuati, and Martin A. Moore. 1994. "Every Mother Is a Working Mother: Breastfeeding and Women's Work." *International Journal of Gynecology and Obstetrics* 47 (Suppl): S33-S39. https://doi.org/10.1016/0020-7292(94)02232-N.

Oken, Emily. 2009. "Maternal and Child Obesity: The Causal Link." *Obstetrics and Gynecology Clinics of North America* 36: 361–77. doi: 10.1016/j.ogc.2009.03.007.

Oken, Emily, and Matthew W. Gillman. 2003. "Fetal Origins of Obesity." *Obesity Research* 11, no. 4: 496–506.

Olshansky, S. Jay, Douglas J. Passaro, Ronald C. Hershow, Jennifer M.D. Layden, Bruce A. Carnes, Jacob M.D. Brody, Leonard Hayflick, Robert N. Butler, David B. Allison, and David S. Ludwig. 2005. "A Potential Decline in Life Expectancy in the United States in the 21st Century." *New England Journal of Medicine* 352 (11): 1138–45.

Olson, Christine M. 2005. "Food Insecurity in Women: A Recipe for Unhealthy Trade-Offs." *Topics in Clinical Nutrition* 20, no. 4: 321–28.

O'Neill, T. 1997. "Carpets, Markets and Makers: Culture and Entrepreneurship in the Tibeto- Nepalese Carpet Industry." PhD diss., McMaster University.

Ontario Government. 2017. *Ontario Basic Income Pilot*. https://www.ontario.ca/page/ontario-basic-income-pilot.

Opie, Iona, and Peter Opie. 1997. *The Oxford Dictionary of Nursery Rhymes*. 2nd ed. Oxford: Oxford University Press.

Ostroff, Joshua. 2015. "The Dutch City of Utrecht Is Doling Out Free Money for a 'Basic Income' Experiment." *Huffington Post Canada*, 10 July. https://www.huffingtonpost.ca/2015/07/10/utrecht-basic-income_n_7770648.html.

Oxfam. 2013. *Behind the Brands: Food Justice and the 'Big 10' Food and Beverage Companies.* 166 Oxfam Briefing Paper.

Paeratakul, Sahasporn, Daphne P. Ferdinand, Catherine M. Champagne, Donna H. Ryan, and George A. Bray. 2003. "Fast-Food Consumption among US Adults and Children: Dietary and Nutrient Intake Profile." *Journal of the American Dietetic Association* 103, no. 10: 1332–38.

Pan, An, and Frank B. Hu. 2011. "Effects of Carbohydrates on Satiety: Differences between Liquid and Solid Food." *Current Opinion in Clinical Nutrition and Metabolic Care* 14: 385–90.

Panter-Brick, Catherine. 1992. "Women's Work and Child Nutrition: The Food Intake of 0–4 Year Old Children in Rural Nepal." *Ecology of Food and Nutrition* 29: 11–24.

Panter-Brick, Catherine, and Malcom T. Smith, eds. 2000. *Abandoned Children.* Cambridge: Cambridge University Press.

Paolella, Giulia, and Pietro Vajro. 2016. "Childhood Obesity, Breastfeeding, Intestinal Microbiota, and Early Exposure to Antibiotics." *Journal of the American Medical Association Pediatrics* 170, no. 8: 735–37. doi: 10.1001/jamapediatrics.2016.0964.

Patel, Raj. 2012. *Stuffed and Starved: The Hidden Battle for the World Food System.* New York: Melville House.

Patico, Janet. 2020. *The Trouble with Snack Time.* New York: New York University Press.

Patico, Janet, and Eriberto P. Lozada Jr. 2019. "Children's Food." In *The Handbook of Food and Anthropology*, ed. Jakob A. Klein and James L. Watson, 200–26, New York: Bloomsbury Academic.

Pelto, Gretel H. 1987. "Cultural Issues in Maternal and Child Health and Nutrition." *Social Science and Medicine* 25, no. 6: 533–39.

Pelto, Gretel H., Darna L. Dufour, and Alan H. Goodman. 2013. "The Biocultural Perspective in Nutritional Anthropology." In *Nutritional Anthropology: Biocultural Perspectives on Food and Nutrition*, ed. Darna L. Dufour, Alan H. Goodman, and Gretel H. Pelto, 1–6. New York: Oxford University Press.

Pelto, Gretel H., Yuanyuan Zhang, and Jean-Pierre Habicht. 2010. "Premastication: The Second Arm of Infant and Young Child Feeding for Health and Survival?" *Maternal Child Nutrition* 6: 4–18.

Pérez-Escamilla, Rafael, Kenda Cunningham, and Victoria Hall Moran. 2020. "COVID-19 and Maternal and Child Food and Nutrition Insecurity: A Complex Syndemic." *Maternal and Child Nutrition* 16: e13036. doi: org/10.1111/mcn.13036.

Peterson-Withorn, Chase. 2016. "How Billionaires Get Rich: Which Industries Make the Most Mega-Fortunes?" *Forbes*, 7 March. https://www.forbes.com/sites/chasewithorn/2016/03/07/how-billionaires-get-rich-which-industries-make-the-most-mega-fortunes/#82dfd6545e16).

Piernas, Carmen, and Barry M. Popkin. 2010. "Trends in Snacking among US Children." *Health Affairs* 29, no. 3: 398–404.

Pietrykowski, Bruce. 2004. "You Are What You Eat: The Social Economy of the Slow Food Movement." *Review of Social Economy* 62, no. 3: 307–21. doi: 10.1080/0034676042000253927.

References

Pike, Ivey L., and Lauren A. Milligan. 2010. "Pregnancy and Lactation." In *Human Evolutionary Biology*, ed. Michael P. Muehlenbein, 338–50. Cambridge: Cambridge University Press.

Piperata, Barbara A., Seungjun Lee, Alba C. Mayta Apaza, Adelaide Cary, Samuel Vilchez, Pallavi Oruganti, Rebecca Garabed, Warren Wilson, and Jiyoung Lee. 2019. "Characterization of the Gut Microbiota of Nicaraguan Children in a Water Insecure Context." *American Journal of Human Biology* 32, no. 10: 1–18.

Piperata, Barbara A., Kammi K. Schmeer, Craig Hadley, and Genevieve Ritchie-Ewing. 2013. "Dietary Inequalities of Mother–Child Pairs in the Rural Amazon: Evidence of Maternal-Child Buffering?" *Social Science and Medicine* 96: 183–91. https://doi.org/10.1016/j.socscimed.2013.07.024.

Pitkin, Roy M. 2007. "Folate and Neural Tube Defects." *American Journal of Clinical Nutrition* 85, no. 1: 285S–8S.

Pollan, Michael. 2006. *The Omnivore's Dilemma*. London: Bloomsbury.

Popkin, Barry M. 2006. "Global Nutrition Dynamics: The World Is Shifting Rapidly toward a Diet Linked with Noncommunicable Diseases." *American Journal of Clinical Nutrition* 84, no. 2: 289–98. https://doi.org/10.1093/ajcn/84.2.289.

Popkin, B.M., C. Corvalan, and L.M. Grummer-Strawn. 2020. "Dynamics of the Double Burden of Malnutrition and the Changing Nutrition Reality." *The Lancet* 395, no. 10217: 65-74.

Poppendieck, Janet. 2010. *Free for All: Fixing School Food in America*. Berkeley, CA: University of California Press.

Poti, Jennifer M., and Barry M. Popkin. 2011. "Trends in Energy Intake among US Children Eating Location and Food Source, 1977–2006." *Journal of the American Dietetic Association* 111, no. 8: 1156–64. doi: 10.1016/j.jada.2011.05.007.

Potvin Kent, Monique, Erika Rudnicki, and Crystal Usher. 2017. "Less Healthy Breakfast Cereals Are Promoted More Frequently in Large Supermarket Chains in Canada." *BMC Public Health* 17: 877–84. doi: 10.1186/s12889-017-4886-3.

Power, Elaine M. 2005. "The Unfreedom of Being Other: Canadian Lone Mothers' Experiences of Poverty and 'Life on the Cheque.'" *Sociology* 39, no. 4: 634–60. doi: 10.1177/0038038505056023.

–. 2008. "Conceptualizing Food Security for Aboriginal People in Canada." *Canadian Journal of Public Health* 99: 95–97.

–. 2014. "Food and Poverty in High Income Countries." In *Encyclopedia of Food and Agricultural Ethics*, ed. Paul B. Thompson and David M. Kaplan, 830–38, Dordrecht: Springer.

–. 2016. "Fat Children, Failed (Future) Consumer-Citizens, and Mothers' Duties in Neoliberal Consumer Society." In *Neoliberal Governance and Health: Duties, Risks, and Vulnerabilities*, ed. Elaine M. Power and Jessica Polzer, 45–65. Montreal and Kingston: McGill-Queen's University Press.

Power, Elaine M., Margaret H. Little, and Patricia A. Collins. 2014. "Should Canadian Health Promoters Support a Food Stamp-Style Program to Address Food Insecurity?" *Health Promotion International* 30, no. 1: 184–93. doi: 10.1093/heapro/dau080.

Prendergast, Andrew J., and Jean H. Humphrey. 2014. "The Stunting Syndrome in Developing Countries." *Paediatrics and International Child Health* 34, no. 4: 250–65. doi: 10.1179/2046905514Y.0000000158.

Prowse, Tracy L., Shelley R. Saunders, Henry P. Schwarcz, Peter Garnsey, Luca Bondioli, and Roberto Macchiarelli. 2008. "Isotopic and Dental Evidence for Infant and Young Child Feeding Practices in an Imperial Roman Skeletal Sample." *American Journal of Physical Anthropology* 137, no. 3: 294–308.

Prowse, Tracy L., Shelley Saunders, Charles Fitzgerald, Luca Bondioli, and Roberto Macchiarelli. 2010. "Growth, Morbidity, and Mortality in Antiquity: A Case Study from Imperial Rome." In Studies of the Biosocial Society, vol. 5, *Human Diet and Nutrition in Biocultural Perspective*, ed. Tina Moffat and Tracy Prowse, 173–96. New York: Berghahn Books.

Qasem, Wafaa, Tanis Fenton, and James Friel. 2015. "Age of Introduction of First Complementary Feeding for Infants: A Systematic Review." *BMC Pediatrics* 15: 107. doi: 10.1186/s12887-015-0409-5.

Racey, Megan, Charlene O'Brien, Sabrina Douglas, Olivia Marquez, Gilly Hendrie, and Genevieve Newton. 2016. "Systematic Review of School-Based Interventions to Modify Dietary Behavior: Does Intervention Intensity Impact Effectiveness?" *Journal of School Health* 86, no. 6: 452–63.

Raine, Kim D., Tim Lobstein, Jane Landon, Monique Potvin Kent, Suzie Pellerin, Timothy Caulfield, Diane Finegood, Lyne Mongeau, Neil Neary, and John C. Spence. 2013. "Restricting Marketing to Children: Consensus on Policy Interventions to Address Obesity." *Journal of Public Health Policy* 34, no. 2: 239–53.

Ramakrishnan, Usha. 2004. "Nutrition and Low Birth Weight: From Research to Practice." *American Journal of Clinical Nutrition* 79, no. 1: 17–21. https://doi.org/10.1093/ajcn/79.1.17

Rao, Deepa P., E. Kropac, M.T. Do, K.C. Roberts, and G.C Jayaraman. 2016. "Childhood Overweight and Obesity Trends in Canada." *Health Promotion and Chronic Disease Prevention in Canada* 36, no. 9: 194–98.

Raulio, Susanna, Eva Roos, and Ritva Prättälä. 2010. "School and Workplace Meals Promote Healthy Food Habits." *Public Health Nutrition* 13, no. 6: 987–92.

Ravelli, A.C., J.H. van der Meulen, R.P. Michels, Clive Osmond, David J.P. Barker, C. Nicholas Hales, and O.P. Bleker. 1998. "Glucose Tolerance in Adults after Prenatal Exposure to Famine." *Lancet* 351, no. 9097: 173–77.

Reiches, Meredith W. 2019. "Adolescence as a Biocultural Life History Transition." *Annual Review of Anthropology* 48: 151–68, https://doi.org/10.1146/annurev-anthro-102218-011118.

Reilly, John J., and Jonathan C.K. Wells. 2005. "Duration for Exclusive Breast-Feeding: Introduction of Complementary Feeding May Be Necessary before 6 Months of Age." *British Journal of Nutrition* 94, no. 6: 869–72.

Ricciardi, Vincent, Navin Ramankutty, Zia Mehrabi, Lariss Jarvis, and Brenton Chookolingo. 2018. "How Much of the World's Food Do Smallholders Produce?" *Global Food Security* 17: 64–72. https://doi.org/10.1016/j.gfs.2018.05.002.

Ristovski-Slijepcevic, Svetlana, Gwen E. Chapman, and Brenda L. Beagan. 2008. "Engaging with Healthy Eating Discourse(s): Ways of Knowing about Food and

Health in Three Ethnocultural Groups in Canada." *Appetite* 50: 167–78. doi: 10.1016/j.appet.2007.07.001.

Roberts, Karen C., Margo Shields, Margaret de Groh, Alfred Aziz, and Jo-Anne Gilbert. 2012. "Overweight and Obesity in Children and Adolescents: Results from the 2009 to 2011 Canadian Health Measures Survey." *Health Reports*, Statistics Canada, Catalogue No. 82–003-XPE 23(3): 37–41.

Roberts, Susan B., and Gerard E. Dallal. 2001. "The New Childhood Growth Charts." *Nutrition Reviews* 59, no. 2: 31–36.

Rodd, Celia, and Atul K. Sharma. 2016. "Recent Trends in the Prevalence of Overweight and Obesity among Canadian Children." *Canadian Medical Association Journal* 188, no. 13: E31–E320. doi: 10.1503 /cmaj.150854.

Rodriguez, Juan Miguel, Kiera Murphy, Catherine Stanton, R. Paul Ross, Olivia I. Kober, Nathalie Juge, Ekaterina Avershina, Knut Rudi, Arjan Narbad, Maria C. Jenmalm, Juliana R Marchesi, and Maria Carmen Collado. 2015. "The Composition of the Gut Microbiota throughout Life, with an Emphasis on Early Life." *Microbial Ecology in Health and Disease* 26: 1. doi: 10.3402/mehd.v26.26050.

Rogers, B.L., and N. Youssef. 1988. "The Importance of Women's Involvement in Economic Activities in the Improvement of Child Nutrition and Health." *Food and Nutrition Bulletin* 10, no. 3: 33–41.

Rosenkranz, Richard R., and David A. Dzewaltowski. 2008. "Model of the Home Food Environment Pertaining to Childhood Obesity." *Nutrition Reviews* 66, no. 3: 123–40.

Rosin, Hanna. 2009. "The Case Against Breastfeeding." *Atlantic Monthly*, April.

Rosser, Sue V. 1997. "Possible Implications of Feminist Theories for the Study of Evolution." In *Feminism and Evolutionary Biology. Boundaries, Intersections, and Frontiers*, ed. Patricia Adair Gowaty, 21–41. New York: Chapman and Hall.

Rozin, Paul, and Theresa A. Vollmecke. 1986. "Food Likes and Dislikes." *Annual Review of Nutrition* 6: 433–56. https://doi.org/10.1146/annurev.nu.06.070186.002245.

Rundle, Andrew G., Yoosun Park, Julie B. Herbstman, Eliza W. Kinsey, and Y. Claire Wang. 2020. "COVID-19–Related School Closings and Risk of Weight Gain Among Children." *Obesity* 28, no. 6: 1008–9. doi: 10.1002/oby.22813.

Rydell, Sarah A., Lisa J. Harnack, J. Michael Oakes, Mary Story, Robert W. Jeffery, and Simone A. French. 2008. "Why Eat at Fast-Food Restaurants: Reported Reasons among Frequent Consumers." *Journal of the American Dietetic Association* 108, no. 12: 2066–70.

Sadegholvad, Sanaz, Heather Yeatman, Anne-Maree Parrish, and Anthony Worsley. 2017. "What Should Be Taught in Secondary Schools' Nutrition and Food Systems Education? Views from Prominent Food-Related Professionals in Australia." *Nutrients* 9, no. 1207: 1–14. doi: 10.3390/nu9111207.

Salanave, Benoit, Sandrine Peneau, Marie-Françoise Rolland-Cachera, Serge Hercberg, and Kata Castetbon. 2009. "Stabilization of Overweight Prevalence in French Children between 2000 and 2007." *International Journal of Pediatric Obesity* 4: 66–72.

Sánchez-Pimienta, Tania G., Carolina Batis, Chessa K. Lutter, and Juan A. Rivera. 2016. "Sugar-Sweetened Beverages Are the Main Sources of Added Sugar Intake in the Mexican Population." *Journal of Nutrition* 146, no. 9: 1888S–96S.

Satter, Ellyn M. 1986. "The Feeding Relationship." *Journal of the American Dietetic Association* 86: 352–56.

Saul, Nick, and Andrea Curtis. 2013. *The Stop: How the Fight for Good Food Transformed a Community and Inspired a Movement.* Brooklyn: Melville House.

Scaglioni, Silvia, Michela Salvioni, and Cinzia Galimberti. 2008. "Influence of Parental Attitudes in the Development of Children and Eating Behaviour." *British Journal of Nutrition* 99, no. S1: S22–S25. doi: 10.1017/S0007114508892471.

Schell, Lawrence M. 2020. "Modern Water: A Biocultural Approach to Water Pollution at the Akwesasne Mohawk Nation." *American Journal of Human Biology* 32: e23348. https://doi.org/10.1002/ajhb.23348.

Schlosser, Eric. 2002. *Fast Food Nation: The Dark Side of the All-American Meal.* New York: Houghton Mifflin.

Schor, Juliet B. 2004. *Born to Buy. The Commercialized Child and the New Consumer Culture.* New York: Scribner.

Schor, Juliet B., and Margaret Ford. 2007. "From Tastes Great to Cool: Children's Food Marketing and the Rise of the Symbolic." *Journal of Law, Medicine and Ethics* 35, no. 1: 10–21.

Scrinis, G. 2012. *Nutritionism. The Science and Politics of Dietary Advice.* New York: University of Columbia Press.

Sela, David A., J. Chapman, A. Adeuya, J.H. Kim, F. Chen, T.R. Whitehead, A. Lapidus, D.S. Rokhsar, C.B. Lebrilla, J.B. German, N.P. Price, P.M. Richardson, and D.A. Mills. 2008. "The Genome Sequence of Bifidobacterium Longum Subsp. Infantis Reveals Adaptations for Milk Utilization within the Infant Microbiome." *Proceedings of the National Academy of Science* 105, no. 48: 18964–69. doi: 10.1073pnas.0809584105.

Selby, Jennifer A. 2011. "French Secularism as a 'Guarantor' of Women's Rights? Muslim Women and Gender Politics in a Parisian Banlieue." *Culture and Religion* 12, no. 4: 441–62.

Seligman, Hilary K., Barbara A. Laraia, and Margo B. Kushel. 2009. "Food Insecurity Is Associated with Chronic Disease among Low-Income." *Journal of Nutrition* 140: 304–10.

Sellen, Daniel W. 2001. "Weaning, Complementary Feeding, and Maternal Decision Making in a Rural East African Population." *Journal of Human Lactation* 17, no. 3: 233–44.

–. 2007. "Evolution of Infant and Young Child Feeding: Implications for Contemporary Public Health." *Annual Review of Nutrition* 27: 123–48.

–. 2010. "Infant and Young Child Feeding in Human Evolution." In *Human Diet and Nutrition in Biocultural Perspective: Studies of the Biosocial Society*, vol. 5, ed. Tina Moffat and Tracy Prowse, 57–88. New York: Berghahn Books.

Shao Mlay, Rose, Barbara Keddy, and Phyllis Noerager Stern. 2004. "Demands out of Context: Tanzanian Women Combining Exclusive Breastfeeding with Employment." *Health Care for Women International* 25, no. 3: 242–54.

Sidaner, Emilie, Daniel Balaban, and Lucienne Burlandy. 2013. "The Brazilian School Feeding Programme: An Example of an Integrated Programme in Support of

Food and Nutrition Security." *Public Health Nutrition* 16, no. 6: 989–94. doi: 10.1017/S1368980012005101.

Sigal, Ronald J., Glen P. Kenny, David H. Wasserman, Carmen Castaneda-Sceppa, and Russell D. White. 2006. "Physical Activity/Exercise and Type 2 Diabetes. A Consensus Statement from the American Diabetes Association." *Diabetes Care* 29, no. 6: 1433–38. doi: 10.2337/dc06–9910.

Simen-Kapeu, Aline, and Paul J. Veugelers. 2010. "Should Public Health Interventions Aimed at Reducing Childhood Overweight and Obesity Be Gender-Focused?" *BMC Public Health* 10, no. 340: 1–7. http://www.biomedcentral.com/1471-2458/10/340.

Simmonds, M., A. Llewellyn, Chris G. Owen, and N. Woolacott. 2016. "Predicting Adult Obesity from Childhood Obesity: A Systematic Review and Meta-Analysis." *Obesity Reviews* 17: 95–107. doi: 10.1111/obr.12334.

Singh, Gopal K., Mohammad Siahpush and Michael D. Kogan. 2010. "Rising Social Inequalities in US Childhood Obesity, 2003–2007." *Annals of Epidemiology* 20: 40–52.

Slater, J., G. Sevenhuysen, B. Edginton, and J. O'Neil, J. 2012. "Trying to Make It All Come Together": Structuration and Employed Mothers' Experience of Family Food Provisioning in Canada." *Health Promotion International* 27, no. 3: 405–15.

Slining, Meghan M., Kevin C. Mathias, and Barry M. Popkin. 2013. "Trends in Food and Beverage Sources among US Children and Adolescents: 1989–2010." *Journal of the Academy of Nutrition and Dietetics* 113, no. 12: 1683–94.

Smith, Chery, and Rickelle Richards. 2008. "Dietary Intake, Overweight Status, and Perceptions of Food Insecurity among Homeless Minnesotan Youth." *American Journal of Human Biology* 20, no. 5: 550–63. doi: 10.1002/ajhb.20780.

Smolin, Lori A., Mary B. Grosvenor, and Debbie Gurfinkel. 2012. *Nutrition: Science and Applications*. Canadian edition. Mississauga, ON: John Wiley and Sons.

Sobal, Jeffery, Laura Kahn, and Carole Bisogni. 1998. "A Conceptual Model of the Food and Nutrition System." *Social Science and Medicine* 47, no. 7: 853–63.

Sonnino, Roberta. 2009. "Quality Food, Public Procurement, and Sustainable Development: The School Meal Revolution in Rome." *Environment and Planning*, A 41: 425–40. doi: 10.1068/a40112.

Soubry, Adelheid. 2018. "POHaD: Why We Should Study Future Fathers." *Environmental Epigenetics* 4, no. 2: 1–7. doi: 10.1093/eep/dvy007.

Statistics Canada. 2015. *Study: Prevalence of Obesity among Children and Adolescents in the United States and Canada, 1976 to 2013*. https://www150.statcan.gc.ca/n1/daily-quotidien/150826/dq150826a-eng.htm.

–. 2017. *Census Brief: Children Living in Low-Income Households*. https://www12.statcan.gc.ca/census-recensement/2016/as-sa/98–200-x/2016012/98–200-x2016012-eng.cfm.

Stephenson, Judith, Nicola Heslehurst, Jennifer Hall, Danielle A.J.M. Schoenaker, Jayne Hutchinson, Janet E. Cade, Lucilla Poston, Geraldine Barrett, Sarah R. Crozier, Mary Barker, Kalyanaraman Kumaran, Chittaranjan S. Yajnik, Janis Baird, and Gita D. Mishra. 2018. *Lancet* 391, no. 10132: 1830–41. https://doi.org/10.1016/S0140-6736(18)30311-8.

Stevens, Emily E., Thelma E. Patrick, and Rita Pickler. 2009. "A History of Infant Feeding." *Journal of Perinatal Education* 18, no. 2: 32–39. doi: 10.1624/105812409X426314.

Stevens, Gretchen A., James E. Bennett, Quenton Hennocq, Yuan Lu, Luz Maria De-Regil, Lisa Rogers, Goodarz Danaei, Guangquan Li, Richard A. White, Seth R. Flaxman, Sean-Patrick Oehrle, Mariel M. Finucane, Ramiro Guerrero, Zulfiqar A. Bhutta, Amarilis Then-Paulino, Wafaie Fawzi, Robert E. Black, and Majid Ezzati. 2015. "Trends and Mortality Effects of Vitamin A Deficiency in Children in 138 Low-Income and Middle-Income Countries between 1991 and 2013: A Pooled Analysis of Population-Based Surveys." *Lancet Global Health* 3, no. 9: e528–e536. https://doi.org/10.1016/S2214-109X(15)00039-X.

Stone, Pamela K. 2016. "Biocultural Perspectives on Maternal Mortality and Obstetrical Death from the Past to the Present." *Yearbook of Physical Anthropology* 159: S150–71.

Subramanian, Meera. 2019. "Anthropocene Now: Influential Panel Votes to Recognize Earth's New Epoch." *Nature News*, 21 May. https://www.nature.com/articles/d41586-019-01641-5.

Swallen, Karen C., Eric N. Reither, Steven A. Haas, and Ann M. Meier. 2005. "Overweight, Obesity, and Health-Related Quality of Life among Adolescents: The National Longitudinal Study of Adolescent Health." *Pediatrics* 115, no. 2: 340–7.

Swinburn, Boyd, Garry Egger, and Fezeela Raza. 1999. "Dissecting Obesogenic Environments: The Development and Application of a Framework for Identifying and Prioritizing Environmental Interventions for Obesity." *Preventive Medicine* 29, no. 6: 563–70. https://doi.org/10.1006/pmed.1999.0585.

Szabo, Michelle. 2011. "The Challenges of 'Re-engaging with Food." *Food, Culture and Society* 14, no. 4: 547–66. doi: 10.2752/175174411X13046092851514.

Tapias, Maria. 2006. "'Always Ready and Always Clean'? Competing Discourse of Breast-Feeding, Infant Illness, and the Politics of Mother-Blame in Bolivia." *Body and Society* 12, no. 2: 83–108. https://doi.org/10.1177/1357034X06064324.

Tarabashkina, Liudmila, Pascale Quester, and Roberta Crouch. 2016. "Social Exploring the Moderating Effect of Children's Nutritional Knowledge on the Relationship between Product Evaluations and Food Choice." *Social Science and Medicine* 149: 145–52. https://doi.org/10.1016/j.socscimed.2015.11.046.

Tarasuk, Valerie. 2017. "A Critical Examination of Community-Based Responses to Household Food Insecurity in Canada." *Health Education and Behavior* 28, no. 4: 487–99. https://doi.org/10.1177/109019810102800408.

–. 2001. *Implications of a Basic Income Guarantee for Household Food Insecurity.* Research Paper No. 24. Thunder Bay, ON: Northern Policy Institute.

Tarasuk, Valerie, Andrew Mitchell, Lindsay McLaren, and Lynn McIntyre. 2013. "Chronic Physical and Mental Health Conditions among Adults May Increase Vulnerability to Household Food Insecurity." *Journal of Nutrition* 143, no. 11: 1785–93. https://doi.org/10.3945/jn.113.178483.

Tarasuk, Valerie, and Andrew Mitchell. 2020. *Household Food Insecurity in Canada, 2017–18.* Toronto: Research to Identify Policy Options to Reduce Food Insecurity (PROOF). https://proof.utoronto.ca/.

Tasch, Barbara. 2017. "Ranked: The 30 Poorest Countries in the World." *Business Insider*, 7 March. https://www.businessinsider.com/the-25-poorest-countries-in-the-world-2017-3?r=UK.

Taveras, Elsie M., Catherine S. Berkey, Sheryl L. Rifas-Shiman, David S. Ludwig, Helaine R.H. Rockett, Alison E. Field, Graham A. Colditz, and Matthew W. Gillman. 2005. "Association of Consumption of Fried Food Away from Home with Body Mass Index and Diet Quality in Older Children and Adolescents." *Pediatrics* 116, no. 4: e518–24. doi: 10.1542/peds.2004-2732.

Taylor, Caroline M., Susan M. Wernimont, K. Northstone, and Pauline M. Emmett. 2015. "Picky/Fussy Eating in Children: Review of Definitions, Assessment, Prevalence and Dietary Intakes." *Appetite* 95: 349–59.

Téchouyeres, Isabelle. 2003. "Eating at School in France." In *Eating Out in Europe*, ed. Marc Jacobs and Peter Scholliers, 373–88. Oxford: Berg.

Thomas, Heather M.C., and Jennifer D. Irwin. 2011. "Cook It Up! A Community-Based Cooking Program for At-Risk Youth: Overview of a Food Literacy Intervention." *BMC Research Notes* 4: 495. http://www.biomedcentral.com/1756-0500/4/495.

Thompson, Amanda L. 2012. "Developmental Origins of Obesity: Early Feeding Environments, Infant Growth, and the Intestinal Microbiome." *American Journal of Human Biology* 24: 350–60.

Tremblay, Mark S., Valerie Carson, Jean-Philippe Chaput, Sarah Connor Gorber, Thy Dinh, Mary Duggan, Guy Faulkner, Casey E. Gray, Reut Gruber, Katherine Janson, Ian Janssen, Peter T. Katzmarzyk, Michelle E. Kho, Amy E. Latimer-Cheung, Claire LeBlanc, Anthony D. Okely, Timothy Olds, Russell R. Pate, Andrea Phillips, Veronica J. Poitras, Sophie Rodenburg, Margaret Sampson, Travis J. Saunders, James A. Stone, Gareth Stratton, Shelly K. Weiss, and Lori Zehr. 2016. "Canadian 24-Hour Movement Guidelines for Children and Youth: An Integration of Physical Activity, Sedentary Behaviour, and Sleep." *Applied Physiology, Nutrition, and Metabolism* 41, no. 6: S311–27. https://doi.org/10.1139/apnm-2016-0151.

Trivers, Robert L. 1974. "Parent-Offspring Conflict." *Integrative and Comparative Biology* 14, no. 1: 249–64.

Tucker, Bram, and Alyson G. Young. 2005. "Growing up Mikea: Children's Time Allocation and Tuber Foraging in Southwestern Madagascar." In *Hunter-Gatherer Childhoods: Evolutionary, Developmental and Cultural Perspectives*, ed. Barry S. Hewlett and Michael E. Lamb, 147–74. London: Routledge.

Tugault-Lafleur, Claire N., Jennifer L. Black, and Susan I. Barr. 2017. "Lunch-Time Food Source Is Associated with School Hour and School Day Diet Quality among Canadian Children." *Journal of Human Nutrition and Dietetics* 31, no. 1: 96–107. https://doi.org/10.1111/jhn.12500.

Tully, Kristin P., and Helen L. Ball. 2013. "Trade-Offs Underlying Maternal Breastfeeding Decisions: A Conceptual Model." *Maternal and Child Nutrition* 9: 90–98. doi: 10.1111/j.1740-8709.2011.00378.x.

Turnbaugh, Peter J., Ruth E. Ley, Michael A. Mahowald, Vincent Magrini, Elaine R. Mardis, and Jeffrey I. Gordon. 2006. "An Obesity-Associated Gut Microbiome with Increased Capacity for Energy Harvest." *Nature* 444: 1027–31. doi: 10.1038/nature05414.

UNESCO. 2010. "Gastronomic Meal of the French." http://www.unesco.org/culture/ich/en/RL/gastronomic-meal-of-the-french-00437.

—. 2013. "Washoku, Traditional Dietary Cultures of the Japanese, Notably for the Celebration of New Year." http://www.unesco.org/culture/ich/en/RL/washoku-traditional-dietary-cultures-of-the-japanese-notably-for-the-celebration-of-new-year-00869.

UNICEF. 2019. *The State of the World's Children 2019. Growing Well in a Changing World*. New York: UNICEF.

UNICEF Canada. 2017. *UNICEF Report Card 14: Canadian Companion, Oh Canada! Our Kids Deserve Better*. Toronto: UNICEF Canada.

United Nations. 2018. "68% of the World Population Projected to Live in Urban Areas by 2050, Says UN." United Nations News, 16 May. https://www.un.org/development/desa/en/news/population/2018-revision-of-world-urbanization-prospects.html.

USDA (United States Department of Agriculture). n.d.a. *Choose My Plate*. https://www.choosemyplate.gov/.

—. n.d.b. *Special Supplemental Nutrition Program for Women, Infants, and Children (WIC)*. https://www.fns.usda.gov/wic.

—. n.d.c. *Supplemental Nutrition Assistance Program (SNAP)*. https://www.fns.usda.gov/snap/supplemental-nutrition-assistance-program.

Vaidya, Abhinav, Suraj Shakya, and Alexandra Krettek. 2010. "Obesity Prevalence in Nepal: Public Health Challenges in a Low-Income Nation during an Alarming Worldwide Trend." *International Journal of Environmental Research in Public Health* 7: 2726–44. doi: 10.3390/ijerph7062726.

Vaitkeviciute, Rimante, Lauren E. Ball, and Neil Harris. 2015. "The Relationship between Food Literacy and Dietary Intake in Adolescents: A Systematic Review." *Public Health Nutrition* 18, no.4: 649–58. doi: 10.1017/S1368980014000962.

Vallianatos, Helen, and Kim Raine. 2008. "Consuming Food and Constructing Identities among Arabic and South Asian Immigrant Women." *Food, Culture and Society* 11, no. 3: 355–73.

van der Horst, Klazine, Denise M. Deming, Ruta Lesniauskas, B. Thomas Carr, and Kathleen C. Reidy. 2016. "Picky Eating: Associations with Child Eating Characteristics and Food Intake." *Appetite* 103: 286–93.

Van Esterik, Penny. 1989. *Beyond the Breast-Bottle Controversy*. New Brunswick, NJ: Rutgers University Press.

—. 1995 "The Politics of Breastfeeding: An Advocacy Approach." *In Breastfeeding: Biocultural Perspectives*, ed. Patricia Stuart-Macadam and Katherine A. Dettwyler, 145–66. New York: Aldine de Gruyter.

—. 2002. "Contemporary Trends in Infant Feeding Research." *Annual Review of Anthropology* 31: 257–78.

Van Esterik, Penny, and Ted Greiner. 1981. "Breastfeeding and Women's Work: Constraints and Opportunities." *Studies in Family Planning* 12: 184–97.

Van Lancker, Wim, and Zachary Parolin. 2020. "COVID-19, School Closures, and Child Poverty: A Social Crisis in the Making." *Lancet Public Health* 5: e243–44. doi.org/10.1016/ S2468-2667(20)30084-0.

Vennemann, Mechtild M., Hans-Werner Hense, Thomas Bajanowski, Peter S. Blair, Christina Complojer, Rachel Y. Moon, Ursula Kiechl-Kohlendorfer. 2012. "Bed Sharing and the Risk of Sudden Infant Death Syndrome: Can We Resolve the Debate?" *Journal of Pediatrics* 160, no. 1: 44–48. doi: https://doi.org/10.1016/j.jpeds.2011.06.052.

Ventura, Alison K., and J. Worobey. 2013. "Early Influences on the Development of Food Preferences." *Current Biology* 23: R401–08. http://dx.doi.org/10.1016/j.cub.2013.02.037.

Vercellotti, Giuseppe, Barbara A. Piperata, Amanda M. Agnew, Warren M. Wilson, Darna L. Dufour, Julio C. Reina, Rosa Boano, Hedy M. Justus, Clark Spencer Larsen, Sam D. Stout, and Paul W. Sciulli. 2014. "Exploring the Multidimensionality of Stature Variation in the Past through Comparisons of Archaeological and Living Populations." *American Journal of Physical Anthropology* 155: 229–42. doi: 10.1002/ajpa.22552.

Vitzthum, Virginia J. 1994. "Causes and Consequences of Heterogeneity in Infant Feeding Practices among Indigenous Andean Women." *Annals of the New York Academy of Science* 709: 221–24.

–. 1997. "The Flexibility and Paradox: The Nature of Adaptation in Human Reproduction." In *The Evolving Female*, ed. Mary Ellen Morbeck, Alison Galloway, and Adrienne L. Zihlman, 242–58. Princeton, NJ: Princeton University Press.

Vos, Miriam B., Jill L. Kaar, Jean A. Welsh, Linda V. Van Horn, Daniel I. Feig, Cheryl A.M. Anderson, Mahesh J. Patel, Jessica Curz Munos, Nancy F. Krebs, Starva A. Xanthakos, and Rachel K. Johnson. 2017. "Added Sugars and Cardiovascular Disease Risk in Children: A Scientific Statement from the American Heart Association." *Circulation* 135: e1017–34. https://doi.org/10.1161/CIR.0000000000000439.

Waage, Jonathan K., and Patricia Adair Gowaty. 1997. "Myths of Genetic Determinism." In *Feminism and Evolutionary Biology. Boundaries, Intersections, and Frontiers*, ed. Patricia Adair Gowaty, 585–614. New York: Chapman and Hall.

Walker, Renee E., Christopher R. Keane, and Jessica G. Burke. 2010. "Disparities and Access to Healthy Food in the United States: A Review of Food Deserts Literature." *Health and Place* 16: 876–84.

Walson, Judd L., and James A. Berkley. 2018. "The Impact of Malnutrition on Childhood Infections." *Current Opinion in Infectious Disease* 31: 231–236. doi: 10.1097/QCO.0000000000000448.

Wan, Lester, Elaine Watson, and Rachel Arthur. 2017. "Sugar Taxes: The Global Picture in 2017." *Beverage Daily.com*, 18 July. https://www.beveragedaily.com/Article/2017/12/20/Sugar-taxes-The-global-picture-in-2017

Wang, Claire Y., Sara N. Bleich, and Steven L. Gortmaker. 2008. "Increasing Caloric Contribution from Sugar-Sweetened Beverages and 100% Fruit Juices among US Children and Adolescents, 1988–2004." *Pediatrics* 121, no. 6: e1604–14. doi: 10.1542/peds.2007-2834.

Warin, Megan, Tanya Zivkovic, Vivienne Moore, and Michael Davies. 2012. "Mothers as the Smoking Guns: Fetal Overnutrition and the Reproduction of Obesity." *Feminism and Psychology* 22, no. 30: 360–75.

Waterlow, Jonathan C. 1973. "Note on the Assessment and Classification of Protein-Energy Malnutrition in Children. *Lancet* 2: 87–89.

Watson, James, ed. 2006. *Golden Arches East: McDonald's in East Asia.* 2nd ed. Stanford, CA: Stanford University Press.

Weller, Chris. 2016. "These 10 Countries Have the Best Parental Leave Policies in the World." *Business Insider,* 22 August. https://www.businessinsider.com/countries-with-best-parental-leave-2016–8.

Wells, Jonathan, C.K. 2012a. "A Critical Appraisal of the Predictive Adaptive Response Hypothesis." *International Journal of Epidemiology* 41: 229–35.

–. 2012b. "Obesity as Malnutrition: The Role of Capitalism in the Obesity Global Epidemic." *American Journal of Human Biology* 24: 261–76.

Wells, Jonathan C.K., and M.S. Fewtrell. 2006. "Measuring Body Composition." *Archives of Disease in Childhood* 91: 612–17. doi: 10.1136/adc.2005.085522.

Westwater, Margaret L., Paul C. Fletcher, and Hisham Ziauddeen. 2016. "Sugar Addiction: The State of the Science." *European Journal of Nutrition* 55 (Suppl 2): S55–S69. doi: 10.1007/s00394-016-1229-6.

Whitaker, Robert C., Shannon M. Phillips, and Sean M. Orzol. 2006. "Food Insecurity and the Risks of Depression and Anxiety in Mothers and Behavior Problems in Their Preschool-Aged Children." *Pediatrics* 118, no. 3: e859–68. doi: 10.1542/peds.2006-0239.

WHO (World Health Organization). 2002. *The World Health Organization's Infant and Young Child Nutrition.* Geneva: World Health Organization. https://apps.who.int/gb/archive/pdf_files/WHA55/ea5515.pdf?ua=1.

–. 2009. *Infant and Young Child Feeding.* Geneva: World Health Organization.

–. 2015. *Guideline: Sugars Intake for Adults and Children.* Geneva: World Health Organization.

–. 2016a. *What Is Malnutrition?* https://www.who.int/features/qa/malnutrition/en/.

–. 2016b. *World Health Assembly Resolution on the Inappropriate Promotion of Foods for Infants and Young Children.* Policy brief. https://www.who.int/nutrition/netcode/WHA-Policy-brief.pdf?ua=1.

–. 2017. *The Double Burden of Malnutrition.* Policy brief. Geneva: World Health Organization.

–. 2019. *Replace Trans Fat: An Action Package to Eliminate Industrially Produced Trans-Fatty Acids.* WHO/NMH/NHD/18.4. https://www.who.int/docs/default -source/replace-transfat/2019-6-17-replace-framework-updated-june-2019.pd.

WHO/UNICEF. 2018. *Implementation Guidance: Protecting, Promoting and Supporting Breastfeeding in Facilities Providing Maternity and Newborn Services: The Revised Baby-Friendly Hospital Initiative.* Geneva: World Health Organization. Licence: CC BY-NC-SA 3.0 IGO. https://www.who.int/nutrition/publications/infantfeeding/bfhi-implementation-2018.pdf.

Widstrom, Ann-Marie, G. Lilja, P. Aaltomaa-Michalias, A. Dahllof, M. Lintula, and E. Nissen. 2011. "Newborn Behavior to Locate the Breast When Skin-to-Skin: A Possible Method for Enabling Early Self-Regulation." *Acta Paediatrica* 100: 79–85.

Wiley, Andrea, S. 1992. "Adaptation and the Biocultural Paradigm In Medical Anthropology: A Critical Review." *Medical Anthropology Quarterly* 6: 216–36.

References 221

–. 2007. "Transforming Milk in a Global Economy." *American Anthropologist* 109, no. 4: 666–77.

–. 2016. *Re-imagining Milk: Cultural and Biological Perspectives.* 2nd ed. New York: Routledge.

–. 2019. "Cow's Milk as Children's Food: Insights from Indian and the United States." In *The Handbook of Food and Anthropology,* ed. Jakob A. Klein and James L. Watson, 227–48. New York: Bloomsbury Academic.

Wiley, Andrea S., and J.S. Allen. 2013. *Medical Anthropology. A Biocultural Approach.* Oxford: Oxford University Press.

Wiley, Andrea S., and Jennifer M. Cullin. 2016. "What Do Anthropologists Mean When They Use the Term *Biocultural*?" *American Anthropologist* 118, no. 3: 554–69.

–. 2020. "Biological Normalcy." *Evolution, Medicine, and Public Health* 2020, no. 1: 11 https://doi.org/10.1093/emph/eoz035.

Wilk, Richard. 2010. "Power at the Table: Food Fights and Happy Meals." *Cultural Studies ↔ Critical Methodologies* 10, no. 6: 428–36.

Willett, Walter, Johan Rockström, Brent Loken, Marco Springmann, Tim Lang, Sonja Vermeulen, Tara Garnett, David Tilman, Fabrice DeClerck, Amanda Wood, Malin Jonell, Michael Clark, Line J. Gordon, Jessica Fanzo, Corinna Hawkes, Rami Zurayk, Juan A. Rivera, Wim De Vries, Sibanda Majele, Afshin Lindiwe, Chaudhary Ashkan, Abhishek, Mario Herrero, Rina Agustina, Francesco Branca, Anna Lartey, Shenggen Fan, Beatrice Crona, Elizabeth Fox, Victoria Bignet, Max Troell, Therese Lindahl, Sudhvir Singh, Sarah E. Cornell, K. Srinath Reddy, Sunita Narain, Sania Nishtar, and Christopher J.L. Murray. 2019. "Food in the Anthropocene: The EAT–Lancet Commission on Healthy Diets from Sustainable Food Systems." *Lancet* 393: 447–92. http://dx.doi.org/10.1016/S0140-6736(18)31788-4.

Williams, Jennifer L. 2016. "Spaces between Home and School: The Effect of Eating Location on Adolescent Nutrition." *Ecology of Food and Nutrition* 55, no. 1: 65–86. doi: 10.1080/03670244.2015.1072816.

Williamson, Iain, Dawn Leeming, Steven Lyttle, and Sally Johnson. 2011. "'It Should Be the Most Natural Thing in the World': Exploring First-Time Mothers' Breastfeeding Difficulties in the UK Using Audio-Diaries and Interviews." *Maternal and Child Nutrition* 8: 434–47.

Willows, Noreen D., Anthony J.G. Hanley, and Treena Delormier. 2012. "A Socioecological Framework to Understand Weight-Related Issues in Aboriginal Children in Canada." *Applied Physiology and Nutritional Metabolism* 37: 1–13. doi: 10.1139/H11–128.

Wilson, Warren, Jillian Milner, Janette Bulkan, and Peter Ehlers. 2006. "Weaning Practices of the Makushi of Guyana and Their Relationship to Infant and Child Mortality: A Preliminary Assessment of International Recommendations." *American Journal of Human Biology* 18: 312–24.

Winson, Anthony. 2004. "Bringing Political Economy into the Debate on the Obesity Epidemic." *Agriculture and Human Values* 21, no. 4: 299–312. doi https://doi.org/10.1007/s10460-003-1206-6.

–. 2008. "School Food Environments and the Obesity Issue: Content, Structural Determinants, and Agency in Canadian High Schools." *Agriculture and Human Values* 25: 499–511. https://doi.org/10.1007/s10460-008-9139-8.

–. 2013. *The Industrial Diet: The Degradation of Food and the Struggle for Healthy Eating.* Vancouver: UBC Press.

Winter Falk, Laura, Jeffery Sobal, Carole A. Bisogni, Margaret Connors, and Carol M. Devine. 2001. "Managing Health Eating: Definitions, Classifications, and Strategies." *Health Education and Behavior* 28, no. 4: 425–39.

Wittman, Hannah, and Jennifer Blesh. 2017. "Food Sovereignty and Fome Zero: Connecting Public Food Procurement Programmes to Sustainable Rural Development in Brazil." *Journal of Agrarian Change* 17, no. 1: 81–105. doi: 10.1111/joac.12131.

Woolhouse, Maxine. 2017. "'The Failed Child of the Failing Mother': Situating the Development of Child Eating Practices and the Scrutiny of Maternal Foodwork." In *Different Childhoods Non/Normative Development and Transgressive Trajectories,* ed. Lindsay O'Dell, Charlotte Brownlow, and Hanna Bertilsdotter-Rosqvist, 57–71. New York: Routledge.

Woolridge, M.W. 1995. "Baby-Controlled Breastfeeding: Biocultural Implications." In *Breastfeeding. Biocultural Perspectives,* ed. Patricia Stuart-Macadam and Katherine A. Dettwyler, 217–42. New York: Aldine de Gruyter.

World Food Programme (WFP). 2013. *State of School Feeding Worldwide.* Rome: World Food Programme.

Xue, Yong, Eva Lee, Ke Ning, Yingdong Zheng, Defu Ma, Hongchong Gao, Baoru Yang, Ying Bai, Peiyu Wang, and Ymei Zhang. 2015. "Prevalence of Picky Eating Behavior in Chinese School-Age Children and Associations with Anthropometric Parameters and Intelligence Quotient: A Cross-Sectional Study." *Appetite* 91: 248–55.

Yamashita, Lina, and Diana Robinson. 2015. "Making Visible the People Who Feed Us: Educating for Critical Food Literacy through Multicultural Texts." *Journal of Agriculture, Food Systems, and Community Development* 6, no. 2: 269–81. http://dx.doi.org/10.5304/jafscd.2016.062.011.

Yan, Jing, Lin Liu, Yun Zhu, Guowei Huang, and Peter Wang. 2014. "The Association between Breastfeeding and Childhood Obesity: A Meta-Analysis." *BMC Public Health* 14: 1267. http://www.biomedcentral.com/1471-2458/14/1267.

Yimyam, Susanha, Martha Morrow, and Wichit Srisuphan. 1999, "Role Conflict and Rapid Socio-Economic Change: Breastfeeding among Employed Women in Thailand." *Social Science and Medicine* 49: 957–65.

Young, Brian. 2003. "Does Food Advertising Influence Children's Choices? A Critical Review of Some of the Recent Literature." *International Journal of Advertising* 22: 441–59.

Yourex-West, Heather. 2017. "More Hospitals in Canada Becoming 'Baby Friendly.'" Global News, 29 September. https://globalnews.ca/news/3777365/more-hospitals-in-canada-becoming-baby-friendly/.

Zagmutt, Francisco, Jane Pouzou, and Solenne Costard. 2019. "Continuing the Dialogue on EAT-Lancet." Epix Analytics. https://www.epixanalytics.com/eat-lancet-criticism-correspondence.html.

Ziegelman, Jane, and Andrew Coe. 2016. *A Square Meal: A Culinary History of the Great Depression.* New York: HarperCollins.

Zimmerman, Michael B., and Richard F. Hurrell. 2007. "Nutritional Iron Deficiency." *Lancet* 370, no. 9586: 511–20. doi: https://doi.org/10.1016/S0140-6736(07)61235-5.

Zong, Geng, Yanping Li, Anne J. Wanders, Marjan Alssema, Peter L. Zock, Walter C. Willett, Frank B. Hu, and Qi Sun. 2016. "Intake of Individual Saturated Fatty Acids and Risk of Coronary Heart Disease in US Men and Women: Two Prospective Longitudinal Cohort Studies." *British Medical Journal* 355 doi: https://doi.org/10.1136/bmj.i5796.

Zuckerman, Molly K., and Debra L. Martin. 2016. "Introduction: The Development of Biocultural Perspectives in Anthropology." In *New Directions in Biocultural Anthropology*, ed. Molly K. Zuckerman and Debra L. Martin, 7–28. Hoboken, NJ: John Wiley and Sons.

Zuk, Marlene. 2013. *Paleofantasy: What Evolution Really Tells Us about Sex, Diet, and How We Live.* New York: W.W. Norton.

Index

Academy of Nutrition and Dietetics, 99
Acquired Tastes: Why Families Eat the Way They Do (Beagan), 152
Adams, Jean, 91
additives, 3, 71, 76, 161. *See also* fortification
adolescence/adolescents: caregiver–self-feeding transition, 55–56; change in dietary habits, 177–78; community food centres and, 178; and fast food, 56; foundational evolutionary approach to, 6; growth during, 45, 55, 66–67; and healthy food, 112; neophobia in, 58; nutrition, 55–57; snack eating, 56; social changes during, 55
adolescent obesity: gender and, 152–53; mental health and, 140; and physical quality of life, 140; socioeconomic inequalities and, 149–50; trends in, 141–42. *See also* obesity, child
adult foods, children eating, 60, 62, 63, 166, 170
advertising: breakfast cereals, 77; children's cognition and, 88–89; food,
72, 99; "health halo" in, 89; of toddler milk, 69
advertising targeted to children: bans/restrictions on, 88, 90–93; breakfast cereals, 76; commercial food products, 88–93; neoliberalism and, 66; new/emerging media and, 92; normalization of sweetened food in, 93–94; processed foods, 3–4; snack foods, 78–80
agriculture: advent of, 179; and environmental change, 179; in Japanese curricula, 106; National School Lunch Program and, 97; Neolithic, 25–26; size of farms, 167; and sustainability, 180. *See also* industrial agriculture; local agriculture/farming
Alberta, school meals in, 113
Allen, Jennifer M., *Medical Anthropology: A Bicultural Approach*, 8
allergies, 37, 38, 52
Allison, Anne, 80, 101
allomothering/-parenting, 20, 42–43, 96

Index   225

American Heart Association: and low-fat products, 86; and sugar, 77, 93
American Medical Association, and infant formula, 27
American Psychiatric Association, *Diagnostic and Statistical Manual of Mental Disorders*, 61
anencephaly, 19
anorexia nervosa, 160
Anthropocene, 178–79
anthropology: biocultural approach in, 7; biological, 7; and breastfeeding, 40; and children/childhood, 12–13; and children's food, 164; feminist, 40; holistic perspective, 6; and obesity, 138; and Paleodiets, 37
antibiotics: breastfeeding and, 158; and child obesity, 155–56, 165
archaeology: bio-, 7
Assari, Shervin, 140
Assman, Stephanie, 105–6
atopy, 38
avoidant/restrictive food intake disorder (ARFID), 61
Azzarito, Laura, "The Rise of the Corporate Curriculum: Fatness, Fitness and Whiteness," 161

Baby-Friendly Hospital Initiative, 28
Ball, Helen L., 41
Ballantyne, Sarah, 36–37
Barker, David, 18–19
Beagan, Brenda L., 11; *Acquired Tastes: Why Families Eat the Way They Do*, 152
Beauvoir, Simone de, 30
behaviours, as learned vs. instinctive, 20
Behind the Brands (Oxfam), 71–72
Belfast (Northern Ireland), adolescent eating/youth clubs in, 56
Belize, meals in, 50
Bellows, Anne C., 135–36
Beneytou, Jean-Paul, 110
biocultural approach, 7–9; to child eating habits, 57–62; to child feeding,

167; to infant feeding, 25; and picky eating, 63
Birch, Leann, 59
Bird, Douglas W., 54
Bisogni, Carole, 9
Black children/people: and food insecurity, 127; and overweight, 149
Blaffer Hrdy, Sarah, 20, 42–43, 163
Blair, Tony, 103
Blaser, Martin, *Missing Microbes*, 155
Bliege Bird, Rebecca, 54
Blumberg, Bruce, 153–54
Bobowski, Nuala K., 82
body mass index (BMI): fried food consumption and, 148; increase in, 143; and obesity, 140–41
body size/shape: culture and, 151–52; ideal type, 160–61
body weight: gender and, 152; health status and, 160; parents and, 152; sugar and, 87. *See also* overweight; underweight children
Bogin, Barry, *Patterns of Human Growth*, 45
Born to Buy (Schor and Ford), 72
bottle feeding: baby bottles and, 26–27; and co-parenting, 38–39; in Nepal, 33; politics and, 38. *See also* infant formula
Bourdieu, Pierre, 107
Bray, George A., 87
Brazil: adolescent eating in Sao Paulo, 56; Food-Based Dietary Guidelines, 176; school food in, 174
breakfast cereals: added adulterants, 76; as children's food product, 164; child-targeted vs. non-child-targeted, 77; coupons, 76; foraging for/self-feeding of, 76, 77; fortification of, 76, 164; history, 75–76; marketing to children/youth, 66, 71, 75–76, 77; sugar in, 77, 164
Breakfast Clubs Canada, 111
breast milk: alternatives, 26; autocrine control of production,

33; as food, 23–24; insufficiency, 33, 35; macronutrients in, 24; micronutrients in, 24; sugar in, 24

breastfeeding: and atopy, 38; "breast is best" movement, 28, 29; and child obesity, 157–59; as choice, 38–39; complementary foods as replacement vs. accompaniment for, 34; co-parenting vs., 38–39; co-sleeping/"breastsleeping" and, 23; on demand vs. scheduled, 33; difficulties, 20–22; and EDCs, 154; employment and, 27, 31–33, 39, 163; evolutionary theory and, 40–41; feminism and, 38–41; and food allergies, 38; in hunter-gatherer foraging societies, 22–23; infant formula use mixed with, 32–33; and infant morbidity, 36; Innocenti Declaration and, 28–29; instinctual aspect, 22; and maternal-infant dyad trade-offs, 41; and microbiome, 158; in Nepal, 20–22, 33, 122; and personal autonomy, 42; politics and, 38; as public health goal, 40; rediscovery of benefits of, 28; structural barriers to, 39; toddler milk and, 69; and type 1 diabetes, 38; wet nursing, 25, 26; and women's productive vs. reproductive work, 29–33; as work, 30. *See also* lactation

The Breastfeeding Book (Sears), 38–39

Brewis, Alexandra, 150–52; *Obesity: Cultural and Biocultural Perspectives*, 138

Bringing up Bébé (Druckerman), 60–61

Broadcast Code for Advertising to Children (Canada), 92

bulimia, 160

Cairns, Kate, 9–10; *Food and Femininity*, 48–49

calcium, 55, 56–57, 67, 68, 131

Canada: Bill S-228, 171; Breakfast Clubs Canada, 111; breastfeeding in, 21; child obesity in, 141; children's eating in, 3; children's food advertising in, 92–93; Coalition for Healthy School Food, 112–13; food banks in, 170; food insecurity in, 4, 127, 134; national food policy, 113, 174; National Longitudinal Survey of Children and Youth, 131; national student food program, 174; parental leave in, 177; school food in, 99, 110–13, 114; trans fats in, 173; Truth and Reconciliation Commission, 151; in UNICEF youth well-being report, 110

Canada Child Benefit, 168

Canada Food Guide (CFG), 12, 174–76

Canada Prenatal Nutrition Program, 135

Canadian 24-hour Movement Guidelines for Children and Youth, 146

Canadian Community Health Survey: on breastfeeding, 32; on food insecurity, 169; and Household Food Security Survey Module, 126

Canadian Medical Association, and school food program, 113

capitalism: anthropological perspective, 6; and global food system, 11; and industrial food system, 143, 167; and modern food system, 9; and obesity, 125; and women breastfeeding at work, 32

carbohydrates, 66, 67, 145

cardiovascular disease: DOHaD and, 18–19; economic cuts and, 96; obesity and, 131; perception of overweight and, 152; trans fats ban and, 173. *See also* heart disease

caregiver-child feeding relationship, 47–53; complexity of, 62–63; emotions expressed in, 49; families in, 50–51; in hunter-gatherer societies, 53–55; immigrants and, 51–53; impact on nutritional status, 62; responsive feeding in, 48; self-feeding in, 53; specialized children's foods in, 76; transition

Index 227

to self-feeding, 55–57, 62, 63; young adults and, 56–57. *See also* parent-child feeding relationship

Center for Science in the Public Interest, 81

Centers for Disease Control and Prevention (CDC) (US): on antibiotics, 155; National Center for Health Statistics growth reference for children, 141

cereals: in infant feeding in ancient Rome, 35; as weaning foods, 36, 70. *See also* breakfast cereals

"Changing Homes, Changing Food," 51–52

Chapman, Gwen E., 11

Charlie and the Chocolate Factory (Dahl), 85

Chee, Bernadine, 81

child feeding: allomothers/ multiple caretakers and, 42–43; anthropological research about, 12–13; biocultural approach to, 167; cultures and, 166; distribution among family/institutions, 163; evolutionary history and, 167; grandmother hypothesis, 42; maternal model in, 42; parental influence in, 59; policies regarding, 166; schools and, 163–64 (*see also* school food/meals); and species health/well-being, 95–96; stages of, 62. *See also* children's eating; children's food(s); infant feeding

child obesity. *See* obesity, child

child overweight. *See* overweight children

childhood: anthropology and, 12–13; body/brain growth, and length of, 46–47; commercialization of, 72; culture and, 4, 164; evolution of, 45–47; human length of time vs. other mammals, 46–47; length of period of, 46, 61; practice theory and, 46; as social construction, 64; as social/cultural construction, 12

"The Childhood Obesity Epidemic: Health Crisis or Social Construction?" (Moffat), 159

children: anthropology and, 12–13; cultural views of, 164; foundational evolutionary approach to, 6

children's eating: of adult foods, 60, 166; family eating vs., 122; in Japanese school curriculum, 106; laissez-faire approach, 122; as more conservative than adults', 58; parental influence in, 59; restraints on, and preoccupation with food/eating, 48; self-regulation of, 48. *See also* eating disorders

Children's Food and Beverage Advertising Initiative (US), 91–92

children's food(s): adult food vs., 4, 70, 166; advertising limits/bans, 171; advertising to children, 88–93 (*see also* advertising targeted to children); anthropological research about, 12–13, 164; caregivers and, 76; in China, 70–71; as commercially produced items, 70; as convenience products, 93; creation/construction of, 64–65, 164; in fast food restaurants, 72–73 (*see also* fast food); food industry and, 65, 71, 93, 164; fruit juice as, 175; future of, 178–81; health effects of, 88; "health halo" in advertising, 89; milk as, 175; in Nepal, 70; nutritional fortification of, 93; in Sarawak, 70; sugar in, 81–82, 164; sweeteners in, 93

China: children's food in, 70–71; fast food in, 73; KFC in, 73–74; picky eating in, 60; school meals in, 98; snack foods in Beijing, 81; transnational food corporations in, 73–74

Chisan Chishō (Local Production for Local Consumption Act) (LPLC) (Japan), 105–6

cholesterol, 85–86, 172

Choose My Plate (USDA), 174, 175–76

climate change, 127, 179
Clinton, Hillary Rodham, 95
Coalition for Healthy School Food (Food Secure Canada), 112–13
Cole, Tim J., 123
Collins, Patricia A., 169, 170
Community Food Centres Canada, 178
community food security (CFS), 135–36
complementary feeding/foods: in ancient Rome, 34–35, 36; anthropological studies and, 34; flexibility, 34–35; as human vs. non-human transitional strategy, 34; intervention programs, 124; in Nepal, 35; as replacement vs. accompaniment for breastfeeding, 34; as transition foods, 34
Constructing and Reconstructing Childhood (James and Prout), 12, 64
Cookin' Up Food Justice, 178
COVID-19 pandemic: and maternal-child nutrition, 168; and school food, 115
critical studies: biocultural, 8–9; food, 9–12; food literacy, 178
Crooks, Deborah, 80
Cullin, Jennifer M., 152
culture(s): and age, 151; and body size, 151–52; and child feeding, 166; and childhood/children, 4, 164; conflation with deprivation among racialized groups, 150–51; events/rituals, and sweet tastes, 85, 125; and food, 4; and gender, 151; and obesity, 151–52
Cummins, Steven, 129
Cunningham, Kenda, 124

Dahl, Roald, *Charlie and the Chocolate Factory*, 85
dairy foods, 11, 37, 68, 156, 175. *See also* milk
daycare centres: in France, 60–61; and nurturing, 6; in obesogenic environment, 147; peer influence in, 59

Delormier, Treena, 151
Denmark, trans fats ban, 173
Descartes, Lara, 84–85
Dettwyler, Katherine, 47
developmental origins of health and disease (DOHaD), 9, 18–19
Diagnostic and Statistical Manual of Mental Disorders (American Psychiatric Association), 61
diarrhea/diarrheal diseases: bottle feeding and, 27; breastfeeding and, 35, 36; and growth retardation, 123; infant malnutrition and, 118; in low-income countries, 35, 36, 118; in Nepal, 36, 122; vitamin A deficiency and, 119
dietary habits. *See* eating/food habits
"Does Child Food Exist for Rural Malays?" (Elliott Cooper), 70
dopamine, 82–83
Drèze, Jean, 116
Druckerman, Pamela, 62; *Bringing Up Bébé*, 60–61
dry nursing, 26
dual energy x-ray absorptiometry (DXA), 140
Dufour, Darna L., 8

early childhood: dependence on adults during, 45, 163; growth during, 45, 66; morbidity in Nepal, 35; mortality rate in Nepal, 120; neophobia in, 58. *See also* childhood; infancy
eating disorders, 153, 159–60; anorexia nervosa, 160; anti-obesity campaigns and, 159; bulimia, 160; obesity stigma and, 165–66
eating outside home: and fast food, 176; increase in, 148; and processed food, 176
eating/food habits: biocultural approach to, 57–62; environmental factors and, 158; experiential modelling of, 112, 114; in Japanese school curriculum, 106; parental role modelling, 99;

Index

school meals, and establishment for life, 114; socioeconomic status and, 150; support for children to develop healthy forms of, 63. *See also* children's eating

EAT-*Lancet* Commission, "Great Food Transformation," 179–80

education about food/nutrition: community organizations and, 177; experiential learning of food skills, 176, 177; experiential learning of nutrition, 104–5; experiential learning/modelling in school meal programs, 105, 173–74; experiential modelling of food habit development, 112; food literacy, 177–78; in France, 61–62; national food guides and, 174–76; school teaching of food skills, 177

Elliott, Charlene, 78, 80

Elliott Cooper, Elizabeth, "Does Child Food Exist for Rural Malays?," 70

employment: balance of domestic and other forms of, 176–77; breastfeeding and, 27, 31–33, 39, 163; hours of work, 177; in Nepal, 30–31; and use of infant formula, 27, 32–33; and work vs. food preparation time, 148

endocrine disrupting chemicals (EDCs), 153–54, 156

environmental stressors, 7, 9

evolutionary approach: and breastfeeding, 40–41; and feeding children, 167; feminism and, 40–41; and food discernment, 57–58; and food/taste preferences, 63; foundational, 6; and lactation, 34; milk in, 68; and paediatric nutrition, 37; and Paleodiets, 37; and weaning, 34

families: and child feeding responsibility, 163; children's participation in food production, 173; community vs., in child feeding/ nutrition, 43; co-sleeping in, 23; food sharing within, 50; government support/policy, 43; home-cooked meals, 3; lone-parent, 127, 133, 135; meals, 50, 90; neoliberalism, and responsibility for child raising, 96; television advertising and meals, 90; women's role in feeding, 42. *See also entries beginning* parent; household food insecurity; intergenerationality; mothers

fast food: adolescents and, 56; ban on advertising, and consumption of, 90–91; and child obesity, 176; children's consumption of, 73; children's meals in restaurants, 72–73; in China, 73; eating outside home and, 176; in France, 62, 107; franchises sponsoring sports teams, 146; growth of industry, 73; healthier meals in restaurants, 75; history of, 72; income/socioeconomic status and, 73; in Japan, 104, 105–6; marketed for children, 71; and nutritional health, 74; and obesity, 104; reasons for consumption, 74–75; restaurants offering child-specific menu items, 93; in South Australia, 74–75; time deficits and, 130; urbanization and, 73

Fast Food Nation (Schlosser), 72

fat, body: measures of, 140; storage of, 139

Fat Chance: Beating the Odds against Sugar, Processed Food, Obesity and Disease (Lustig), 144–45

The Fate of Food (Little), 180

fat(s), dietary: in breast milk, 24; and coronary heart disease, 86; fear of, 85–86; hydrogenated/trans fats, 86; as macro-adulterant, 71; as macronutrient, 66, 67; in milk, 24; nutrition transition and consumption of, 143; and obesity, 144–45; saturated, 144; in school lunches, 108; sugar replacing, 86; trans, 86, 144, 172–73

Fear of Food (Levenstein), 85–86
Federal Communications Commission (US), 92
Feeding China's Little Emperors (Jing), 13, 70–71
"The Feeding Relationship" (Satter), 48
feminism: and breastfeeding, 38–41; evolutionary theory and, 40–41; and gender, 39–40; liberal, 39; and life history approach, 41; multivocality of, 39; postmodern third wave, 39–40
Fildes, Valerie, 26, 36
Finland: breastfeeding, and infant BMI in, 158; school meals in, 98; sweet tastes in, 84
"The First 1,000 Days" (UNICEF), 156
Fitchen, Janet, 128–29
folic acid supplementation, 19, 171
Food and Agriculture Organization (FAO), on food security, 126, 130
Food and Drug Administration (FDA), 173
Food and Femininity (Cairns and Johnston), 48–49
food banks, 134, 135, 169–70
food deserts, 129–30, 147
Food Guide to Healthy Eating (Canada), 134
food industry: Canada Food Guide and, 175; and food visual cues, 148; and HFCS, 164; and national food/dietary guides, 11; policies regarding, 166; revenues, 71–72; and snacking, 78; and specialized children's foods, 65; and uniquely children's food, 71
food insecurity: access to food and, 132; among vulnerable groups, 169; and calcium, 131; in Canada, 127; and child obesity, 149, 150; children's accounts of experiences with, 132; and chronic, nutrition-related diseases, 131; in circumpolar regions, 127; EAT-*Lancet* Commission diet and, 180; food assistance programs, 169; food banks and, 134, 135, 169–70;

guaranteed income programs and, 133–34, 169; health effects, 130–32; in high-income countries, 168–70; households in Canada/US, 4; income and, 127–30, 132–33; as income vs. food issue, 170; income/cash transfers for alleviation of, 168–69; intergenerationality of effects of, 131; lone parent families and, 135; and mental health, 132; mothers buffering children from, 150; in Nunavut, 127; and obesity/overweight, 131–32; policies/programs, 132–35; quality of food and, 129; refugees and, 168; reported for households vs. children, 150; seniors and, 133; sociodemographics of, 127–28; in US, 127; in US compared to Canada, 135; US programs addressing, 134. *See also* food security
Food Politics (Nestle), 65
Food Revolution (Oliver), 108–9
Food Secure Canada, Coalition for Healthy School Food, 112–13
food security: access to food and, 127–30; availability of food and, 126–27; climate change and, 179; community, 170; "country food" and, 168; foraging and, 167–68; four dimensions of, 126–30; hunting and, 167–68; quality of food and, 127; stability of government and, 168; utilization of food and, 130. *See also* food insecurity
food sharing: within families, 50; intergenerational, in foraging societies, 54–55
food sovereignty: in Japan, 105; in low-income countries, 168; school meal programs and, 104
food swamps, 147, 148
food system(s): about, 9; activist stance toward, 11; industrial agriculture and, 9; industrialization of, 26–27; interdisciplinary approaches to, 9;

Index 231

political economy and, 9–10; sustainable, 179–80; technology in, 180. *See also* global food system; industrial food system

Food-Based Dietary Guidelines (Brazil), 176

food(s): advertising, 99; assistance benefits, 169; children's engagement in preparation of, 176; culture and, 4; decline in skills regarding, 148; elasticity as commodity, 128–29; energy-dense, 143–44; equitable distribution of, 180; foodscapes around schools, 112; French investment in production, 98; globalization of commodities, 4; government oversight of supply, 170–71; as individual choice, 10; Japanese investment in production, 98; literacy, 130, 177–78; meanings/ importance of, 166; national guides, 11–12, 174–76; new, 58–59, 60; nutrients vs., 6–7; preferences, 59, 63; prepared away from home, 148; school meals and production methods, 98; trends in, 144; visual cues, 147–48; women's role in providing to family, 42. *See also* education about food/nutrition; local food

FoodShare, Good Food Café program (Toronto), 113

foraging: for breakfast cereals, 76; theory, and obesogenic environment, 147–48. *See also* hunter-gatherer forager societies; self-feeding

Ford, Doug, 133

Ford, Margaret, *Born to Buy*, 72

fortification: of breakfast cereals, 76, 164; of children's processed food products, 93; of infant formula, 27; legislation regarding, 171. *See also* additives

France: adult food as children's food in, 62, 63; appreciation of French

food culture, 63; children's eating in, 60–62; education regarding food in, 61–62, 63; fast food in, 62; new foods in, 60; school meals in (*see* school food/meals (France)); wet nursing in, 25

Free for All: Fixing School Food in America (Poppendieck), 108

Freedhoff, Yoni, 112

French Kids Eat Everything (Le Billon), 60

Friedan, Betty, 38

fructose, 87

fruit, 3; adolescents and, 56; babies and, 37; in *Canada Food Guide,* 175; fast food and, 74, 75; food insecurity and, 129; in French meals, 60, 74, 101, 105; Fruit Roll Ups, 80, 81; in Iqaluit school food, 113; in Japanese food, 106; in school meals, 112, 113; snacks and, 78, 79; sweet taste/sugars and, 82, 83, 85

Fujita, Masako, 24

Fulkerson, Jayne A., 51

gakkō kyūshoku (Japan), 100, 106–7

Galen, 25, 35

Galloway, Tracey, 151

gastro-citizenship, 107–8

gender: culture and, 151; feminism and, 39–40; and healthy eating, 153; and obesity, 152–53; and physical activity, 152–53; and reproductive vs. productive work, 31–32

Gendron, Danielle, 96, 98, 101, 106, 107, 114

General Mills, 77, 81; Lucky Charms Leprechaun, 76

genetics: and childhood obesity, 142–43; inheritance, 7

germ theory of disease, 27

Gettler, Lee, 23

ghrelin, 24

global food system: anthropological perspective, 6; capitalism and, 11;

and community food security, 135–36; and double burden of malnutrition, 117; neoliberalism and, 11; and overweight/obesity, 136; as shaping/constraining access/appetites, 11. *See also* multinational companies

globalization: and culinary nationalism, 105–6; of food commodities, 4; industrial food system and, 4; of media, 94, 171; of multinational food companies, 4

Gluckman, Peter D., 18

glucose, 18–19, 46–47, 87, 158

Godfrey, Keith M., 18

Golden Arches East (Watson), 73

Goldman, Jane A., 84–85

Good Food Café program, Toronto, 113

Goodall, Jane, 21

Goodman, Alan H., 8

Gortmaker, Steven, 89–90

governments: family support, 43; family vs., in responsibility for food, 109; oversight of food supply, 170–71; responsibility for nutritional health/well-being, 10. *See also* legislation; policies

Great Depression: and national school lunch program, 97; and US food insecurity programs, 134

"Great Food Transformation" (EAT-*Lancet* Commission), 179–80

Greece, ancient, wet nursing in, 25

Greenberg, Julia, 92

Greenhalgh, Susan, 159–60

growth: during adolescence, 45, 55, 66–67; CDC/National Center for Health Statistics reference for children, 141; during early childhood, 45; environmental conditions and, 45–46; during infancy, 66; during middle childhood, 45; in Nepal, 164–65; quantitative differences, and timing of childhood stages, 46; WHO reference for children, 119, 120–21, 141

growth failure/retardation: diarrheal diseases and, 123; disease and, 123; in low-income countries, 35; micronutrient deficiencies and, 119; responsive feeding and, 48; stunting, 116. *See also* stunting; wasting

Grün, Felix, 153–54

guaranteed income programs, 133–34, 169

Guthman, Julie, 148–49, 161

Hadza (Tanzanian people), 23, 53, 54, 76

Hagenaars, Luc Louis, 172

Hamilton (Ontario): Community Food Centre, 178; snack foods in, 80; young adults' nutritional perceptions in, 57

Hamm, Michael W., 135–36

Hanley, Anthony J.G., 151

"Hansel and Gretel," 84

Hanson, Mark A., 18

Harris, Jennifer L., 89

Hawkes, Kristen, 42, 54

Headey, Derek D., 120, 124

Health Behaviour in School-Aged Children, 149

Health Canada, on trans fats, 173

Health Measures Surveys (Canada), 141

healthy food/eating: in adolescence, 55–56; adolescents and, 112; *Canada Food Guide* and, 12; discourses regarding, 11–12; gender and, 153; reader's perspectives on, 12; school cooking classes, and obesity, 114; unhealthy food/eating vs., 12; young adults and, 56–57

Heart and Stroke Foundation of Canada: and low-fat products, 86; sugar intake guidelines, 93

heart disease: anorexia nervosa and, 160; fat and, 86; increasing prevalence of, 66; physical activity and, 146; predictive adaptive response and, 18; SSBs and, 171. *See also* cardiovascular disease

Index

Hernandez, Kimberley, 174
Hewlett, Barry S., *Hunter-Gatherer Childhoods*, 53
Hicks, Kathryn, 8
high-fructose corn syrup (HFCS), 84, 87, 88, 164
high-income countries: breastfeeding in, 38; child obesity in, 141; food insecurity in, 168–70; food insecurity-malnutrition connection in, 130–31; parent-child feeding relationship in, 48; rise in human height/stature, 167
Hill, Andrew, 99
Hinde, Katie, 25
Hoddinott, John, 120, 124
homeless people, and food utilization, 130
household food insecurity: in Canada, 4; defined, 126; increase in, 168; and obesity, 150; in US, 4; wealth disparities and, 168
Household Food Security Survey Module (HFSSM), 126
hunger: as cognitive, 129; in malnutrition in, 4; obesity vs., 4; residential schools and, 151. *See also* food insecurity; undernutrition
Hunter-Gatherer Childhoods (Hewlett and Lamb), 53
hunter-gatherer forager societies: breastfeeding in, 22–23; children's participation in, 173; and food security, 167–68; intergenerational food sharing in, 54–55; and practice theory, 46; self-feeding in, 53–55; variation in children's procuring/preparing/self-feeding among, 62

IBIS-World, 73
If Men Breastfed (Naya Health), 32
immigrants: feeding relationships with children, 51–53; and food banks, 170; and food use, 130; school lunches, 52–53; traditional foods, 51–53

immunoglobulins, 24
income: child tax benefit program and, 133; disparities in, 168–69; and fast food consumption, 73; and food insecurity, 127–30, 132–33, 168–69, 170; guaranteed income projects, 133–34, 169; industrial food system and, 168; lone-parent families and, 133; stability of government and, 168. *See also* high-income countries; low-income countries; poverty
India. *See* South Asia
Indigenous communities (Canada): child obesity among, 151; "country" foods, 127; and environmental injustices, 151; food availability, 127; and food insecurity, 127; and residential schools, 151
industrial agriculture: agrofoods industry in France, 107; food procurement through, 168; food system based on, 9; in France, 107
The Industrial Diet (Winson), 71
industrial food system: agrofoods industry in France, 107; capitalism and, 143, 167; and child obesity, 167; and construction of children's food, 65; creation of children's food products, 93, 164; globalization of, 4; history, 26–27, 71; influence of, 65; and legislation, 171; and malnutrition, 167; and sweetness, 83
infant feeding: animals' milk, in Neolithic age, 25–26; biocultural practice of, 25; in Paleodiets, 36–37; politics and, 38; softened/premasticated foods, 36. *See also* bottle feeding; breastfeeding; complementary feeding; weaning
infant formula: American Medical Association and, 27; and child obesity, 157–59; considered as superior to breast milk, 27; development of, 27; and employment, 32–33; fortification

with micronutrients, 27; in hospitals, 29; in low-income countries, 27–28; multinational companies, 29; toddler milk and, 69; use mixed with breastfeeding, 32–33. *See also* bottle feeding

infant mortality: bottle feeding and, 27; infectious diseases and, 118; malnutrition and, 118; in Nepal, 120

Innocenti Declaration, 28–29

insulin, 18–19, 87, 145, 154

intergenerationality: of child obesity, 165; of effects of food insecurity, 131; of food sharing in hunter-gatherer foraging societies, 54–55; of low birthweight, 118; and transmission of obesity, 150. *See also* families

International Obesity Task Force, 141

interventions: behaviourally based, 159; complementary feeding, 124; and obesity, 114; physical activity in, 146; school meals and, 98, 105, 114; in schools/child-care settings, 99; and short-term behaviour modifications vs. system change, 178

intrauterine environment: about, 18–20; and DOHaD, 18–19; micronutrients in, 19; and NCDs, 19; nutritional, 19. *See also* pregnancy

Inuksuk High School, Iqaluit, 113

iron deficiency, 37

Italy, school meals in, 98

James, Allison, *Constructing and Reconstructing Childhood*, 12, 64

Jamie's School Dinners (Oliver), 103

Janssen, Ian, 149

Japan: *Chisan Chishō* (Local Production for Local Consumption Act) (LPLC), 105–6; *gakkō kyūshoku*, 100, 106–7; *obentōs* (boxed lunches) in, 80. *See also* school food/meals (Japan)

Jing, Jun, *Feeding China's Little Emperors*, 13, 70–71

Johnson, Lyndon B., "War on Poverty," 97

Johnston, Josée, 9–10; *Food and Femininity*, 48–49

junk food: advertising, 88, 89–90; in school cafeterias, 112. *See also* snack foods

Keith, Scott, "Putative Contributors to the Secular Increase in Obesity," 153

Kellogg (company), 77; Corn Flakes, 75; Snap, Crackle and Pop, 76; Tony the Tiger, 76

Kellogg, John Harvey, 75

Kellogg, Will Keith, 75

Kennedy, Gail E., 33–34

Keys, Ancel, 85–86

KFC, 73–74

Khan, Laura Kettel, 9

Kirkpatrick, Sharon I., 128, 170

Kline, Stephen, 90

Knodel, John, 27

Kogan, Michael D., 149

Konner, Melvin, 23

!Kung San, 22–23, 53, 54

Kuzawa, Christopher W., 47

La Leche League International, 29

lactase/lactose, 68–69

lactation: biology of, 22; and children's food preferences, 59; evolutionary aspects, 34; instinctual aspect, 22; as learned skill, 20–22; maternal/child competition/trade-offs in, 24–25. *See also* breastfeeding

Lamb, Michael E., *Hunter-Gatherer Childhoods*, 53

Landecker, Hannah, 166

Le Billon, Karen, *French Kids Eat Everything*, 60

Leatherman, Thomas L., 8

legislation, 170–73. *See also* governments; policies

Leonard, William R., 8

LePen, Marine, 110

leptin, 24, 87

leptogenic environment, 148–49

Levenstein, Harvey, 75–76; *Fear of Food,* 85–86

Levine, Susan, *School Lunch Politics,* 97

Leynse, Wendy, 62

Lieberman, Leslie Sue, 147–48

life history/lifecourse approach: and DOHaD, 9; feminism and, 41; and intrauterine environment, 18; to maternal-infant dyad trade-offs, 41; and weaning, 34

Little, Amanda, *The Fate of Food,* 180

Little, Margaret H., 169, 170

local agriculture/farming: community food security and, 135; and school food/meals, 98, 99, 104, 114, 174

local food: markets, 135; movement, 180; and school food/meals, 99, 105–6, 114, 174

lone-parent families: and food insecurity, 127, 135; in low-income households, 133

Loopstra, Rachel, 168–70

low birthweight (LBW): effects, 118; incidence of, 118; intergenerationality of, 118; undernutrition of mothers and, 118. *See also* underweight children

low-income countries: BMI increases in, 141–42; bottle feeding in, 27–28; child obesity in, 141; co-sleeping in, 23; EAT-*Lancet* Commission diet and, 180; and food sovereignty, 168; growth retardation in, 35; malnutrition in, 4, 118–26; maternal feeding emphasis in studies of, 47–48; parent-child feeding relationship in, 47–48; school meals in, 97; stunting/underweight in, 46; trans fats in, 173

Lozada, Eriberto P., 73–74

Ludwig, David S., 145

Lunchables, 80

Lustig, Robert, *Fat Chance: Beating the Odds against Sugar, Processed Food, Obesity and Disease,* 144–45

Macintyre, Sally, 129

macronutrients, 24, 66–67. *See also* carbohydrates; fat(s), dietary; protein

Maher, Vanessa, 32

Mali, self-feeding in, 47

malnutrition: biocultural determinants of, 123; bottle feeding and, 27; catastrophic events and, 118; causes of, 124; characteristics in infancy, 118; chronic, 118–19; defined, 117; double burden of, 117, 125–26, 165; incidence of, 116; Indigenous peoples and, 151; industrial food system and, 167; intervention programs and, 124; lack of resources and, 124; low energy/protein intakes and, 119; in low-income countries, 4; and overweight, 117; poverty and, 124, 165; prenatal, 118; in residential schools, 151; and Second World War, 97. *See also* undernutrition

Marlowe, Frank, 54–55

maternal capital, 18

Mbogoni, Lawrence, 95

McDade, Thomas W., 41

McDonald, Maurice, 72

McDonald, Richard, 72

McDonald's, 72–73; Golden Arches, 148; Happy Meal, 72–73, 75; toys, 72–73

McKenna, James, 23

media: children as consumers of, 72; food product marketing on, 72; globalization of, 94, 171; new/emerging, 92, 94, 171; and school food program, 113

Medical Anthropology: A Bicultural Approach (Wiley and Allen), 8

Mennella, Julie A., 82

mental health: eating disorders and, 160; food insecurity and, 132; and obesity, 140

Mexico: diabetes in, 172; food swamps in, 148; National Health Nutrition

Survey, 172; obesity/overweight in, 172; tax on SSBs, 172
microbiota, 155; breastfeeding and, 158; and children's well-being, 123
micronutrients: deficiencies, and growth failure, 119; and growth/development, 67; in intrauterine environment, 19; supplementation, 119
middle childhood, growth during, 45
middle-income countries: BMI increases in, 142; child obesity in, 141; EAT-*Lancet* Commission diet and, 180; trans fats in, 173
milk: about, 20; from animals, 25–26; animals' as baby food, in Neolithic age, 25–26; calcium in, 68; in Canada Food Guide, 175; cows', 26, 67–68; digestibility of, 68–69; drinking in East Asia, 69; evaporated, 26–27; in Japanese school meals, 107, 108; normalization of drinking, 68; nutrients in, 68; pasteurization, 27, 171; as special children's food, 67–69, 175; toddler milk, 69; Vitamin D fortification, 171. *See also* breast milk
Milligan, Lauren A., 25
Mintz, Sidney, 164; *Sweetness and Power,* 81–82
Missing Microbes (Blaser), 155
Mitchell, Andrew, 127, 128
Moffat, Tina, 30–31; "The Childhood Obesity Epidemic: Health Crisis or Social Construction?," 159
Moore, Henrietta L., 39–40
Mosby, Ian, 151
Moss, Michael, *Salt Sugar Fat,* 83
mothers: allomothers, 42–43; child health/socialization agendas and, 49–50; "foodwork," 48–50, 176–77; responsibility for child feeding, 163. *See also* parent-child feeding relationship
multinational companies: advertising to children, 136; in China, 73–74; globalization of, 4; infant formula,

29; influence of, 65; localization by, 73–74; in Nepal, 125; and obesity, 125; partnerships/sponsorships, 74; school food outsourcing to, 107. *See also* global food system

National Farmers Union (France), 61–62
National Food Policy (Canada), 113, 174
national food/dietary guides, 11–12, 174–76
National Health and Nutrition Examination Surveys (US), 145
National Longitudinal Study of Adolescent Health (US), 140
National Longitudinal Survey of Children and Youth (Canada), 131
National School Lunch Program (NSLP) (US), 134; civil rights activism and, 97; and defence nutrition, 97; Great Depression and, 97; a la carte foods sold in, 108; origins of, 97; stigma in, 108; subsidization of, 108; "War on Poverty" and, 97
Naya Health, *If Men Breastfed,* 32
neoliberalism: and advertising food products to children, 66; and family responsibility for child raising, 96; and family responsibility for food, 109; and global food system, 11; and personal responsibility, 49; and state vs. individual responsibility for food, 10
Neolithic age, animals' milk as baby food, 25–26
Nepal: bottle feeding/infant formula in, 33; breast milk insufficiency in, 35; breastfeeding in, 20–22, 33, 122; carpet-making industry in, 30–31, 120; child growth in, 164–65; child nutrition improvement in, 168; complementary foods in, 35; Demographic Health Surveys, 123–24; gastrointestinal diseases in, 122; infant morbidity in, 35; infant

mortality in, 120; as low-income nation, 119–20; multinational fast food companies in, 125; overweight/obese children in, 125; specialized children's foods in, 70; stunting in, 120–21, 123, 124; underweight children in, 120–21, 123; weaning in, 33, 122; women's reproductive vs. productive work in, 30–31

Nestlé, 27–28, 29, 136

Nestle, Marion, *Food Politics,* 65

Nestlé-General Mills, 77

Netherlands, Winter Famine, 18–19

Neumark-Sztainerl, Dianne, 51

neural tube defects (NTDs), 19

New Brunswick, food insecurity government funding in, 134

new foods: in France, 60; and neophobia, 58–59, 63

newcomers. *See* immigrants

Newton, William, 26

Nisbett, Nicholas, 9

noncommunicable diseases (NCDs): adolescent nutrition and, 55; child obesity and, 139; economic cuts and, 96; increasing prevalence of, 66; predictive adaptive response and, 18; school meals and, 114; sugar and, 164

North, Canadian, "country food" in, 168

northern circumpolar regions, food availability/insecurity in, 127

Notley, Rachel, 113

Nunavut: food insecurity in, 127; school lunches in Iqaluit, 113

nurturing: responsibility for, 6; school food and, 113–14; women's role in, 42

nutrition: body weight and, 160; caregiver-child feeding relationship and, 62; COVID-19 pandemic and maternal-child, 168; crisis, 3; defence, 97, 109; experiential learning of, 104–5; foods vs. nutrients, 6–7; human evolution and, 37; improvement in Nepal, 168; in Japanese school curriculum, 106; lessons in France,

104–5; lessons in Japan, 104; maternal, and child obesity, 156–57; nutrient deficiencies, 116; overweight and, 160; parental feeding style and, 47; school meals as intervention sites for, 98; stability of government and, 168; transition, 73, 143–44; young adult awareness of, 56–57. *See also* education about food/nutrition; macronutrients; micronutrients

nutritionism: and construction of children's food, 65; and food/feeding vs. nutrition, 6–7; and manipulation of health through diet, 166

Nutritious Food Basket (Canada), 128

obesity: anthropology and, 138; capitalism and, 125; and cardiovascular disease, 131; complexity of, 138; culture and, 151–52; defined, 138–39; dietary fats and, 144–45; in double burden of malnutrition, 117; environmental/behavioural variables in, 153; as epidemic, 159; food insecurity and, 131–32; gender and, 152–53; global food system and, 136; HFCS and, 87; household food insecurity and, 150; increasing prevalence of, 138, 149, 153; intergenerational transmission of, 150; in Mexico, 172; and NCDs, 131; physiological perspective on, 138–39; in South Asia, 125; stigmatization, 151–52; stunting, and metabolic susceptibility to, 125–26; sugar and, 145, 164; and type 2 diabetes, 131

obesity, child: among Indigenous peoples (Canada), 151; antibiotics and, 155–56, 165; anti-obesity campaigns, 159; behaviourally based interventions in, 159; BMI and, 140–41; breastfeeding and, 157–59; causes of, 138, 142–46; colonization and, 151; co-morbidities associated with, 139–40; diet and, 143–45; early life environment and, 156–57; environmental toxins and, 165; as epidemic, 114; fast food and, 104, 176; food advertising and, 89–90; food insecurity and, 149, 150; in France, 104; gender and, 152–53; genetics and, 142–43; ghrelin/leptin as preventing, 24; healthy cooking school classes and, 114; hunger vs., 4; increase in, 3, 138, 139, 141, 149, 153, 165; industrial food system and, 167; infant formula and, 157–59; intergenerationality of, 165; in Japan, 104; maternal nutrition and, 156–57; maternal pregnancy weight and, 156–57; and moral panic, 159; multinational food companies and, 125; and NCDs, 139; in Nepal, 125; and nutrition crisis, 3; obesogens in, 153–54, 158; over-emphasis on, 165; physical activity and, 114, 145–46; racial inequalities in, 149; school meals and, 98, 104, 114; social/cultural determinants of, 149–53; socioeconomic status and, 149, 158; SSBs and, 145, 171; stigmatization, 165–66; sugar and, 145, 164; systems perspective, 161–62; television watching and, 89–90; tracking into adulthood, 139; trends in, 141–42; in UK, 114; underweight children vs., 141–42; in US, 149. *See also* adolescent obesity

Obesity: Cultural and Biocultural Perspectives (Brewis), 138

obesogenic environment: built environment and, 147–48; and environmental injustices, 151; food deserts and, 147; food swamps and, 147, 148; increase in consumption of food prepared away from home, and, 148; leptogenic environment vs., 148–49

obesogens, 153–54, 158; EDCs, 153–54; PFASs, 154

Oliver, Jamie: *Food Revolution,* 108–9; *Jamie's School Dinners,* 103

Ontario: guaranteed basic income pilot project in, 133–34; Quebec ban on children's advertising, and, 90–91

osteoporosis, 55, 57, 131, 160

overweight: diet and, 144–45; in double burden of malnutrition, 117; food insecurity and, 131–32; increasing prevalence of, 153; malnutrition and, 117; in Mexico, 172; and nutrition, 160; perception of, 152

overweight children: BMI and, 140–41; in Central Asia, 117; diet and, 143–45; in Eastern Europe, 117; food advertising and, 89–90; in France, 104; global food system and, 136; Hispanic, 149; increasing prevalence of, 138, 153, 165; in Nepal, 125; racial inequalities in, 149; stigmatization of, 159; television watching and, 89–90

Oxfam, *Behind the Brands,* 71–72

oxytocin, 22

Paleodiets, 36–37

parasitism, 122, 130

parent-child feeding relationship: child self-regulation in, 48; as emotionally charged, 48; fathers in, 50; in high-income countries, 48; in low-income countries, 47–48; modelling in, 59; as nutrition determinant, 47, 48; parental influence in, 59; poverty and, 62. *See also* caregiver-child feeding relationship

parents: alloparenting, 20, 42–43, 96; conflicting advice given to, 5; parental leave, 177. *See also* families; mothers

partially hydrogenated oils. *See* fat(s)

Pasteur, Louis, 27

Patel, Raj, *Stuffed and Starved,* 11, 117

Patico, Janet, *The Trouble with Snack Time,* 13

Patterns of Human Growth (Bogin), 45

Pelto, Gretel H., 8

Perfluoroalkyl substances (PFASs), 154

physical activity: *Canadian 24-Hour Movement Guidelines for Children and Youth* and, 146; and child obesity, 145–46; and chronic diseases, 146; environmental factors and, 158; gender and, 152–53; in intervention programs, 146; and obesity, 114; socioeconomic status and, 150

picky eating: and avoidant/restrictive food intake disorder, 61; children's eating in France vs., 60–62; as construction, 166; cultural food practices and, 63; and family meals, 50; in France, 61, 62; neophobia and, 58–59, 63; as pathological, 61, 62; as socially/culturally constructed vs. innate, 44–45; in UK, 61; in US, 61

Piernas, Carmen, 78

Piperata, Barbara, 123

pneumonia, 118, 123

policies: policy-maker apathy, 3; regarding child feeding, 166; regarding food industry, 166. *See also* legislation

Pollan, Michael, 50, 57, 176

Popkin, Barry M., 73, 78, 143

Poppendieck, Janet, *Free for All: Fixing School Food in America,* 108

Post, 77; Grape-Nuts, 75

poverty: alleviation of, 180; and child obesity, 149; and malnutrition, 124, 165; and parent-child feeding relationship, 62; "poverty diets," 129. *See also* food insecurity; socioeconomic status

Power, Elaine M., 128–29, 169, 170

predictive adaptive response, in rapidly developing economies, 18

pregnancy: diet during, and children's food preferences, 59; intrauterine environment, 18–20; outside influences on diet during, 163

processed food(s): cheapness compared to fresh, 3–4; eating outside home and consumption of, 176; and environmental unsustainability of food production, 179; hydrogenated oils in, 173; marketed to children, 3

productive work. *See* employment

Programme National Nutrition Santé (National Nutrition and Health Program) (France), 104–5

prolactin, 22

protein, 66–67

Prout, Allan, *Constructing and Reconstructing Childhood,* 12, 64

puberty, 46, 55

public health system: breastfeeding as goal of, 40; and micronutrient supplementation, 119; and obesogenic environment, 147; role of schools, 164; school meals and, 114

"Putative Contributors to the Secular Increase in Obesity" (Keith), 153

Quaker Oats Company: Life cereal, 76; Puffed Rice/Wheat, 75

Quebec: ban on children's advertising in, 90–91; food insecurity and hyperactivity/inattention in, 132; food insecurity government funding in, 134

racial inequalities: in health, 149. *See also* Black children/people; Indigenous communities (Canada)

Raine, Kim, 52, 92–93

rapidly developing economies, predictive adaptive response in, 18

Reed, Danielle R., 82

Reilly, John J., 36

Reimagining Milk (Wiley), 68–69

respiratory system: babies and, 27; diseases, 36, 123

"The Rise of the Corporate Curriculum: Fatness, Fitness and Whiteness" (Azzarito), 161

Ristofski-Slifjepcevic, Svetlana, 11
Robinson, Diane, 178
Rome, ancient: complementary foods in, 34–35, 36; wet nursing in, 25
Roosevelt, Franklin D., 97
Rosin, Hanna, 38–39
Rozin, Paul, 7

salt: advertising restrictions regarding foods high in, 91; in Canadian/US diets, 3; in children's food products, 88; iodization of, 171; as macro-adulterant, 71; and NCDs, 88; in snacks, 78, 81
Sarawak, specialized children's foods in, 70
Satter, Ellyn, "The Feeding Relationship," 48
Schlosser, Eric, *Fast Food Nation*, 72
School Breakfast Program (US), 134
School Food and Beverage Policy (Canada), 112
The School Food Revolution, 98
school food/meals: advantages of, 112–13; in Canada (*see* school food/meals (Canada)); children's perspectives on, 108; in China, 98; COVID-19 and, 115; and defence nutrition, 109; dietary restrictions and, 109–10; experiential learning/ modelling in, 105, 173–74; in Finland, 98; as food-based social safety net, 98; in France (*see* school food/meals (France)); and gastro-citizenship, 107–8; history of, 96–97; immigrants and, 52–53; in India, 98; in Italy, 98; in Japan (*see* school food/meals (Japan)); and learning about significance/ history of dishes, 106; and local agriculture/food, 98, 99, 114, 174; in low-income countries, 97; mainstream media and, 113; in national public health programs, 114; and nationalism, 109; and NCDs, 114; and nurturing, 113–14; and obesity, 114; Oliver and,

103; self-sourced from hydroponic towers, 113; social exclusion from, 109–10; traditional foods in, 52–53; in UK, 98, 103; unavailability during holidays/summer vacation, 134; in US (*see* school food/meals (US)); worldwide programs, 97–98
school food/meals (Canada): in Alberta, 113; breakfast, 111, 134; cafeterias, 112; food insecurity and, 111; history of, 110–13; home-packed lunches, 111; in Iqaluit, 113; lack of publicly funded/managed, 110, 114; national movement toward, 112–13; student food program, 174; in Toronto, 113
school food/meals (France): administration, 100; courses, 60–61; and dietary/physical activity behaviours, 99–100; and education about healthy eating/ food literacy, 99; equitability of, 109; food in national culture/heritage, and, 105; as intervention site, 98; *laïcité* and, 109–10; local farmers/ food production and, 99, 105–6, 174; monthly menus, 104; numbers eating, 100; as obesity prevention/ nutrition interventions, 105; outsourcing to multinational food production companies, 107; personal account, 101–2; *restauration scolaire*, 100; subsidization of, 100; and teaching about French food/culture, 107; varying quality/authenticity of food in, 107–8; vegetarian meals/ items, 109, 110
school food/meals (Japan): and chopstick use, 107; compulsoriness of, 100; and education about healthy eating/food literacy, 99; equitability of, 109; food in national culture/ heritage, and, 105; *gakkō kyūshoku*, 100, 106–7; as intervention site, 98; local farmers/food production and, 99, 105–6, 174; and obesity,

104; as obesity prevention/nutrition interventions, 105; personal account, 102–3; subsidization of, 100–101; teaching meal-time behaviours, 106–7; varying quality/authenticity of food in, 107–8

school food/meals (US): breakfast, 134; history, 97; quality of food, 98, 108–9. *See also* National School Lunch Program (NSLP) (US)

School Lunch Politics (Levine), 97

schools: foodscapes around, 112; historical role in feeding children, 163–64; and nurturing, 6; in obesogenic environment, 147; public health role, 164; snack foods and funding of, 80; teaching of food skills in, 177

Schor, Juliet, *Born to Buy,* 72

Sears, Martha and William, *The Breastfeeding Book,* 38–39

Second World War: and defence nutrition, 97; Dutch Winter Famine, 18

self-feeding: breakfast cereals and, 76, 77; in hunter-gatherer forager societies, 53–55; laissez-faire approach and, 47; in Mali, 47; nonhuman primates and, 53; transition from caregiver-child feeding relationship to, 55–57, 62, 63; young adults and, 56–57

Sellen, Daniel, 33–34

La Semaine du Goût, 62

Sen, Amartya, 116

Shokuiku Kihon Hō (Japan), 104

Siahpush, Mohammad, 149

Simen-Kapeu, Aline, 152–53

Singh, Gopal K., 149

Slining, Meghan M., 144

Slow Food Movement, 105

snack foods: about, 78; adolescents and, 56; in Beijing, 81; family food-sharing vs., 50; "fruit," 81; in Hong Kong, 81; increasing intake of, 78; marketing to children, 71, 78–80; nutritional value in, 80–81; and school funding, 80

Sobal, Jeffery, 9

socioeconomic status: and adolescent obesity, 149–50; attunement to, 11; and child obesity, 149, 158; and dietary habits, 150; embodiment in individuals/communities, 11; and family meals, 51; and fast food consumption, 73; and physical activity, 150; and processed food, 3. *See also* poverty

soft drinks/soda pop: HCFS in, 87; sugar in, 77; taxes, 136

Somali immigrants, 52–53

Soranus, 25, 35

South Asia: child malnutrition in, 120; obesity in, 125; school meals in, 98; stunting/wasting in, 119; underweight children in, 141; vitamin A deficiency in, 119. *See also* Nepal

Special Milk Program (US), 134

spina bifida, 19

state. *See* governments

State of School Feeding Worldwide (World Food Programme), 97–98

sterilization, 26–27

stigma/stigmatization: child obesity and, 165–66; food banks and, 170; National School Lunch Program and, 108; obesity and, 151–52, 160

Story, Mary, 51

Stuffed and Starved (Patel), 11, 117

stunting: about, 46, 119; decrease in, 116; and metabolic susceptibility to obesity, 125–26; in Nepal, 120–21, 123, 124; in sub-Saharan Africa, 119; undernourishment and, 164; in West/Central Africa, 116

sub-Saharan Africa: famines in, 118; stunting in, 119; vitamin A deficiency in, 119; wasting in, 119

sucrose, 87

sudden infant death syndrome, 23

sugar: about, 164; addictiveness of, 83, 93; as additive, 82; amount in food, 84; beets, 82; and body weight, 87; in breakfast cereals, 77, 164; in breast milk, 24; cane, 82; in children's food products, 164; as common ingredient in children's foods, 81–82; and diet-related diseases, 164; health effects of, 85–88, 93; history of, 82; intake guidelines, 86–87; as macro-adulterant, 71; in milk, 24; in NSLP foods, 108; and obesity, 145, 164; replacing fats, 86; in soda pop, 77; taste for, 93; taxes, 136; in toddler milk, 69. *See also* sweet taste/ sweetness

sugar-sweetened beverages (SSBs): and obesity, 126, 145, 171; taxes on, 171

Summer Food Service Program (US), 134

supermarkets: breakfast cereals in, 76–77; increased access to, 143; in obesogenic environment, 147; snack foods in, 78, 81

Supplemental Nutrition Assistance Program (US) (SNAP), 134, 169

sustainability: agriculture and, 180; community food security and, 135–36; critical food literacy and, 178; environmental, 180; food systems and, 179–80; French investment in, 98; Japanese investment in, 98; local agriculture in school meal programs, and, 99, 174; school food and, 99, 114; Sustainable Development Goals, 110, 180; unhealthy vs. healthy foods and, 179–80

Sustainable Development Goals (UNICEF), 110

Sweden, restrictions on children's advertising in, 91

sweet taste/sweetness: added sweeteners, 85; babies/children and, 83; children and, 93; cultural associations between children and, 84–85; industrial food and, 83; innate preference for, 57; sweeteners in children's processed food products, 93; taste receptors, 82–83. *See also* sugar

Sweetness and Power (Mintz), 81–82

Szabo, Michelle, 177

Tapias, Maria, 40

Tarasuk, Valerie, 127, 128, 132–33, 169–70

teenagers. *See* adolescents

television: nutritional effects of advertising on, 90; watching, and obesity, 89–90. *See also* media

Thompson, Amanda, 157, 158

Time Magazine, 86

Toronto: Nutritious Food Basket in, 128; school meals in, 113

transnational food corporations (TFCs). *See* multinational companies

The Trouble with Snack Time (Patico), 13

Trudeau, Justin, National Food Policy, 113

Truth and Reconciliation Commission (Canada), 151

Tucker, Bram, 54

Tully, Kristin P., 41

type 1 diabetes, breastfeeding and, 38

type 2 diabetes mellitus (T2DM): DOHaD and, 18–19; economic cuts and, 96; food insecurity and, 131; and health care systems, 165; increasing prevalence of, 66; obesity and, 131, 139–40; physical activity and, 146; predictive adaptive response and, 18; SSBs and, 171

undernutrition: in double burden of malnutrition, 117; of mothers, and low birthweight, 118; responsive feeding and, 48; and underweight children, 164. *See also* hunger

underweight children: about underweight, 46; in East Africa, 141;

in Nepal, 120–21, 123; obese children vs., 141–42; in South Asia, 141; undernourishment and, 164. *See also* low birthweight (LBW); wasting

UNESCO, Intangible Cultural Heritage, 105

UNICEF: and Baby-Friendly Hospital Initiative, 28; "The First 1000 Days," 156; report on Sustainable Development Goals, 110

United Kingdom: child obesity in, 114; childhood conceptions in, 64; food banks in, 170; food insecurity and emotional problems in, 132; picky eating in, 61; restrictions on children's advertising in, 91; school lunches in, 103; school meals in, 98

United States: adolescent eating in Minneapolis–Saint Paul, 56; child obesity in, 141; children's accounts of food insecurity in Mississippi, 132; children's eating in, 3; Children's Food and Beverage Advertising Initiative, 91–92; Food and Drug Administration (FDA), 173; food banks in, 170; food insecurity in, 4, 127, 134; Food Pyramid, 11; health risks of food-insecure infants/ toddlers in, 131; National Health and Nutrition Examination Surveys, 145; National Longitudinal Study of Adolescent Health, 140; picky eating in, 61; school meals in, 97, 98; trans fats in, 173; in UNICEF youth well-being report, 110

United States Department of Agriculture (USDA): *Choose My Plate*, 174, 175–76; Household Food Security Survey Module, 126; programs addressing food insecurity, 134; School Breakfast Program (US), 134; Special Milk Program, 134; Summer Food Service Program, 134; Supplemental Nutrition Assistance Program, 74, 134, 169; Women,

Infant, and Children Program, 134. *See also* National School Lunch Program (NSLP) (US)

urbanization: and fast food, 73; increase in, 167–68; and nutrition transition, 143

Vallianatos, Helen, 52

Van de Walle, Etienne, 27

Van Esterik, Penny, 28, 29, 30, 31–32, 40, 42

vegetables, 3; babies and, 37; Brassicaceae, 58, 59; fast food and, 74; in French food, 60, 61, 105; in Iqaluit school food, 113; in Japanese food, 106; modelling eating, 59; picky eating and, 58, 61; poverty diets vs., 129; sweet taste vs., 83, 85

Veugelers, Paul J., 152–53

vitamin A, 119

vitamin D, 27, 55, 56–57, 171

Vollmecke, Theresa A., 7

"War on Poverty" (US), 97

wasting, 119; in sub-Saharan Africa, 119; undernourishment and, 164

Watson, James, *Golden Arches East*, 73

weaning: anthropological studies, 34; evolutionary aspects, 34; life history theory and, 34

weaning foods: cereal grains, 36; diet in Nepal, 122; in Nepal, 33; pabulums, 33, 37; panadas, 36; paps, 36; solid, 37

Wells, Jonathan C.K., 36, 125

Widstrom, Ann-Marie, 22

Wiley, Andrea S., 8, 24, 67–68, 152; *Medical Anthropology: A Bicultural Approach*, 8; *Reimagining Milk*, 68–69

Wilk, Richard, 50–51

Williams, Jennifer, 56

Williamson, Iain, 21–22

Willows, Noreen D., 151

Winson, Anthony, 65; *The Industrial Diet*, 71

Women, Infant, and Children Program (US), 134
World Food Programme (WFP), *State of School Feeding Worldwide*, 97–98
World Health Organization (WHO): and Baby-Friendly Hospital Initiative, 28; on breastfeeding, 35, 36; on cardiovascular disease, 173; code for marketing of breast milk substitutes, 28, 29; cross-national study of adolescents, 149; growth reference for children, 119, 120–21, 141; on malnutrition, 117; sugar intake guidelines, 86–87, 93; on trans fatty acids, 173

Worthman, Carol M., 41

Yamashita, Lina, 178
Young, Alyson G., 54
young adults: caregiver–self-feeding transition, 55–56; community food centres and, 178; nutritional awareness, 56–57; self-feeding, 56–57

Zero Hunger, 110